Mammographic Imaging

A Practical Guide

Mammographic Imaging

A Practical Guide

Valerie Fink Andolina, R.T.(R)
Breast Clinic of Rochester
Rochester, New York

Shelly Lillé, R.T.(R)
Healthcare Analysts
Arlington Heights, Illinois

Kathleen M. Willison, R.T.(R)
Breast Clinic of Rochester
Rochester, New York

J. B. Lippincott Company
Philadelphia

Acquisitions Editor: Charles McCormick, Jr.
Sponsoring Editor: Kimberley Cox
Production Manager: Robert D. Bartleson
Production: Bermedica Production, Ltd.
Compositor: Compset, Inc.
Printer/Binder: Arcata Graphics

6 5 4 3 2

Library of Congress Cataloging-in-Publication Data

Andolina, Valerie.
    Mammographic imaging : a practical guide / Valerie Fink Andolina,
Shelly Lillé, Kathleen M. Willison.
      p.   cm.
    Includes bibliographical references and index.
    ISBN 0-397-51096-9
    1. Breast—Radiography. 2. Screen-film radiography. I. Lillé,
Shelly. II. Willison, Kathleen M. III. Title
    [DNLM: 1. Mammography—methods.   WP 815 A552m]
RG493.5.R33A23 1992
618.1'907572—dc20
DNLM/DLC
for Library of Congress   91-45981
                                                                         CIP

The authors and publisher have exerted every effort to ensure that drug selection and dosage set forth in this text are in accord with current recommendations and practice at the time of publication. However, in view of ongoing research, changes in government regulations, and the constant flow of information relating to drug therapy and drug reactions, the reader is urged to check the package insert for each drug for any change in indications and dosage and for added warnings and precautions. This is particularly important when the recommended agent is a new or infrequently employed drug.

Foreword

Breast cancer kills more women than any other cancer. Because it victimizes women in every walk of life, breast cancer has become the modern women's scourge. No other cancer terrorizes women as much as breast cancer. No other routine screening procedure engenders as much fear in women as the annual mammogram. A kind, compassionate, knowledgeable technologist can foster the patient's confidence and trust, but an abrupt hurried, abrasively indifferent technologist can make the patient vow never again to return for another mammogram.

Yet radiologists, in the main, are insufficiently aware of how dependent they are on the radiographic technologist's expertise. Nowhere is this dependence more evident than in mammography. Physicians talk about the need for the "team approach" to the diagnosis of breast cancer. The archetypal team includes the radiologist, the pathologist, and the surgeon. At our clinic, the mammographic technologist is an equally essential part of the diagnostic team. Her information and opinions merit equal attention and respect from the rest of the team.

The mammographic technologist is in the frontline of interaction with the patient. When a woman consults a radiologist for a mammogram, she spends most of her time with the technologist. It is the technologist who must win her confidence and create an atmosphere of mutual trust. The technologist must convince the patient that the contortions of pulling the breast onto the film are necessary, that vigorous compression is in the patient's own best interest. No matter how many patients she or he sees in a day, the technologist must act as though each patient is the only one in the office. As a radiologist who performed her own mammograms in the first five years of her practice, I particularly appreciate what a tall order that can be.

With the ever-increasing statistical incidence of breast cancer, with radiologists striving to educate women and their physicians to the need for routine mammographic screening for all eligible women, with the rapidly growing number of breast imaging facilities, it is crucial that the technologist obtain the best mammographic images possible. The technologist is the linchpin in assuring and maintaining the quality of a mammographic facility. The technologist can never relax her or his vigilance to mammographic detail. At the same time, the technologist must talk to the patient, obtain and record any pertinent history, look for and report significant physical signs, such as a mole on the skin or a scar from an earlier biopsy, to help the radiologist come to a more accurate interpretation of the mammogram. The technologist's knowledge of mammary anatomy, her or his understanding of mammography's myriad technical aspects, adeptness at technique and positioning and ability to reassure the patient and influence her to accept any discomfort attendant on vigorous compression are vital.

As the first textbook on breast imaging that specifically addresses the concerns and problems of students of screen-film mammographic technology, *Mammographic Imaging: A Practical Guide* answers an important need. Its purpose is to help budding screen-film mammographic technologists, recent technologist graduates, and more experienced mammographic technologists understand the basic tenets of mammography, as well as other imaging procedures, and so to improve and expedite their own handling of all aspects involved in the diagnosis of breast imaging.

Screen-film mammographic technology differs radically from ordinary radiologic technique, yet until the advent of this book, no textbook has been available to guide the novice through its cardinal principles and help new or experienced technologists find ways of improving their technical proficiency and communication with patients.

With their astute insights and eminently practical suggestions, their particular emphasis on mammographic technique and positioning, Valerie Andolina, Shelly Lillé, and Kathleen Willison have provided vital information on establishing and bettering the ways and means of mammography. Technologists, radiologists, and patients alike will benefit from their having performed this valuable service for breast imaging.

The Breast Clinic of Rochester is proud of its long association with these dedicated technologists. We congratulate them on transferring their commitment to the highest standards of mammographic technology to the printed page.

Wende Westinghouse Logan-Young, M.D.

Breast Clinic of Rochester
Rochester, New York

Preface

In this text we have tried to incorporate all aspects of the technology and the art of mammography. It will enable the experienced technologist to broaden his or her base of knowledge, as well as provide the novice with basic information.

Because we are certain that most people will not read this book from cover to cover, there are certain points that we feel must be made clear to the reader of segments of the text. First, all aspects involved in producing the final mammogram are equally important; the radiograph will only be as good as the poorest aspect of the entire system. Second, there are many schools of thought on positioning, problem solving, technique, biopsy localization, and the like. We have drawn from our collective experiences as mammographers to present the methods that we know will work, and that we ourselves use to produce quality mammograms. All information contained herein was current at the time of writing; however, the technology of mammography and testing procedures are constantly changing and improving.

In reference to the text itself, it must be stated that *the actual degree of angulation used for positioning the breast may change* from one patient to the next. For example, the 45° oblique view may actually constitute a 40° angle of the C-arm for some women. Additionally, although many brands and models of radiographic equipment are shown in photographs within this book, this is not meant as an endorsement of any brand name. Likewise, we regret that we have been unable to use photographs of all equipment that we feel is competitive in the mammographic market.

It is our hope that mammographers will continue to explore new methods of producing quality in their films. It is hoped that this book will be a source of inspiration to technologists, as they were the inspiration for this book.

This book is dedicated to all technologists who, in their quest for knowledge, inspired us to write this guide.

Acknowledgments

There are many people whom we must thank wholeheartedly; without their inspiration, teachings, support, and encouragement we would not have been able to complete this text. To the people who helped us technically, we say a special thank you. Without your time and effort we would not have been able to accomplish all that has been done. Our thanks to:

Dr. Wende Logan-Young for passing on to us your knowledge, your enthusiasm, and your dedication to improving mammography and the detection of breast cancer. Most of all, we thank you for your time (a precious commodity in your life) to guide us and answer questions.

Angie Cullinan, FASRT, whose dedication to the field of radiologic technology and mammography has inspired us to do our best.

Jack Cullinan, FASRT, for putting the idea of this text into our heads, and for his encouragement along the way.

The technologists of the Breast Clinic of Rochester—Kathy Barnsdale, Peggy Bishop, Yvonne Piccarreto, Sue Good, Olena Haber, Amy Kupski, Judy LaBella, Joanne Malchoff, Renee Morgan, and Pam Nordin—for many helpful comments and suggestions, and for having so much patience with us!

Denise Sigel and Nancy Wayne for cheerfully spending their time typing and retyping manuscripts.

Diane Cubit for illustrations in Chapters 10 through 15.

Nathaniel Horenstein and Scot Gordon, Biomedical Photography students at Rochester Institute of Technology, for clinical photographs and mammography prints in Chapters 10 through 15, and additional photographs in Chapters 7 and 8.

Steve Grauman of the Photo Illustration Lab of the Breast Clinic of Rochester for photography and prints in Chapters 3, 7, and 8 and additional work in Chapter 5.

Phyllis and Moore Anderson for illustrations in Chapter 5.

Jim Princehorn of Transworld Radiographic X-Ray Systems, and Nicola Yanaki of Eureka X-Ray Tubes, Inc. for instruction, suggestions and drawings in Chapter 5.

Dr. Joyce Janus of the University of Rochester for taking time to read and comment on manuscripts.

The Cytopathology Department of The University of Rochester for their help.

Charles McCormick, Jr., Kimberley Cox, and the J. B. Lippincott Company for their help and patience, and for providing us with the opportunity to create this book.

Gayla Dieball, Kathy Durrell, Susan Jaskulski, and Bob Pizzutiello for their comments, suggestions, and support.

Bonnie Kissel, Cathy Snyder, Barb McAvinney, and Shivaun Featherman for their time and energy.

Our families, for their patience and support, and for giving of themselves so that we could put this text together:

Charlie Willison
Erik Willison
Katy Willison
Patricia Eisner
Michele Gervase
Gene Andolina
Nicole Fink
Thomas Andolina
Sam Andolina
John and Daphne Fink
Ken Lillé

Contents

I

General and Background Information

1 Shelly Lillé

History of Mammography

Those who cannot remember the past are condemned to repeat it.

George Santayana

"I remember the exact moment I found my breast cancer. Time stood still as my heart pounded. My brain tried to rationalize away this new-found lump in my breast" the woman sobbed. So many times, as the radiologic technologist performing a mammogram on such a woman, I've wanted to ask, "Why . . . why did you *wait* to have a mammogram?"

Breast cancer is emotional. Breast cancer is biological. Technologists must continue to search for a better understanding of both aspects of the disease in order to improve the technical skills necessary to detect disease and to strengthen interpersonal skills to help the patients. This book is written by radiologic technologists for radiologic technologists. The authors share their experiences, collect information about mammography and present it from a practical viewpoint that is useful to the radiologic technologist.

The biologic aspects of breast cancer are addressed from many vantage points in this book. These include materials on the etiology of breast disease and its appearance, the anatomy of the breast, how breast tissue affects and is affected by the design and performance of dedicated mammography machines, the appearance of breast tissue on a screen-film image, and positioning of the breast. The emotional aspects also are addressed in many ways, including the initial meeting with the patient, history taking, teaching breast self-examination, allaying patient fears of firm compression during the mammogram, and dealing with patient emotions that range from a mild case of embarrassment to hostile resistance.

Three points must be made clear from the start:

1. Breast cancer continues to be a major killer of women in the United States.
2. Early detection is necessary to improve the survival rate for patients with cancer.
3. Knowledge of breast disease coupled with improved technical skills and greater personal care can help the radiologic technologist to detect disease and to educate patients toward better breast care.

The Oldest Story in Mammography

Legend has it that the concept of mammography was first proposed in 1924 when a group of male radiol-

3

ogists in Rochester, New York, were assembled around a view box "admiring" the chest x-ray of a very buxom woman. After a brief discussion including playful as well as serious remarks, the radiologists' thoughts and discussion turned to speculation about the ability to x-ray the breast itself for localization of a tumor. Articles detailing radiography of mastectomy specimens were published prior to 1930. Stafford Warren, M.D. published the first article on mammography in 1930.[1] Warren described the use of double emulsion film and intensifying screens, a moving grid, a 60 kVp, 70 mA, 2.5-second exposure, and a 25-inch source–image detector distance.

The Father of Mammography

It was not until the 1960s that the "father of mammography"—Robert Egan, M.D., then at M. D. Anderson Hospital in Houston—began widespread teaching of his mammographic technique with the assistance of the American College of Radiology. Training centers for radiologists and technologists were established throughout the United States.

"Not all in the medical community were as impressed with mammography and its potential as were those in the field of radiology. Many surgeons were concerned that a negative mammogram might delay or prevent an exploration suggested on clinical grounds. Experts . . . protested that if a cancer was present, their fingers would find it, and that the 'newfangled' modality was not only unnecessary but perhaps insidious. Many radiologists furtively attempting the new technique were effectively suppressed by blown x-ray tubes, much less than 98% accuracy, and the supercilious sneers of their surgical colleagues.

But a few radiologists persisted, buoyed up by the potential of mammography. After all, there was a great need for improved diagnosis in breast disease, especially in that gray area of 'fibrocystic disease.' Also, an occasional cancer was detected when clinical findings were questionable and, even more remarkably, completely non-palpable cancers which turned out to have a high degree of no axillary nodal involvement were often discovered."[2]

It is with deep appreciation for their efforts that we acknowledge doctors Stafford Warren, Jacob Gershon-Cohen, Raul Leborgne, Robert Egan, Phillip Strax, Charles Gros, Gerald Dodd, John Martin, and John Wolfe as well as countless others who valiantly held on to their belief in mammography. Any new procedure will undergo initial scrutiny, and comparisons will be made to current detection modalities. If the new procedure can endure the initial doubts cast upon its integrity, and if the basic tenets upon which the examination is based prove to be sound, those who helped evolve the examination's principles deserve our gratitude.

Compared to the images we produce today with dedicated equipment, high-contrast screen-film combinations, and dedicated processing of the latent image, these initial attempts in mammography generally were of limited value and today are considered archaic. However, to put things into perspective, in the not-too-distant future when breast cancer is detected in its earliest cellular stage, today's mammography will be considered primitive.

Pioneers, Tires, and Dedicated Equipment

Modern-day mammography began in France in the mid 1960s. Charles Gros, M.D. and the CGR Company developed the first dedicated mammographic unit. The heart of the new unit—the molybdenum target tube—was an application of technology developed for quality control efforts in automobile and truck tire production. The molybdenum target tube was initially used by a tire manufacturing company to produce high-contrast images of their tires to search for imperfections upon final inspection. Until Gros' adaptation of this invention, the ceiling-mounted, tungsten target diagnostic x-ray unit used for chest films and other general radiologic studies also was used for mammograms.

The new mammography unit, introduced commercially into the United States in 1969, used a molybdenum target, had an integral device for compressing the breast, and employed low kVp's. These were three important contributions that solved a major shortcoming of early mammography: low-contrast images. At this time, direct exposure film (whether medical or industrial) was used and required hand processing. Also, 8–12 R was a typical patient dose; this issue became an easy target for the early critics of mammography.

The development of a dedicated unit was the first significant step taken toward the use of mammography as a tool for mass screening, a goal advocated in articles and books written by the proponents of mammography. The following 15 years was a period of significant change as the results of research and improvements in related fields were applied to mammography. Improvements came rapidly in equipment, accessories, film, and techniques to better image fibrocystic tissue, breast cancers, and calcifications.

To See More Clearly: A Decade and a Half of Change

1971

Although its use was reported in the literature as far back as 1960, xeroradiography was not introduced commercially until 1971. Many physicians preferred its lower x-ray dose (2–4 R) and its blue powder/white paper images over the available film systems. Xeroradiography also afforded the hospital the ability to use one of its existing diagnostic x-ray machines; thus it was not necessary to purchase a special machine to perform mammography. However, it was necessary to acquire the specialized processing and conditioning units.

1972

In 1972, R. E. Wayrynen, Ph.D. and the Dupont Company developed the LoDose I screen-film imaging system, a specially designed mammographic cassette employing a single calcium-tungstate intensifying screen in conjunction with a single-emulsion film. The radiation dose with this system was approximately 1–1.5 R, another improvement over all other existing systems. The development of this imaging system was the major improvement needed to realize the potential benefits from dedicated mammography units. Mass screening was considered by many to be on the horizon.

1973 and 1974

Three new dedicated units were introduced in 1973: the Siemens Mammomat, Philips' Mammo Diagnost, and Picker's Mammorex. In 1974, General Electric introduced their MMX unit. The variety of dedicated mammography units on the market coupled with the availability of lower dose screen-film systems widened the gap between mammographers with dedicated units versus those attempting mammography with standard x-ray equipment and industrial or medical film. Clinical practice began to change as xeroradiography and the new dedicated screen-film units replaced the older equipment and methods for producing mammograms.

1976

In 1976, Kodak introduced a rare earth screen-film combination—the Min-R-System—with a dose measurement of approximately 0.08 R. At the same time Dupont began to market their improved LoDose II system. Agfa-Gevaert also entered the film and cassette market during this period. In response to concern regarding the x-ray dosage for mammography, those performing xeroradiography increased the filtration and the recommended kVp settings to lower the dose to approximately 0.5 R.

1977

In 1977, Xonics manufactured an x-ray machine that utilized electron radiography. The Radiologic Science Inc. unit (later known as Pfizer and then as Elscint) introduced the microfocus tube (a 0.09-mm round focal spot) to allow for magnification. Techniques that allowed clearer, bigger, brighter, and better images were a major focus of equipment research and design at this time, as clinicians and researchers sought to emulate successes in other types of imaging. Systems that used the new electronics and computer-based technologies began to influence the designs and directions taken by later generations of mammographic systems.

1978

Philips introduced a moving grid with special carbon fiber interspace material for low absorption of the soft x-ray beam necessary for screen-film mammography.

1984

Liebel-Flarsheim began marketing a fine-line stationary grid. This was an acceptable alternative for machines that could not be retrofitted with a moving grid. Also, LoRad Medical Systems introduced the high-frequency/constant-potential generation of dedicated mammography machines.

1986

In 1986, Kodak introduced Min-R-T screens and film—two intensifying screens within a cassette combined with a double-emulsion film. This system offered increased speed and reduced dosage, but with slightly less resolution and contrast; for use with younger or infirm patients.

Continuing Advancements in Mammography

Improvements in dedicated mammographic equipment, accessories, films, cassettes, screens, and processors are expected to continue. Chapter 5 addresses the features and benefits of the newer technologies that are employed in modern mammography.

The Influence of Plastics

Two plastics, silicone and Lexan, have had a significant influence on the history of mammography. Treatment of breast cancer by modified radical mastectomy is advocated by many surgeons, and silicone breast implants became a favored approach to help restore a woman's image and confidence. Cosmetic surgery, also gaining in popularity, resulted in many women with healthy breast tissue obtaining silicone implants to increase their breast size. Currently, each year some 250,000 women in the United States have such implants. Mammography had to respond with newer techniques to image these altered breasts. (Chapter 13 addresses how to image the breast with implants.) Lexan is a strong, thin, clear, hard plastic that allows the compression device on the mammographic unit to flatten and immobilize the breast without a great deal of attenuation of the x-ray beam. Modern mammography would be difficult without its presence.

Summary

The history of mammography began with good natured discussion and scientific curiosity in 1924. From the start of modern mammography in the 1950s, the field progressed slowly during the 1950s and 1960s with help from the industrial sector. More recently, mammography has benefited from the rapid technological advances in electronics, computer sciences, and plastics and the emergence of other sophisticated medical imaging devices over the 20-year period from 1970 through 1990. This history is not yet completed. The interdependence between the recording system and x-ray system continues to be a major factor in producing the best image at the lowest dose. This relationship is central to the efforts of the manufacturers of equipment, accessories, and film as they strive to make the next breakthrough. The newer technological advances in manufacturing, materials development and design, computer sciences (medical imaging without film) and biologic sciences (use of DNA technology), also have potential applications for the detection of breast cancer.

References

1. Warren SL: Roentgenologic study of the breast. *AJR* 1930; 24: 113.
2. Strax P: Evolution in techniques in breast screening, in Strax P (ed): *Control of Breast Cancer Through Mass Screening*. St Louis, MO, Mosby-Yearbook Inc, 1978, p 167.

2

Shelly Lillé

Background Information and the Need for Screening

Breast Cancer in America

Empirical data concerning breast cancer and mammography are both instructive and discomforting. The American Cancer Society (ACS) projected that 191,000 new cases of breast cancer would occur in the United States in 1991 and that an additional 44,800 women would die from the ravages of their disease.[1] This means that every 13 minutes four American women will develop breast cancer and one will die from this disease. Currently, breast cancer averages 191,000 new cases (in situ + invasive) a year with a 98% 5-year survival rate with early detection of a minimal breast cancer. The survival rate is reduced to 55% if positive lymph nodes are found. By comparison, cervical cancer averages 63,000 new cases a year (in situ + invasive) with an 86% 5-year survival rate with early detection.[1–3] Despite the higher survival rate for breast cancer with early detection, women routinely have Pap smears yet will refrain from having a mammogram until they are placed in a "high-risk" category or become symptomatic. Many reasons are given for this underusage of mammography (Tables 2-1 and 2-2).

A survey conducted by Sarah Fox, Ph.D., while in training at the University of Michigan–Ann Arbor supports the findings of the two polls reported in Tables 2-1 and 2-2. "Findings showed that while more than half of the participants—53% to 69%—performed a monthly breast self exam, only 22% of the 40–49 year olds and 25% of the women older than 50 had at least one baseline and one repeat mammogram. Furthermore, 60% of the women younger than 50 and 51% of women older than 50 had not obtained one baseline screening mammogram. Physician referral was the primary reason why women sought mammography in the first place, Fox said. Yet only 9% cited maintenance or prevention as the reason for having been sent to mammography; almost half of the referrals were sent because of clinical findings.

Given these findings, Fox said that the underuse of mammography appears to be due largely to lack of acceptance by the primary care physician for the purpose of mass screening. The group that needs to be persuaded is the one that controls mammography as a referral procedure."[6] In 1987, Howard cited an ACS retrospective study of primary care physicians and their preventive maintenance habits.[7] At the bot-

7

TABLE 2-1   Statistics on the Use of Mammography*

Never had a mammogram	59%
Had a mammogram 0–1 yr ago	22%
1–2 yr ago	8%
2–5 yr ago	4%
5 + yr ago	2%
Reasons:	
Physician did not suggest	56%
Did not know the need for exam	27%
Expense	26%
Inconvenience	15%
X-ray exposure	9%
Fear of finding cancer	7%
Won't change the outcome	6%
Fear of pain	5%

*Data from a May 1988 Roper Organization Poll of women age 45 and older.[4]

TABLE 2-3   Incidence of Naturally Occurring Breast Cancers by Age*

Age	Annual Incidence/ Million Women
40	800
45	1,400
50	1,800
55	2,050
60	2,400
65	2,700
70	2,950

*Data from Siedman and Mushinski.[10]

tom of the list of recommended exams/procedures to prevent advanced illness/disease was the flu immunization shot, with mammography holding the next to the bottom ranking!

The incidence of breast cancer increased 17% between 1975 and 1985.[8,9] In 1973 there were 82.3 cases of breast cancer per 100,000 American women; in 1987 the rate was 110 per 100,000.[4] The death rate from breast cancer increased by 5% between 1979 and 1986 after almost two decades of decline. "This finding suggests women are not taking advantage of screening techniques that could detect breast cancer at a stage when cure is more likely, although detection of breast cancer is at the highest rate in history."[8]

As women age the likelihood of developing breast cancer increases. Table 2-3 illustrates the rates of naturally occurring breast cancer cases per million women per year at various ages. An earlier study of the incidence of breast cancer for all ages of women also indicated that breast cancer is truly a disease of advancing age (Table 2-4). Therefore, as women age the need for mammography becomes more critical; the

current guidelines from several professional and medical associations (ACS, the American College of Radiology, the National Cancer Institute, the American Medical Association, the American College of Obstetricians and Gynecologists) reflect this thinking (refer to Chapter 3 for a listing of the guidelines).

The data from Table 2-4 are also presented as a bar graph (Fig. 2-1) to illustrate the dramatic increase in the incidence of breast cancer as age increases. It is apparent from the bar graph that during the ages of 25 to 49 there are particularly sharp increases in the number of cancers. From age 50 on, the number of cancers per 100,000 women continues to increase but at a much slower rate. We now take a different ana-

TABLE 2-2   Use of Mammography versus Pap Smears

62% of women age 40 + have never had a mammogram
17% did not know the exam existed
6.5% of women 40 + had a mammogram in past year
75% of women age 18 + had a Pap smear within the past 3 years

*National Cancer Institute Study data cited in ref. 5.

TABLE 2-4   Average Annual Age-Specific Breast Cancer Incidence Rates (per 100,000 Females)*

Age Group	Incidence per 100,000
15–19	0.2
20–24	1.1
25–29	8.3
30–34	26.7
35–39	57.2
40–44	106.2
45–49	173.8
50–54	195.9
55–59	228.9
60–64	251.2
65–69	282.9
70–74	302.2
75–79	338.0
80–84	350.0
85 +	376.3
(All ages adjusted to 1970 population)	85.4

*From Young et al.[11]

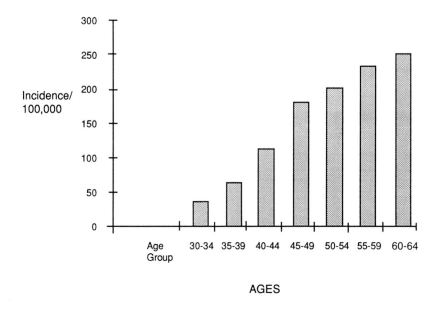

FIGURE 2-1   The information from Table 2-4 is presented as a column graph to show the precipitous rise in breast cancer cases from ages 30 through 49.

lytic approach to these numbers and couple this to the ease of detecting a breast cancer due to the parenchymal pattern of each woman's breast. In addition, recent studies have found that cancers detected in women in the 40 to 50 year age group are generally more aggressive, with a faster growth rate. The guidelines for mammography need to be altered as our knowledge of this disease process becomes better defined.

Factors in Early Detection

Early detection of any cancer is critical to successful treatment and the quality of the patient's life. Screening mammograms of asymptomatic women are vital in the battle against breast cancer. However, before the discussion of *how* to obtain a good image begins, it must first be understood *why* technical expertise and interpretation are so vital in mammography.

White on White

Screen-film mammography images the cancers in white: either as white microcalcifications or as a white mass (1) whose borders are irregular, (2) that is new when compared with previous mammograms, or (3) that is increasing in size when compared with

previous mammograms. The glandular tissue from which the cancers arise also appears white on the mammogram. As women with varying parenchymal patterns age, all but one of these patterns will experience a decrease in the amount of glandular tissue. Each pregnancy greatly displaces the amount of glandular tissue remaining, while each month during the menstrual cycle a much smaller scale replacement will occur. The white-appearing glandular tissue is replaced with dark-appearing adipose tissue. However, contemporary use of estrogen replacement therapy throughout the postmenopausal years results in retention of more of the glandular tissue. When looking for a cancer in the typical young woman's breast, we are looking for a white dot on a white background; in the typical postmenopausal, adipose replaced breast we are looking for a white dot on a dark background.

Guidelines

Clinical specialists with extensive experience in mammography now advocate that screening mammograms be done yearly on women in their 40s and every 1–2 years after age 50,[12–14] depending on the individual risk factors and ease of interpreting the films. This differs from the current guidelines of the associations cited above. "Tumors in the 40–49 year age population grow more rapidly than in the 50+

population," stated Myron Moskowitz, M.D., of the University of Cincinnati. Moskowitz "contends that the every other year guideline was intended as a compromise. It certainly wasn't chosen on any kind of scientific basis. We think it's important to screen 40 to 49 year olds every year, because that's where you're going to catch the early cancers."[13] The Health Insurance Plan in New York State (1963–1969) and the W-E Study (Swedish screening trials conducted from 1977 to 1982 and 1977 to 1984) confirmed that "breast cancer mortality could be reduced by using mammography as the only examination method. . . . Regular mammographic examinations are highly recommended on asymptomatic women aged 40–70. The optimum interval time between two consecutive mammographic examinations is one year for women aged 40–49 years, while it is 18–24 months in women 50–70 years of age."[12]

Over the past 60 years there has been no substantial reduction in the mortality rate from breast cancer even though the ability to detect occult lesions exists (Fig. 2-2). "You can survive breast cancer if it is detected early, and you can detect it early through monthly breast self exams (BSE) and periodic mammograms."[4]

If a woman develops cancer of the cervix, the Pap smear will detect it at an early, more curable stage. The same approach should exist for breast cancer. In order to save lives, mammography should not be performed only on women who present with symptoms or are considered "high risk" candidates; it should be done on a screening basis just as the Pap smear is done, since the average time it takes for a breast cancer to grow large enough to feel (approximately 1 cm) is 10–12 years.[13,15–17] If mammography is done well technically, with a qualified radiologist reading the films, the average breast cancer should be detected 2–4 years before it becomes palpable. Often, this will be a minimal breast cancer, for which the cure rate approaches 95%.[18,19]

Lesion Size and Survival Rates

By the time a 0.5-cm lesion increases in size to a palpable 1 cm, its mass has increased eight times. A 1-cm tumor contains from 100 million to 1 billion cells. By the time they reach 2 cm in size, these lesions often have metastasized. For patients with metastatic le-

sions, the median time of survival is 2 years. As the tumors increase in size, the cell types become more heterogeneous and will respond less predictably to various drugs, to radiation therapy, and to biologic markers. This is why it is so important to detect the smallest lesion possible.

The average size palable tumor detected by a woman is 2–3 cm (Fig. 2-3), by which time axillary lymph node involvement has already occurred in 50–60% of the cases; the 5-year survival rate is 60%.[2,20,21] The survival rate is approximately 95% if mammography detects an occult lesion at an earlier stage. In general, the duration of the patient's survival is inversely related to the size of the tumor; thus the larger the tumor the lower the survival rate. Survival of those women with lesions whose borders are smooth (such as medullary carcinoma) are better than for those whose lesions have irregular borders (such as the typical scirrhous carcinoma)—80% versus 38% at 10 years.

An informative European study concerned with survival rates was conducted in the Netherlands. "Dutch data in which the five year survival rate of patients whose cancers were detected at the first examination is better than 90%. Of those cancers detected between the first and second examinations (1–23 months after initial screening) the five year survival rate is less than 90%. For the cases detected either at or after the second examination, the 5 year survival rate is around 80% and decreases sharply."[22]

Decreases in the mortality rate from a cancer are dependent upon early detection through mass screening as in the use of the Pap smear to reduce cervical cancer deaths. Screening for breast cancer is becoming more prevalent in the United States, although current levels are far below that of the Pap smear. Current United States population data indicate there are an estimated 56 million women who are age-eligible for a mammogram (according to ACS guidelines), yet only 5–15% actually have a mammogram.[15,17,18,23,24] For example, if 10% of these 56 million age-eligible women had mammograms done, with half (5%) symptomatic and the other half (5%) asymptomatic, then only 5% of this 56 million population had a screening mammogram.

Cervical cancer mortality rates have been reduced by 70% since the introduction of the Pap smear. If Pap smears were performed on only 5% of all eligible

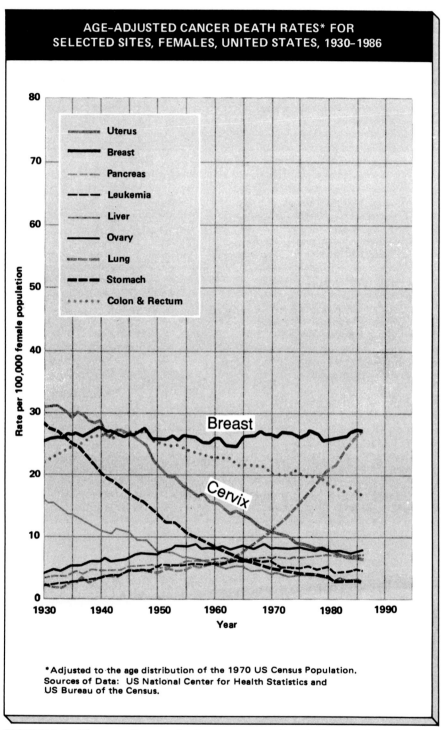

FIGURE 2-2   The mortality rates for breast cancer and cervical cancer. Mortality rates for cancer of the cervix declined by 70% since the Pap smear gained nationwide acceptance. The mortality rate for breast cancer has increased in the mid-1980s. (From Boring CC et al., ref. 1.)

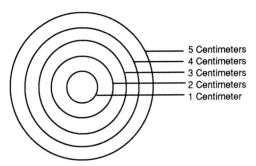

FIGURE 2-3   Size of breast lumps.

women, the mortality rate from cancer of the cervix would not have fallen by 70% (see Fig. 2-2).

The great disparity in the mortality rates for breast and cervical cancers can be attributed to misconceptions regarding the efficacy of mammography. "A recent survey by the ACS of primary care physicians' attitudes and practices concerning breast cancer detection revealed some disturbing statistics. 'We found that while 49% of all primary care physicians said that they have ordered screening mammography on their asymptomatic people, only 11% actually followed our guidelines' said Diane Fink, M.D., American Cancer Society Vice President for Professional Education."[25] The reasons stated for noncompliance with the guidelines were: (1) cost, (2) lack of appreciation of the benefits of screening, and (3) fear of excessive radiation.

The Economics of Early Detection

The cost of medical care in America has become as important an issue as the need for care. A renewed emphasis on disease prevention, patient participation in health decisions, and trade-offs in medical care are actively proposed because of economic considerations. The true cost of treating a disease in its later stages is staggering. The economics of screening and early detection of cervical cancer with the Pap smear are understood and accepted on the basis of the future costs, in lives and money, that can be avoided. The cost of screening mammography for breast cancer can be compared favorably to the true costs of screening for cervical cancer.

Using statistics from the HIP study (New York City 1963–1969), if a mammogram cost $45.00, the cost for each cancer identified by screening would be $23,403.00. If no screening examination was done and a woman subsequently developed breast cancer, it would cost $60,000.00 for treatment of her disease; this figure increases to $150,545.00 when disability costs to industry are added. "It has recently been estimated that the cost per cervical cancer detected was $17,000.00. Renal dialysis costs have been estimated to run between $23,000.00 and $32,000.00 per year. The cost of the first year of coronary bypass surgery has been estimated at $13,500.00. It has been estimated that the cost per day for the last month of life of a terminal cancer patient ranges around $1,200.00 to $1,500.00."[26] The cost-effectiveness of screening for breast cancer compares favorably.

The reports on patient use of mammography suggest that some primary care physicians may not recommend mammography for their patients because of the current costs (averaging $50 to $150) and the lack of insurance coverage for screening. Reports on utilization indicate very low compliance rates with the guidelines the various national medical groups have established.[15,23,27] The Federal Government has recognized the merits of mammography, since it is the only screening examination paid for by Medicare. However, the current criteria only allow reimbursement for one study every 2 years after age 65. A more affordable cost to the patient, as suggested by Moscowitz, may offer a mechanism to screen more women at earlier ages and improve the opportunities for early detection of breast cancers.

Lack of Appreciation of the Technology

Primary care physicians familiar only with mammography as it was performed in past years may hold outmoded beliefs regarding the radiation dose and the ability to detect nonpalpable tumors, and as a result may avoid ordering routine mammograms. These ideas are obsolete where modern mammography is available. However, the occasional lack of availability of modern mammography helps perpetuate these old perceptions.

Fortunately, modern mammography (a good screen-film image, performed on a quality mammographic unit by a qualified technologist, processed in a dedicated film processor, and interpreted by a qualified radiologist) is being practiced throughout more and more of the United States. Updated training for physicians and technologists, newer dedicated mammographic units, improved x-ray film and processing techniques, and new positioning techniques have contributed to improved diagnostic accuracy. Accuracy and specificity rates for radiologists are improving each year.

One perception and reservation about mammography *is* currently justified. Unlike the Pap smear, which can detect cervical cancer at the cellular level, a mammogram cannot detect breast cancer at the cellular level. Mammography today is much better than it was just a few years ago, but it could improve in this respect. On average, occult lesions detected by mammography are 8 years old. Currently there is ongoing research to allow detection of breast cancer at the cellular stage.

Fear of Excessive Radiation

Physicians who are more familiar with mammography performed on older general diagnostic x-ray equipment had a valid concern about the amount of radiation used. However, with the current recording systems and x-ray equipment that have been specifically designed for mammography, this fear has been largely dispelled.

The ACS estimates the natural incidence of breast cancer to be 7% over a lifetime. On the basis of the 1972 BIER report, it has been estimated that 1 rad of absorbed radiation to the tissue of the breast would increase the risk of cancer by 1%, to yield a total risk of 7.07% over a lifetime. Extrapolating from that estimate, a 1977 National Cancer Institute (NCI) study headed by Upton stated that if an average glandular dose were 80 mR/exposure (a reasonable dose for today's exam) then a woman could have 180 mammograms done before her natural risk would increase by that same 1%.[28] The lifetime risk of death from developing a breast cancer due to radiation received during routine mammograms is cited as being equivalent with the risk associated with traveling 2,500 miles by air, 1,500 miles by train, or 220 miles in a car or smoking 1.5 cigarettes.[14]

Supporting the theory that radiation *can* induce cancer are studies of Japanese women in Hiroshima and Nagasaki who survived the atomic bomb[29–31] and of sanatorium patients from Massachusetts[32] and Canada[33,34] who were repeatedly fluoroscoped while undergoing treatment for tuberculosis. Also, in the late 1940s and early 1950s in Rochester, New York, 606 women were treated for postpartum mastitis with 75–1,000 R of radiation; these women now show a two times greater incidence of breast cancer in the treated breast.[35,36] These reported levels of radiation are from 100 to 4,000 times that currently used for a full mammographic examination. Also, the age of the populations involved in these early studies tended to be below 30, at which time the breasts are radiosensitive. "To our knowledge, no woman has ever been shown to have developed breast cancer as a result of undergoing mammography."[14]

Misses and Other Mistakes

Mammographic procedures are highly "operator dependent." The knowledge and skills of the radiologic technologist will be severely tested to produce high-quality diagnostic images and to do so consistently. In 1991, the Federal Government began to regulate facilities that perform mammography for Medicare patients; in the near future technologists will be required to obtain certification in order to perform mammography. Mammography has generally taken a back seat to some of the "high-tech" radiologic procedures, but conditions are changing. Within the last 5 years there has been a national trend to upgrade existing mammography services with better dedicated mammography equipment.

Mammography is not 100% accurate, nor should it be 20% inaccurate. "Patients typically regard their radiological tests as infallible. This formidable expectation stands in vivid contrast to research that reported 20% to 41% of all radiologic interpretations are in error."[37] The American College of Radiology wishes for no more than a 10% false-negative rate by any radiologist who interprets mammograms, which is optimistic when compared to inaccuracy rates reported in the literature.[4,17,39–43] For example, Young et al. "analyzed 342 women who had suspicious breast lumps to determine if preoperative mammography could improve the malignancy yield of biopsy procedures. The number of women with cancer of the breast and false-negative mammography reports ranged from 11% to 25%, depending on how equivocal mammographic reports were interpreted."[43]

This inaccuracy rate is not always due to an inaccurate interpretation by the radiologist; there is a long list of variables that could influence the ability to detect a cancer on the radiograph. Each variable could distort the image or in combination render a radiograph that is difficult to interpret. Major factors that will influence the quality of the image include: the knowledge and skill of the person who performed the mammographic examination, the equipment used, the film-screen combination used, the processing conditions of the latent image, the positioning technique employed, the amount of breast compression the patient could tolerate, the type of breast cancer, and the radiographic appearance of the tissue.

A missed diagnosis counts as a false-negative statistically, and at one level represents merely a misinterpretation of a radiograph. To a referring physician who sees surgeons remove a cancerous lump from a patient whose mammogram was "negative," a missed diagnosis represents a great deal more. It does not take many misses for a primary care physician to stop believing in the value of mammography.

A missed diagnosis also influences the attitudes of many patients toward mammography. Every technologist has undoubtedly had a patient relate a personal story, or one that involves a friend or relative, in which mammography did not find a cancer when there was a lump present—these patients see no reason to trust the exam when there is no lump. In response to such a patient, the technologist cannot say "I am a better technologist than the one who did your exam last year" or "My radiologist has a better than 80% accuracy rate" or "We have a new machine this year," but the list of variables that could have influenced the failed exam is long. In reality there is little that can be said to this patient that will not sound defensive or be considered a lame excuse for a mistake that could cost the patient her life. The best response is, through conscientious effort, to make this mammogram the best this woman has ever had, and to reassure her that this is so. The difficult diagnoses that are made may not always be appreciated at the time, but the misses will long be remembered.

Expectations

Mammography is not appropriate for everyone. For women below the age of 30, mammography generally is not a recommended procedure. First, younger women's breasts are more radiosensitive. Second, the incidence is too low in this group to make screening

economically feasible; women in this age group have an incidence of only 8 cases per 100,000 women (Table 2-4). Third, mammography is not 100% accurate, and the white-on-white image in the younger woman's mostly glandular breasts would further compound the inaccuracy rate. When a young woman is clinically symptomatic, she is better advised to see a surgeon before seeking a mammogram.

At Risk for Breast Cancer

During 1991, approximately 190,000 females in the United States will develop breast cancer—and 900 males. Males with Kleinfelter's syndrome (an extra X chromosome) are 66 times more likely to develop breast cancer than are other males and represent approximately two-thirds of cases. According to these statistics, being female is the single highest risk factor. Aside from being female, the next highest risk factor is having had breast cancer. Because there is a genetic predisposition to developing breast cancer, another risk factor is having a positive family history of breast cancer in a premenopausal mother, sister, or daughter; as always, bilateral cancer in such instances presents a higher risk than unilateral cancer.

In a humorous description of "the woman at highest risk for breast cancer," Henry Leis, Jr. combined all the known risks for developing breast cancer in our society in one unfortunate hypothetical woman. "Perhaps the best way to summarize all the currently known risk factors for breast cancer is to view them in terms of the ultimate search for the woman at highest risk. Such a search would culminate in the finding of a 58-year-old, wide body-type, hypertensive, diabetic, hypothyroid, Caucasian, Jewish convert nun, taking reserpine for hypertension and estrogens for severe climacteric symptoms, living in a cold climate in the western hemisphere, whose mother and sister had bilateral premenopausal breast cancer, who has a wet type of ear wax, a low estriol titer and subnormal androgen excretion levels, who had previous endometrial cancer and cancer in one breast, who nursed from her mother who had B viral particles in her milk, whose menarche was at the age of 9, whose remaining breast reveals precancerous mastopathy on the random biopsy, a DY parenchymal pattern on X-ray, and an abnormal thermogram, who received multiple fluoroscopies for tuberculosis therapy when she was 19 years of age, who had severe hepatitis and now has liver dysfunction, and who lives on a high-fat, high-beef, low-fish diet, deficient in both vitamin C and B complex, and who drinks an excessive amount of coffee and dyes her hair."[44]

Unfortunately, according to Strax a "statistical study by the ACS teaches us that less than 25% of cancers develop in women with any of these [risk] factors. The vast majority, up to 75% of breast cancer, occurs in women with none of the known risk factors. The sad truth is that we have to consider all women over the age of 30 at risk for this disease."[17] We must not *wait* until a woman meets certain risk profiles, nor should we *wait* until someone (the woman or her doctor) feels something in the breast in order to justify having a mammogram. What are we "waiting" for?

Physical Examination of the Breast

Three reports on who first detects palpable breast cancers are highly consistent:

"[Ninety percent] of breast cancer is first detected by women themselves."[17]

"Accidental discovery of a lump by the woman continues to be the principal manner in which breast cancer is found [50%]. Another 30% of the victims find their cancer by routine breast self examination, so that the patient herself finds her own cancer 80% of the time."[3]

"About 90 percent of breast tumors today are discovered by women themselves, not their doctors."[45]

If a woman practices breast self-examination (BSE), the lesion found is on average 0.75 cm smaller than that found by the nonpractitioner.[46] However, estimates in the literature indicate that the number of women who regularly examine their breasts is low. A recent Gallup Poll found that only one in three women examines her own breasts[47] and an article in *U.S. News and World Report* estimates that only 15–40% of women examine their breasts.[4] Rabinowitz and Adler stated that "Research has shown that only 24% of all women use this self-examination technique."[48]

1" or about 2.5 cm

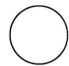
3/4" or about 2 cm

1/2" or about 1.2 cm

1/4" or about .5 cm

FIGURE 2-4 The average size of a tumor detected by a woman practicing occasional BSE is 2.5 cm (1 inch); mammography can detect cancers as small as 0.50 cm (¼ inch).

These statistics attest to the fact that the vast majority of breast cancers will not be detected until they have advanced in their growth to a size at which the victims accidentally discover them or they are purposefully detected through BSE or physical examination by a physician. Mammography is capable of detecting cancer at a much smaller size (Fig. 2-4). BSE or a physical examination by a physician is very important since some cancers (e.g., lobular carcinoma) will be felt before they can be imaged on film. Also,

TABLE 2-5 Characteristics of Malignant and Benign Breast Lumps

Malignant*	Benign†
Hard	Soft
Immobile	Spongy
Fixed to the skin	Easily movable
Skin dimpling	Smooth contour
Nipple retraction	

*These characteristics are typical of an advanced carcinoma.
†A lump with these characteristics may truly be a benign lesion, or it may be a minimal tumor that in time will grow to an advanced stage at which time its characteristics will fit the profile of a malignant tumor.

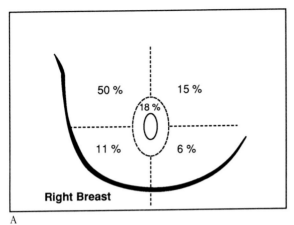
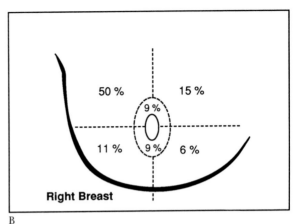

A   B

FIGURE 2-5   **A.** The frequency of breast cancers by location: upper outer quadrant (UOQ) = 50%; central region = 18%; upper inner quadrant (UIQ) = 15%; lower outer quadrant (LOQ) = 11%; and lower inner quadrant (LIQ) = 6%. **B.** The frequency of breast cancers in the upper and lower halves of the breast: superior aspect = UOQ + UIQ + ½ central region = 74%; inferior aspect = LOQ + LIQ + ½ central region = 26%. (Redrawn from *The Breast Cancer Digest*.[49])

women should perform BSE to compensate for any inaccuracy on the part of the mammographic findings.

Medical literature for the public still cites the traditional "warning signs" when examining the breast for lumps (Table 2-5). It must also be remembered that the breasts are symmetrical; that is, they are mirror images of one another. If a lump is discovered, there should be a matching lump in the same location in the opposite breast. The lumps may be of different sizes because the left breast tends to be approximately 10% larger than the right; therefore a lump in the larger breast might be expected to be slightly larger. If there is not a "twin" in the opposite breast, a lump that "feels" benign should be treated as suspicious of carcinoma.

Many physicians perform a cursory examination of the breasts, generally with the woman supine; they may make only a visual inspection of the breasts and examine the axillae when the woman is upright. However, approximately 74% of all breast cancers are in the upper half of the breast[49] (Fig. 2-5). Cancers in the upper half will often be felt best when examined in the upright position, whereas cancers in the lower half of the breast will be felt best when the patient is supine. Therefore, the breasts should be examined in both the upright and supine positions.

Summary

The prevention, detection, and treatment of breast cancer continues to be a major goal in the health care of women. This disease strikes one in every nine American women and is a major cause of death. We cannot prevent this disease at this time; we can, however, detect it at an earlier stage at which the word "cure" can be more than something the woman hopes for. The radiologic technologist's knowledge and personal interest in helping patients will go a long way in educating women to care for their breasts and to encourage their female family members and friends to have a mammogram.

References

1. Boring CC, Squires TS, Tong T: Cancer statistics, 1991. *CA* 1991;1(1):19.
2. Kalisher L, Feig S, McLelland R: *Mammography in Clinical Practice,* American College of Radiology Audiovisual Subcommittee, 1983.
3. Eckley A: Early detection major theme at breast cancer conference. *Diagn Imag* 1984;6(5):100.
4. Silbner J: How to beat breast cancer. *U.S. News & World Report,* 11 July 1988, p 52.
5. Laxity abounds in having test. *Chicago Tribune,* 21 August 1988, p 2.
6. Mammography underused despite ACR guidelines. *Diagn Imag* 1985;7(11):24.
7. Howard J: Using mammography for cancer control—an unrealized potential. *CA* 1987;37(1):33.
8. Some setbacks, some gains in war on cancer. Arlington Heights, IL *Daily Herald,* 2 February 1988, p 1.
9. *1980 NCI Division of Cancer Prevention and Control Surveillance Program: Cancer Statistics Review 1970–1986,* National Institutes of Health publication No. 89-2789. Bethesda, MD, National Cancer Institute, 1989.
10. Siedman H, Mushinski MH: Breast cancer incidence, mortality, survival, prognosis, in Feig SA, McLelland R (eds): *Breast Carcinoma: Current Diagnosis and Treatment.* New York, Masson, 1983, p 9.
11. Young JL, Percy CL, Asire AJ (eds): *Surveillance, Epidemiology, End Results: Incidence and Mortality Data, 1973–1977,* U.S. Department of Health and Human Services publication No. (NIH) 81-2330. Government Printing Office, 1981.
12. Tabar L: The control of breast cancer through regular mammographic examinations. *Hospimedia* Nov/Dec 1987;47.
13. Dakins D: Diagnostic problem-solving takes a back seat in breast screening. *Diagn Imag* 1987;9(11):372.
14. Feig SA, Ehrlich SM: Estimation of radiation risk from screening mammography: Recent trends and comparisons with expected benefits. *Radiology* 1990;174(3):638.
15. Vinocur B: The breast cancer battle: Screening with mammography. *Diagn Imag* 1986;8(7):84.
16. Self-exams, mammograms recommended. *USA Today,* 19 October 1987, p 12A.
17. Strax P: Control of breast cancer. *Administrative Radiology,* September 1989, p 30.
18. Subtle mammographic signs disclose presence of early breast cancer. *Radiology Today* 1987;4(4):4.
19. Egan R: The new age of breast care. *Administrative Radiology,* September 1989, p 9.
20. Wertheimer M, et al: Increasing the effort toward breast cancer detection. *JAMA* 1986;255(10):1311.
21. Wanebo HH, Huvos AG, Urban JA: Treatment of minimal breast cancer. *Cancer* 1974;33:349.
22. Moskowitz M: Breast cancer: Age-specific growth rates and screening strategies. *Radiology* 1986;161:37.
23. ACR and ACS conduct national breast cancer detection program. *Radiology Today* 1987;4(4):1.
24. Glassman L: Letters to the Editor. *Administrative Radiology,* November 1987, p 12.
25. Fisher L: Mammography holdouts. *Medicenter Management,* October 1987, p 31.
26. Moskowitz M: Cost-benefit determinations in screening mammography. *Cancer* 1987;60(7):1680.
27. New focus on screening for breast cancer. *Changing Times,* March 1986, p 16.
28. Upton AC, Beebe GW, Brown JM, et al: Report of the Ad Hoc Working Group. *JNCI* 1977;59:481.
29. McGregor DH, Land CE, Choi K, et al: Breast cancer incidence among atomic bomb survivors, Hiroshima and Nagasaki, 1950–1969. *JNCI* 1977;59:799.
30. Tokunaga M, Land CE, Yamamoto T, et al: Incidence of female breast cancer among atomic bomb survivors, Hiroshima and Nagasaki, 1950–1980. *Radiat Res* 1987;112:243.
31. Preston DL, Kato H, Kopecky KF, et al: Studies of the mortality of atomic bomb survivors. Cancer mortality 1950–1982. *Radiat Res* 1987;11:151.
32. Boice JD, Land CE, Shore RE, et al: Risk of breast cancer following low-dose radiation exposure. *Radiology* 1979;131:589.
33. Howe GR, Miller AB, Sherman GJ: Breast cancer mortality following fluoroscopic irradiation in a cohort of tuberculosis patients. *Cancer Detect Prev* 1982;5:175.
34. Miller AB, Howe GR, Sherman GJ, et al: Mortality from breast cancer after irradiation during fluoroscopic examinations in patients being treated for tuberculosis. *N Eng J Med* 1989;321:1285.
35. Mettler FA, Hempelmann LH, Dutton AM, et al: Breast neoplasma in women treated with x-rays for acute postpartum mastitis: A pilot study. *JNCI* 1969;43:803.
36. Shore RE, Hildreth N, Woodard ED, et al: Breast cancer among women given x-ray therapy for acute postpartum mastitis. *JNCI* 1986;77:689.

37. Bartlett E: Talk to your patients to avoid trouble later with malpractice. *Diagn Imag* 1987;9(11):179.
38. Haight D, Tsuchiyama S: Radiologists spread their wings: A look at the possibilities in stereotactic breast biopsy. *Administrative Radiology,* November 1987, p 89.
39. Dakins D: Attention to practical concerns can improve mammographic quality. *Diagn Imag* 1988;10(12):75.
40. Physicians reaffirm mammography for breast screening. *Diagn Imag* 1985;7(6):22.
41. Mammography should be read in clinical context. *Radiology Today* 1987;4(4):7.
42. Dempsey P: Ultrasound's distinctive role in breast cancer diagnosis. *Diag Imag* 1985;7(2):59.
43. Young JO, Sadowsky NL, Young JW, et al: Mammography of women with suspicious breast lumps. *Arch Surg* 1986;121:807.
44. Leis Jr HP: Risk factors for breast cancer: An update. *Breast Disease* 1980;6(4):24.
45. James F: Fear barrier. *Chicago Tribune,* 25 March 1990, sect 6, p 4.
46. Penneypacker H, et al: Toward an effective technology of instruction in BSE. *J Mental Health* 1982;11(3):102.
47. Guide prompts men to support breast cancer screening. *Radiology Today,* November 1987, p 38.
48. Rabinowitz B, Adler D: Tough choices. *Administrative Radiology,* September 1989, p 44.
49. *The Breast Cancer Digest,* ed 2, National Institutes of Health publication No. 84-1691. Government Printing Office, 1984.

Valerie Fink Andolina

In Consideration of the Patient

In almost every other chapter of this book the patient is referred to by components in some way—her breast, her position, the relationship of the tube target material to her tissue. This chapter deals with the person who is coming for this exam, and what each facility can do to make her feel more comfortable. Taking a few extra minutes will ultimately be rewarding for everyone involved: the patient, the technologist, and the facility.

When a woman's physician requests that she have a mammogram, her first reaction is usually fear that her doctor has found a problem. Even if she has been reassured that it is for routine purposes, the fear of cancer is still there—that is, after all, what a mammogram is supposed to find. In addition, some of her friends have undoubtedly told her how humiliating the exam was for them, and how painful, elevating her fear even more. By disproving these anxieties through treating her well and with respect, informing her of the exam's purpose, and, most importantly, educating her in breast health, it is hoped that she will find it to be a worthwhile experience that she will intend to repeat yearly.

The Examination Environment

Atmosphere

When a mammogram is first suggested to any woman, she imagines the setting will be much like the traditional radiographic exams that she has had—cold and sterile with huge machinery hanging overhead. Thoughts of being left alone in this intimidating room while the technologist hides behind a lead wall bring even more anxiety.

Making the atmosphere of both the waiting room and the examination room as comfortable and as relaxing as possible is half the battle in winning the patient's confidence and making her feel better about the exam (Fig. 3-1). Comfortable furniture, soft pastel colors, wallpaper, and relaxing artwork on the walls all contribute to a more casual setting. Soft lighting from table lamps has a more calming influence than harsh lighting from overhead fluorescent fixtures. The availability of coffee and tea (decaffeinated, of course) and shawls to help ward off chills are

19

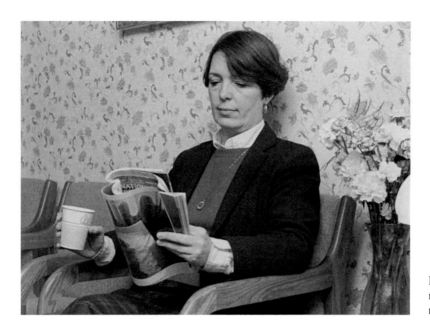

FIGURE 3-1   A comfortable waiting room helps make the patient feel more at ease.

extra personal touches that women appreciate. Many offices have fresh flower arrangements, and some even give patients a flower to take home at the end of their appointment. There are many "homey" touches that can help the ambiance to be more casual, soothing, and personable.

To make the exam more comfortable, many facilities try to warm the breast tray of the x-ray unit with a heating pad or hot water bottle. However, this can interfere with the reliability of some automatic exposure control (phototiming) devices. Check with the manufacturer of the unit before attempting this or any other alterations or modifications to the x-ray unit that may affect its performance in an effort to increase the patient's comfort.

Personality of the Staff

As important as the physical setting in which the mammogram is performed, the personality and friendliness of the staff are what most patients will remember. Before she ever sees the wallpaper of the office, the patient will be talking with a faceless person on the phone to make an appointment. The charm and character of this person is as important as his or her efficiency; first impressions do count. The secretary who schedules appointments must be friendly, helpful, and patient while gathering all the necessary information from the caller prior to her exam. If not, the woman may feel harassed and inconvenienced, and will have negative feelings toward the facility before she has even been there.

The appointment secretary will need to gather a great deal of information from the caller, and if possible he or she should speak directly to the patient because some of the information may be personal. Other than the usual name, address, and phone number, some facilities request additional information such as:

The patient's birthdate.
Whether she has ever had a mammogram before, and if so, when and where.
Name of the referring physician.
Date of the patient's last menstrual period.
Type of medical insurance the patient has.
Whether the appointment is for a screening mammogram, or if the patient has a lump or other problem with her breasts.

Discerning if the patient has a clinical finding before having her mammogram is most important. Some women will try to conceal the fact that they found a lump in their breast, thinking that if a problem exists the mammogram will find it. Because the mammogram is not 100% accurate in finding all cancers, any lump or other symptoms identified by the patient or her physician should be addressed specifically. Questioning the patient about possible problems should be done by the appointment secretary, the receptionist, and the technologist.

The next person the woman coming for a mammogram encounters will be the receptionist. Again, a polite and courteous as well as friendly demeanor is essential. At this point the patient feels very vulnerable—she is here, there is no turning back, and she is in the staff's hands. She needs to trust the people who will be taking care of her.

Most importantly, she needs to trust the technologist. This relationship will be intimate; however, it must remain professional. Conversing about general topics such as the weather or some local news item helps the patient feel a common bond with the person performing her exam. Before the exam begins, the technologist should explain the exam to the patient, especially if she has not previously had a mammogram. This helps to alleviate the woman's fears, or at least acknowledge them, as well as establish the fact that the technologist is a competently trained professional.

Patient Preparation

At the time that a woman makes her appointment, there are usually some demands placed upon her. Two frequent requests are to restrict her intake of caffeine and to not wear deodorant when she comes for her exam. The patient is likely to be much more compliant if she knows the reasons behind the request. These and other such demands should be explained to her, either in literature mailed to her home prior to the exam or by the appointment secretary. She may have many questions, some which may never be asked, but the office staff should be prepared to answer them.

Caffeine Ingestion

Since the publication of a paper by Minton et al.[1] concerning the theory that caffeine, usually considered a diuretic, caused breast tissue to retain fluid, many mammography facilities have requested that their patients refrain from consuming products containing this substance. The pressure from this fluid

buildup within the breast tissue combined with compression during the exam can add to the discomfort that many women feel during a mammogram.

There are many products that contain caffeine. Table 3-1 lists a number of them. It should be stressed to the patient that prescription drugs or necessary medications containing caffeine should not be

TABLE 3-1 Sample List of Foods and Drugs Containing Caffeine*

Food or Drug	Caffeine Content (mg)†
Hot beverages (5-oz cup)	
Coffee, percolated	110
Coffee, drip	150
Coffee, instant	66
Tea, brewed 5 min	45
Cocoa	13
Cold beverages (12-oz glass)	
Coke	42
Pepsi	35
Sunkist Orange	NA
Jolt	NA
Some root beers	NA
Mountain Dew	49
Royal Crown	36
Tab	45
Nonprescription drugs	
Actifed	NA
Anacin	32
APC's	NA
Appedrine	100
Coryban D	30
Dexatrim	200
Empirin	NA
Excedrin	65
Midol	32
No Doz	100
Triaminicin	30
Vanquish	33
Prescription drugs	
APC with Codeine	32
Aminophylline	NA
Cafergot	100
Darvon Compound	32
Emprazil	30
Ephedrine	NA
Fiorinal	40
Migral	50
Repan	40
Synalgos Capsules	30

*Adapted from Logan-Young W: *Breast Self Examination.* Rochester, NY, Logan-Young, 1989.
†NA indicates caffeine amount not available.

stopped or altered without first consulting with their physician. The patient should also be advised that suddenly terminating the use of caffeine may cause severe withdrawal headaches; gradually cutting down her intake will alleviate this problem.

The effect of caffeine on breast tissue is subjective, and no studies have been performed concerning this topic since Minton et al.'s controversial paper was released in 1979. However, after speaking with thousands of women who have abstained from caffeine for at least 2 weeks prior to having a mammographic examination, the authors of this book have concluded that as many as 85% of women do feel considerably less discomfort from the exam when caffeine is restricted. The majority of women are usually those with microcystic breast tissue, rather than those with severe fibrocystic disease or women with adipose-replaced breast tissue.

Many other factors can cause discomfort in the breast tissue: the patient's own hormonal changes, blood pressure and heart medications, hormone therapy, and stress are major causes. Caffeine ingestion and dosage of hormone therapy medications are usually the only controllable factors. Hormone therapy changes should only be made under the direction of the patient's own physician, but caffeine consumption may be changed at the discretion of the woman.

Deodorants and Powders

Many facilities request that their patients refrain from wearing deodorant and body powders on the day of their mammographic exam. This request arose with the advent of xeromammography. Some personal hygiene products contain minute particles of metal (such as aluminum chlorhydrate and zinc) or calcium-like particles (as in talcum powder). These are readily visualized on a xeromammogram, and sometimes simulate the calcium of a breast carcinoma. Even when these particles are recognized as artifacts, large areas of breast tissue may be obliterated by xerography's edge enhancement, and actual cancers could be missed.

Screen-film mammography does not rely on edge enhancement, and the usually discernible low-density specks on the image are not as much of a problem. Deodorants and powders are usually seen on a film within skinfolds or creases, where perspiration has

caused them to become caked. These artifacts can be differentiated from calcifications that typify carcinoma. Calcium from powders is usually seen as lines that run laterally to medially, whereas cancer calcifications will run in a ductal pattern toward the nipple (Fig. 3-2).

The decision to request that patients refrain from using these products is dependent upon the radiologist's preference and expertise. Whether a facility requires this of a patient or not, it is a good idea to have spray cans of deodorant available in the dressing rooms for patients to use after their exam.

Explaining the Examination

It is extremely important for the technologist to take time with each patient to explain exactly what the examination entails and why screening is performed (Fig. 3-3). Having knowledge of the procedure beforehand helps to alleviate the fear of the unknown. Women who have had a mammogram in the past may also need a review of the procedure. In most cases it has been at least a year since her last exam, and the memory of what is expected of her may be vague.

Before explaining the procedure, ask the woman if she is having the exam because of a problem with her breasts, such as a lump or thickening, pain, discharge, or discoloration of the skin. Ask if she has ever had surgery on her breasts, and the reason for the surgery. Her answers may be cause for a deviation from the routine views normally taken, and the exact procedure can then be explained. For example, a woman who has had cosmetic breast augmentation surgery will be positioned differently than a woman who has not (see Chapter 12), and she will want to know what will be done for her specific situation. (See also Chapters 13 and 15 for further discussion.)

Prior to the exam let the patient know how many views will be taken of each breast, but be certain she knows from the start that additional films may be necessary after the routine views have been checked, and that this does not necessarily indicate any pathologic findings. Explain that her breast will be manipulated and pulled in an effort to view as much of her tissue as possible and that her breast will be com-

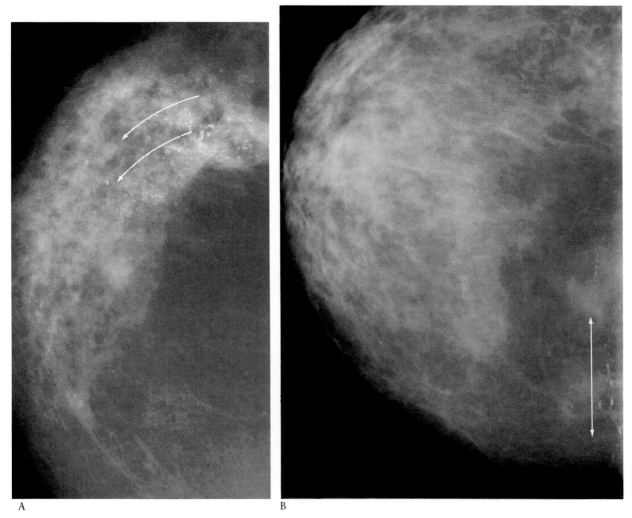

A   B

FIGURE 3-2   **A.** Calcifications typifying a carcinoma follow a ductal pattern toward the nipple. **B.** Calcifications that indicate caked talcum powder at the inframammary crease will be visualized in a lateral-medial pattern. (*Figure continues.*)

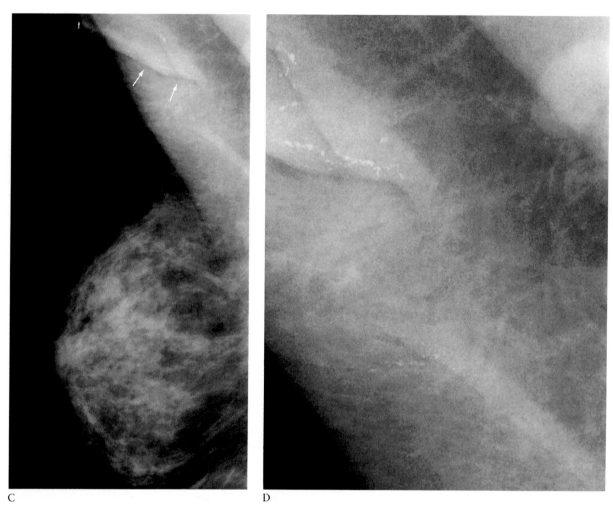

C

D

FIGURE 3-2   (*Continued*) **C.** Deodorant, if visualized, will be seen within skinfolds of the axilla. **D.** Close-up of the axilla showing detail of deodorant within skinfolds.

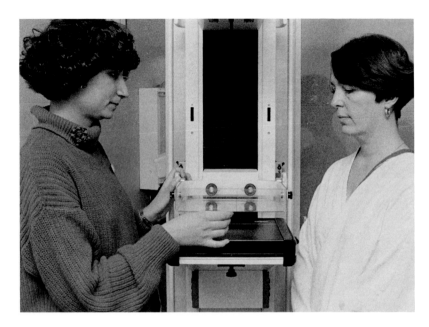

FIGURE 3-3   It is important for the technologist to explain the exam to the patient, along with the need for vigorous compression, before the exam begins.

pressed during the exposure; it may be uncomfortable, but lasts only a few seconds. Indicate that it is very important for her to remain still, and that she will be asked to not breathe as the mammogram is taken to prevent any motion.

Compression is usually the most feared part of the mammogram. It is advisable, when referring to compression, to use the term "discomfort" rather than "pain." A recent study has indicated that only 1% of women who have the exam find mammography to be a painful experience.[2] This low statistic can be maintained by asking the patient to tell the technologist if the compression is painful or too uncomfortable, and reassuring her that the compression will be lowered to an amount that is no more than she can tolerate. This allows the patient to feel she has some control, and she is usually more willing to tolerate the necessary amount of compression. It is better to ensure that the patient will return for another mammogram, wherever she may choose to go, rather than vow never to have another because it was too painful.

Once the basic steps have been outlined to the patient and the exam has begun, it helps to talk her through the steps. Tell her everything that is being done as it is happening. This way, she will know what is expected of her, and will be able to cooperate more knowledgeably, making the mammogram a more pleasant experience for both the patient and the technologist.

Concerns about Dosage

Three fears are usually associated with mammograms: that a cancer will be found, that the compression involved will be painful, and that the radiation involved will cause a cancer that she would not otherwise have. Professionals in the field of radiology realize that this last fear is negligible as a result of the technological advances that have occurred within the last 15 years. Many women in the general public, however, remember the media hype of the 1970s that suggested that mammography was actually dangerous.

Today, we can reassure our patients that the amount of radiation involved in a mammographic exam is safe. The American College of Radiology suggests that a single-view screen-film mammogram should measure less than 300 mrads average glandular dose when a grid is employed. Compared to the 8 to 12 rads of exposure that was received by the patient in the early 1970s, there has been a substantial reduction of radiation dosage to the breast tissue during a mammographic exam.

These figures are impressive; however, to most patients they are just numbers with no meaning. To place the risk of developing a breast cancer from the amount of radiation received from the mammogram into a framework of relative risk, the following comparisons have been made, to which a patient can more easily relate.

The risk of death from developing a breast carcinoma due to radiation received during routine mammograms throughout a woman's lifetime is the same risk that is involved when:

Traveling 220 miles by automobile (New York to Boston).
Traveling 2500 miles by airplane (New York to Los Angeles).
Traveling 1500 miles by train (New York to Miami).
Smoking 1.5 cigarettes.[3]

As with any radiographic examination, unnecessary exposure should be avoided. Most women over the age of 40 should have no more than one mammographic examination within a year's time, but there will always be some exceptions to the rule (e.g., suggested 6-month rechecks of areas suspicious of carcinoma, or radiation therapy rechecks). Women under the age of 35 should be referred by a physician for mammography; the ever-changing cellular structures of younger patients may be more susceptible to radiation changes.

Guidelines for Mammography

Recommendations from the American Cancer Society, the American Medical Association, and the American College of Radiology state that screening mammograms be performed on women as follows:

A baseline mammogram at age 35
A mammogram every 1–2 years between ages 40 and 50
A mammogram every year after age 50

Symptomatic patients need to be diagnosed using a logical protocol taking into consideration both age and length of time since the last mammogram. Chapter 15 gives some insight to these parameters.

Patient Education

A woman who is informed of the benefits of mammography is generally a more cooperative patient.

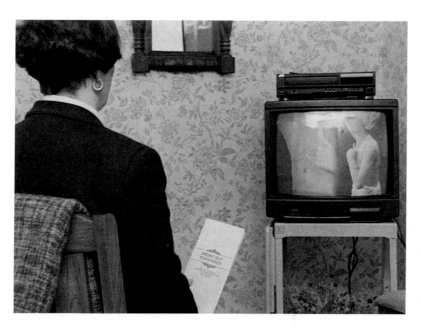

FIGURE 3-4 Mammographic facilities are urged to provide their patients with some type of program for breast self-examination training and breast health education. This can be accomplished with videotapes and pamphlets, as well as personalized training or group classes.

Hówever, mammography is not 100% accurate in finding all breast cancers; approximately 7% of breast cancers are found through clinical breast examination or breast self-examination alone.[4] Therefore, mammographic facilities are urged to take some time to educate all patients in breast self-examination and breast health (Fig. 3-4).

Patient education can take many forms, from a structured class on mammography and breast self-examination to a simple pamphlet handed to a patient. Many facilities show videotapes, and others employ a nurse or other professional to teach breast self-examination personally to each patient. Any of these methods, or a combination of them, are suitable and necessary. Each hospital, clinic, or office should decide which is the best method for its clientele.

References

1. Minton J, Foecking M, Webster D, et al: Caffeine, cyclic nucleotides, and breast disease. *Surgery* 1979;86(1): 105–109.
2. Stomper P, Kopans D, Sadowsky N, et al: Is mammography painful? A multicenter patient survey. *Arch Intern Med* 1988;148:521–524.
3. Feig S, Ehrlich SM: Estimation of radiation risk from screening mammography: Recent trends and comparison with expected benefits. *Radiology* 1990;174(3): 638–647.
4. Seidman H, Gelb S, et al: Survival experience in the Breast Cancer Detection and Demonstration Project. *CA* 1987;37(5):258–290.

Bibliography

Feig S, McClelland R (eds): *Breast Carcinoma, Current Diagnosis and Treatment.* Chicago, American College of Radiology, 1983.

Fox S, Klos D, et al: Improving the adherence of urban women to mammography guidelines: Strategies for radiologists. *Radiology* 1990;174:203–206.

Gold R: Painless mammography [editorial]. *Arch Intern Med* 1988;148:517.

Helvie M, Rebner M, Sickles E, Oberman H: Calcifications in metastatic breast cancer axillary lymph nodes. *AJR* 1988;151:921.

Hill D, et al: Self examination of the breast: Is it beneficial? Meta-analysis of studies investigating breast self examination and extent of disease in patients with breast cancer. *Br Med J* 1988;297:271–275.

Logan-Young W: *Breast Self Examination.* Rochester, NY, Logan-Young, 1989.

Mammography—A User's Guide, NCRP Report No. 85. Bethesda, MD, National Council on Radiation Protection and Measurement, 1986.

Minton J, Foecking M, Webster D, et al: Response of fibrocystic disease to caffeine withdrawal and correlation of cyclic nucleotides with breast disease. *Am J Obstet Gynecol* 1979;135(1):105–109.

Policy Statement. Chicago, American College of Radiology, 1982.

Strax P: Film-screen experience in the screening center, in Logan W (ed): *Breast Carcinoma, The Radiologist's Expanded Role.* New York, John Wiley, 1977.

4

Shelly Lillé

The Radiologic Technologist

Experienced physicians are in agreement about the technical complexity of good mammography and the need for skilled technical support. "Mammography is one of the most technically difficult radiographic examinations. Both proper, specialized equipment and correct use of that equipment are essential to the achievement of satisfactory results."[1] Technologists have an important responsibility in the early detection of breast cancer. Technical expertise is often the determining factor in the localization of a lesion, because if the lesion is not demonstrated it cannot be detected and reported. A statement by Milbrath emphasizes this point: "A technologist can make or break you. If you have a technologist who takes care and is interested, you will have an excellent program. If you have a technologist who does not care, you will get horrible results" (J. Milbrath, personal communication).

Snyder stated that "Good mammography depends not only on excellent technique and low absorbed dose, but also on an intelligent approach to the individual examination as well. The technologist must be able to establish rapport with her patient to obtain her cooperation, must know if there is a particular problem, must develop an appreciation of the type

of breast with which she is dealing in order to establish optimal technique, and must be certain that all areas of concern have been demonstrated" (R. Snyder, personal communication). McLelland stated, "Mammography is a special procedure that requires experienced, skillful, meticulous interpretation and thorough clinical correlation. It is a special procedure no less than neuro-radiology, angiography, CT, sonography, etc., and merits the commitment of radiologists and radiologic technologists equal to the challenge. The results clearly are related to those commitments."[2]

There is general agreement among radiologists that a mammogram is very difficult to interpret. This is one of the few radiology exams that frequently is afforded the luxury of double reading. Within a large group of radiologists, there are usually one or two physicians who are more adept at interpreting a mammogram, whether because of personal experience or because they have an interest in mammography. Such specialization is the key to good interpretation . . . and also to producing a good image. The more consistently one performs a task, the easier the task becomes and the better the results will be. If there are 10 radiologic technologists on staff and a different technologist is assigned to the mammography rotation each day, then 1 day every 2 weeks each will have a turn at trying to produce consistent, high-quality, diagnostic mammograms. In mammography, it is easy for the radiologist to miss a subtle lesion even on a series of technically excellent films. Mammograms performed by many technologists with differing abilities to position and image the breast may not always provide the radiologist with the best possible image every time.

The goals of excellent mammography are high accuracy and specificity rates. It is unrealistic to expect a radiologist to achieve and maintain high accuracy and specificity rates if he or she is allowed to interpret mammograms only once every 10 days, and it is equally unrealistic to expect radiologic technologists to produce their best results with limited experience and occasional practice. Advocates for excellence in mammography recommend that specialized training in mammography and the daily responsibility for taking mammographic images be limited to a few technologists within a department. However, just as there is a potential for future problems in training all technologists in a particular department to perform mammography, there is a clear danger at the other extreme—training only one technologist. If for any reason that individual left the facility or was unavailable, mammography services surely would be downgraded.

Doctor Ferris Hall of Beth Israel Hospital in Boston recommends that a small cadre of radiologic technologists be developed in every hospital or clinic who would be responsible for producing the mammographic films and correlating the clinical picture of the patient with the films. Hall calls these technologists "supertechs."[3] Although it is recommended that a radiologist be readily available, the services of such supertechs are especially helpful in situations where no radiologist is on the premises when a mammogram is done or, if in a busy institution, where the radiologist may not be available to follow up the mammographic study with a clinical exam. The radiologic technologist could (1) perform ultrasound, which would determine if a mass is cystic or solid; (2) supply magnification views or different degree oblique views of a suspicious area; and (3) correlate the physical exam/clinical history with any findings on the mammogram. The technologist would perform these problem-solving tasks while the patient is there, perhaps saving the patient from needless worry and the inconvenience of again taking time off from work to reschedule additional tests when the radiologist is present.

In the 1970s, Strax of the Guttman Institute in New York utilized such paraprofessionals.

Evaluation of the use of allied health personnel, especially the radiologic technologist, in the preliminary reading of mammograms indicates that such personnel can be used successfully in prescreening. They respond readily to the challenge, find the work exciting, seldom become bored, and are prepared to examine large numbers of mammograms. Usually young and with good eyesight, they can be taught to follow details of the interpretive process. In the course of training, paraprofessional readers of mammograms are taught only to choose the obviously normal, the possibly abnormal, and the definitely abnormal. They are not taught to make a histopathologic diagnosis. . . . *The primary function of the paramedical trainee in mammography interpretation is to isolate the obviously normal cases which can then be checked rapidly by the radiologist. Those listed as doubtful or positive are studied more carefully.* Experience to date indicates that a nonmedical reader will overcall about 10 times, i.e., if there is one cancer in a group of 100 mammograms, he or she will call 10 abnormal and 90 negative, but, more importantly, the cancers will usually be present in the abnormal group.[4] [emphasis added]

It is not unusual for radiologists today to have a specificity rate of 1:10 or 1:8; the American College of Radiology advocates a goal of 1:5. However, the luminaries in the mammography community are, generally, able to specify two cancers for every three biopsies recommended (2:3).

Paraprofessionals are utilized to routinely assist professionals in business, law, and medicine. We are all familiar with administrative assistants in large corporations, paralegals in law firms, medical laboratory technicians assisting pathologists, nurse practitioners and physician assistants to aid physicians, and the use of emergency medical technicians (EMTs) to replace nurses and/or physicians on ambulances. In mammography, a "supertech" trained in breast imaging will be an asset to the radiologist.

References

1. *Mammography—A User's Guide,* NCRP Report No. 85. Bethesda, MD, National Council on Radiation Protection and Measurements, 1986.
2. McLelland R: Mammography 1984: Challenge to radiology. *AJR* 1984;143:1.
3. Vinocur D: The breast cancer battle: Screening with mammography. *Diagn Imag* 1986;9,7:84.
4. Strax P (ed): In: Use of allied personnel. Control of Breast Cancer Through Mass Screening. St Louis, MO, Mosby-Yearbook, 1978.

II

Technical Considerations

5 Shelly Lillé

Selection and Use of Equipment

The National Council on Radiation Protection and Measurements (NCRP) has established guidelines that require the use of a dedicated unit when performing screen-film mammography.[1] A dedicated mammographic unit is the only equipment specifically designed to adequately visualize the components of the breast from which breast cancers arise.

There is a wide variety of equipment available today ranging from basic low-cost mammographic units with few features to high-cost units with many built-in features. Many units offer compatibility with a choice of optional peripheral add-on accessories. While the objective of all dedicated mammography units is to produce clinically useful information on x-ray film, manufacturers may choose to engineer and design their equipment with slight differences to accommodate the unique technical demands of screen-film mammography.

The choices of film and processing techniques and the differences in technologists' skills and knowledge of mammography, along with the variables possible with patients of all ages, shapes, and sizes, add up to a very large number of factors that every manufacturer will attempt to accommodate. Some equipment may offer automated features, whereas other units may be sufficiently adjustable to provide acceptable solutions to accommodate most key operating variables. Each facility must select the equipment that best meets its needs and budget. The perfect mammography unit—one that will do everything for everybody all of the time—does not exist at any price. There are trade-offs that must be accepted. This chapter will help in understanding the important design and operating features of a mammographic unit and their relationships to screen-film mammography.

Equipment Selection Considerations

What factor(s) should be considered when selecting a dedicated mammographic unit?

Performance

The technical factors in the design of the equipment that affect production of the image are discussed in detail in this chapter. It is the ability to produce consistent, high-contrast, diagnostic images that is most important. Other equipment selection considerations

35

that reflect a concern for "ergonomics" or "human engineering" features designed into the equipment such as color, style, number and location of foot pedals, etc. are mentioned but not discussed in detail. These features do not directly affect production of the image. Equipment selection is a trade-off between the relative merits of the equipment in addressing these variables and the budget alloted for the dedicated mammography unit. Price alone should not be the major determinant in the selection of equipment.

The basic considerations for equipment should include:

Space

The minimum space for an examination room should accommodate the unit with its shield and enough room for the technologist to move and assist the patient for proper positioning. Additional space may be required to accommodate patients in wheelchairs and for storing some supplies and/or equipment accessories in the examination room.

Portability

Some units are on wheels while others must be anchored to the floor or the wall. If the unit is to be used at various locations (a truly mobile environment), be sure to "test drive" the machine in a realistic setting.

Electrical Requirements

Some machines plug into existing wall outlets while others require three-phase or 220 wiring to be installed. In either case, a dedicated line is recommended.

Ergonomics

User friendliness to the patient and the operator is important. The basic components of a standard dedicated mammography unit are shown in Figure 5-1.

The C-Arm The C-arm's range of vertical movement should accommodate very tall patients (approximately 6 feet) as well as those who need to be seated. There should be no encumbrances under the receptor tray that would interfere with the patient should she

need to be seated for the exam. There should be at least 180° of rotation of the C-arm.

The point at which the C-arm connects to the tower (called the "collar") should be isocentrically designed so that when going from the craniocaudal position to the oblique position no adjustment in height needs to be made. Almost all current units require the C-arm to be lowered several inches when changing to the oblique position.

Electronic Controls Electronic controls on both sides of the C-arm provide easy access for the technologist while the patient is being positioned.

Grips or Handles Handles should be available for the patient to hold onto in order to maintain a difficult or awkward position. These handles should be different from the technologist's handles, on which switches for operating the C-arm movements are located.

Compression Device–to–Receptor Distance This distance (with the compression device raised as far away from the film holder as possible) should allow adequate space when positioning the obese woman for an oblique view, when magnifying an area in a large breast, or when raising the compression device over the needle during preoperative localizations. The minimum measurement should be approximately 20 cm.

Tube Housing or Face Shield This area of the machine should be kept as small as possible in order to facilitate positioning of the patient's head for the craniocaudal view as well as during magnification views.

Foot Controls Remote foot controls for vertical movement of the C-arm and the compression device free the hands of the technologist during patient positioning. The amount of compression able to be exerted by the foot pedal control should be minimal, with final compression of the breast accomplished with a hand-controlled device.

Film Tray The receptor tray should permit fast and easy exchange of different size film cassettes and grids. When imaging a small breast on a 24 × 30-cm receptor tray or a large breast on an 18 × 24-cm tray,

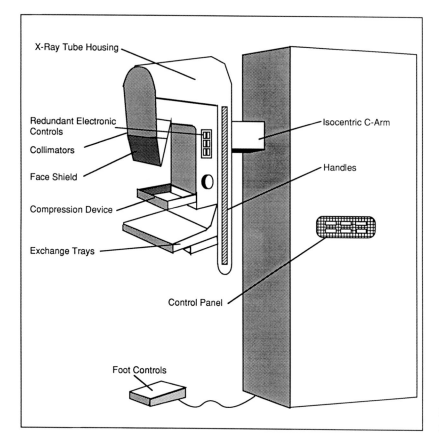

X-Ray Tube Housing

Redundant Electronic Controls

Collimators

Face Shield

Compression Device

Exchange Trays

Isocentric C-Arm

Handles

Control Panel

Foot Controls

FIGURE 5-1   Dedicated screen/film mammographic unit.

the technologist works harder and the patient is more uncomfortable. Additional films that may be necessary under these circumstances will increase the dosage to the patient. Both 18 × 24-cm and 24 × 30-cm grids should be available; match the size of the receptor tray to the size of the breast being imaged.

Control Panel   It should be easy to read and to make adjustments to the control panel. A compression release device must be located on or near this panel. This release must have the ability to be disengaged during needle localizations. Units with automatic exposure control (AEC) should have an mAs readout available after the exposure has been terminated.

Technical Capabilities

Density Selection   Note the percentage of change that occurs with each station. The maximum differ-

ence from one setting to the next should be no greater than 15%. A total of ± 50% change in density from "0" is recommended.

Peak Kilovoltage   One-step increments must be available for peak kilovoltage (kVp) selection.

Milliamperage Selection   Milliamperage (mA) selection may be fixed or variable. If the mA value automatically decreases with increasing kVp, this should occur outside the range of settings routinely used for screen-film mammography.

Time Selection   What is the range of time (from shortest to longest) allowed for an exposure? At the shortest exposure end of the scale, be sure the grid will not be "caught in motion" if using a grid on a thin adipose-replaced breast. At the longest end of the scale, the time setting must be able to surpass the reciprocity law failure of the recording system.

Source–Image Detector Distance The source–image detector distance (SID) may be fixed or it may be variable. In either case the size of the focal spot must match the SID of the unit to provide good resolution as well as to allow the use of acceptable technical factors when dealing with the inverse square law.

Collimators Three designs are currently used: fixed apertures, a set of interchangeable cones of various sizes, and an internal set of collimating blades.

Needle Localization Capability If the equipment has preoperative needle localization capabilities, a side-loading cassette holder or Bucky tray is required. The compression device for needle localization will have either a series of concentric holes or a large rectangular cutout. The concentric hole compression device will hold the breast in place as the needle is inserted, but care must be taken when raising the device over the hub of the needle. With the cutout sys-

tem, the breast will "pillow" through the opening and be less stable during needle placement, and adequate compression for visualizing small or low density lesions cannot be obtained, but there will be no problem in raising the compression device over the hub of the needle.

Image Production Factors

While the space a mammography unit occupies, the ease with which one can exchange imaging receptor trays, or the availability of redundant electronic controls may be important considerations, none of these has a direct influence in actually producing the latent image. *The ability to produce a good image is the single most important consideration in selecting and using equipment.* A summary of the six design/imaging features considered to be the most important in the production of a good image is presented in Table 5-1, and each is discussed more completely in this

TABLE 5-1 Equipment Design Factors in Producing Good Screen-Film Images*

Design Feature	Affects	Design Feature	Affects
Electrical requirements and efficiency	Exposure time SID RLF† Contrast Scatter Filtration Space requirements kVp + mAs selection Screen-film combination Dose HVL† Ripple	Magnification	kVp + mAs selection Exposure time Dose Radiographic sharpness RLF SID Contrast Scatter
Grids	Exposure time Contrast Scatter Dose RLF kVp + mAs selection	X-ray tubes	Filtration Magnification Dose Collimation kVp + mAs selection Exposure time Radiographic sharpness Contrast Scatter Heel effect HVL SID Size
Compression and compression devices	Exposure time Scatter Radiographic sharpness kVp + mAs selection RLF Dose Contrast	Automatic exposure control	RLF Exposure time Dose kVp + mAs selection RLF

*Each equipment design feature influences several imaging factors; for example, x-ray dose is influenced by all six design features while the HVL will be influenced only by two. If the manufacturers were to change any one of the six features listed here, the impact of this modification would be felt in other areas as well.
†RLF, reciprocity law failure; HVL, half-value layer.

chapter. An understanding of the interrelationships between these six features will enable the technologist to use a machine's strengths and minimize its deficiencies.

Electrical Requirements and Efficiency

The method by which electrical power is used in dedicated mammography equipment has an influence on several important operating features, such as efficiency. The output of a mammographic unit should be at least 1000 mR/s at 25kVp, measured 2 cm above the image plane. A short discussion of basic electricity is presented here to aid the reader in understanding the key role electrical power has in producing a useful clinical image.

An alternating voltage or current is usually defined as voltage or current that changes its strength according to a sine curve. Alternating voltage reverses its polarity on each alternation, and an alternating current (AC) reverses its direction of flow on each alternation. The point of maximum voltage, also called the crest voltage or peak voltage of the sine curve, occurs at 90° (Fig. 5-2). Effective voltage (the beginning and ending portion of the usable waveform during the production of x-rays) starts at 45° and continues to 135° (Fig. 5-3).

The frequency of the alternating voltage or current is the number of cycles (completed sine waves) per second (c/s). In the United States the standard is 60 c/

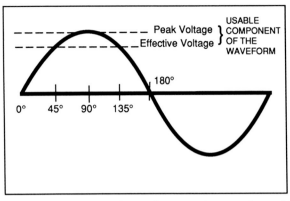

FIGURE 5-3   During the prodruction of x-rays, the useful portion of a sine wave is from the effective voltage up to the peak voltage and down to the effective voltage. The rest of the waveform is unused.

s or 60 Hz. However, *electronic circuits require direct current (DC power)*. The effective voltage component of the AC waveform is equal to the DC power. Half-wave rectification changes alternating current to direct current by using only the positive (+) alternation (from 0° to 180°) of the input voltage, thus effectively cutting off the alternating waveform (Fig. 5-4). The resulting output is fluctuating DC voltage with the same frequency as the AC input. This is extremely inefficient because the output power is much less than the input. Greater efficiency is gained with full-wave rectification. This reverses the polarity of one

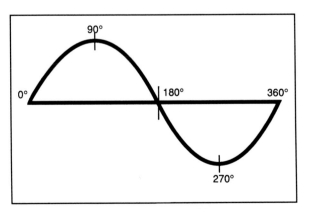

FIGURE 5-2   The highest portion of the sine wave occurs at 90°. An electrical measurement taken here indicates the peak voltage being supplied.

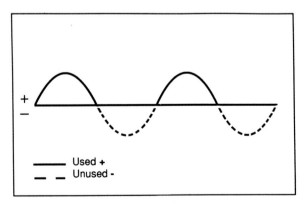

FIGURE 5-4   Half-wave rectification is an inexpensive means of converting AC to DC; however it is very inefficient (50%). Use of half-wave rectification would result in exposure times twice that of full-wave rectification, or almost three times the exposure of a constant potential unit.

alternation of the input sine wave. Thus the resulting output is fluctuating DC voltage with a frequency two times that of the input sine wave (Fig. 5-5). This delivers an average or effective voltage twice as large as that of half-wave rectification; however the peak output voltage is still the same.

A filtered circuit will smooth the fluctuating DC output so the equipment can assure satisfactory operation even though the output voltage is not completely smooth. These small fluctuations are known as *ripple,* which is measured by frequency and amplitude. A filtered circuit is used to compress the peaks of the individually fluctuating DC pulses and to fill in the valleys between the pulses. Capacitors store energy and then release this energy between the pulses (into the valleys) to smooth out the ripple. Tremendously large capacitors (so large in fact that this is impractical) would be required to achieve near-DC power for mammography units operated at a 60-Hz line frequency. *Thus when operating a mammography machine one has always had to account for the effects of this ripple* (Fig. 5-6).

One method of achieving pure DC power (0% ripple) would be use of a *battery*. However, with the kVp values required for mammography, this would be impractical. The battery would have to be even larger than the very large capacitors that would be required for smoothing the waveform at 60 Hz to produce DC in a filtered circuit. Another method, constant potential generation, *is* practical. It will produce this efficient and desirable energy state by rap-idly turning the waveform on and off and utilizing only the peaks of each waveform. By using a microprocessor chip to control the on-off action, pure efficient power is delivered.

Some manufacturers produce mammography units utilizing both high-frequency inverter technology (meaning over 10,000 Hz) and constant potential output (meaning less than 13.5% ripple). However, a further distinction must be made: the most efficient constant potential units will have less than 5% ripple; the less efficient units will have between 5% and 13% ripple. The amount of ripple should remain essentially equal for small and large focal spot operation.

The significant point of this discussion is that *mammography units operate differently and should be used according to their ripple content.* Because of the varying ripple, different mammography units require the use of different kVp settings. Without proper kVp settings, the exposure times might become prohibitively long. Table 5-2 lists the proper settings when comparing dedicated mammography units with varying ripple.

There are several advantages to high frequency/constant potential units. Weigl compared a conventional single-phase generator with a high-frequency/constant potential generator (a multi-pulse generator) also supplied by a single-phase line.[2] He noted the following primary differences:

1. Dose yield and exposure times. We have already seen that dose yield of a three-phase generator is approximately 60% higher than the dose yield of a single-phase generator. This means that a multi-pulse generator [high frequency/constant potential] also has a higher dose yield than a conventional single-phase generator. Figure [5-7] shows the comparison between a conventional single-phase generator, a new multi-pulse generator and a conventional 12 pulse generator. . . . The dose yield of the multi-pulse generator is equivalent to that of a 6 to 12 pulse three-phase generator. Therefore, approximately 40% shorter exposure times than with a conventional single-phase generator are achieved. Or in other words, a tube current of 500 mA on a high-frequency generator results in the same dose output as 800 mA on a conventional single-phase generator.
2. Skin dose. Comparative depth dose measurements illustrate that the skin dose for the same film dose is considerably less from a high frequency generator than the skin dose from a conventional single-phase generator, due to the different high voltage wave shapes. Figure [5-8] shows the relationship of the skin dose of a high frequency generator to a conventional single-phase gen-

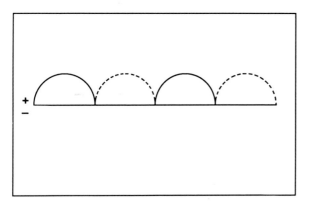

FIGURE 5-5   Full-wave rectification is twice as efficient as half-wave but 30% less efficient, with respect to time, as power produced by constant potential.

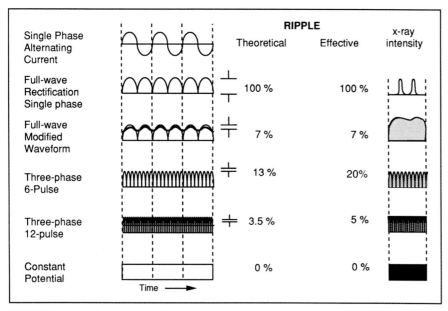

FIGURE 5-6   Tube current and x-ray intensity diagrams. Alternating voltage output from the x-ray transformer is converted into direct current by means of full-wave rectification. Single-phase, single-phase with modified waveform, 3-phase/6-pulse, 3-phase/12-pulse, and constant potential circuits show progressively less variation with time of the voltage curve (decreased "ripple effect"). Short pulses of x-ray intensity are produced by the single-phase generator, whereas steady x-ray intensity results from the constant potential system. (From Feig SA: Mammography equipment: Principles, features, selection. *Radiol Clin North Am* 1987;25(5):897.)

erator as a function of the x-ray tube voltage. . . . The soft x-ray radiation component responsible for the different skin dose is considerably less with the high frequency generator—due to low ripple—than with a conventional single-phase generator. The high frequency technique ensures minimum radiation exposure to the patient also if the generator is connected to a single-phase power supply. . . .

3. Space requirements. A further advantage of high frequency technology is the reduced size. . . . This means the generator is extremely space saving and consists

only of the control desk and the single tank tube unit; no additional high tension transformer or electronics cabinets are necessary.[2]

The advantages of high-frequency/constant potential units are:

1. The ability to use lower kVp settings—thus contrast is increased.
2. Shorter exposure times—more mR/mAs means

TABLE 5-2   Power Variations in Mammography Units*

Generator Setting		Constant Potential Generator Ripple		3-Phase, 6-Pulse Generator, 20% Ripple	Single-Phase Generator (Filtered), 25% + Ripple
		5%	13%		
25 kVp	=	24.4 kV	23.4 kV	22.5 kV	21.9 kV
28 kVp	=	27.3 kV	26.2 kV	25.2 kV	24.5 kV
32 kVp	=	31.2 kV	29.6 kV	28.8 kV	28.0 kV

*Discussion of kilovoltage (kV) rather than peak kilovoltage (kVp) settings is more appropriate when making comparisons between machines. Kilovoltage factors in the inefficiency (or ripple content) of a machine. The average (or effective) kilovoltage equals peak kilovoltage minus one-half ripple.

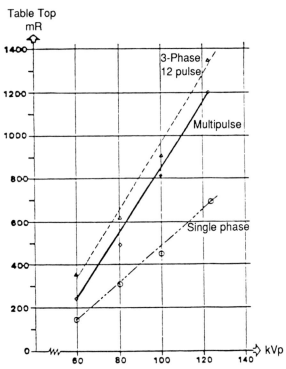

FIGURE 5-7   Comparison of dose yield of a conventional single-phase generator, a multipulse generator (high frequency/constant potential), and a conventional 12-pulse generator. [Three-phase, 12-pulse units have never been available for mammography, although 3-phase, 6-pulse units are commonplace. The line signifying 3-phase, 6-pulse would lie between the multipulse and single-phase lines.] (From Weigl.[2])

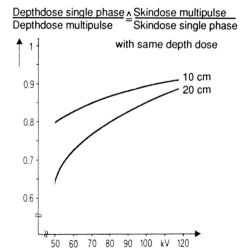

FIGURE 5-8   Comparison of depth doses (skin doses) of conventional single-phase and multiphase generators (high frequency/constant potential). (From Weigl.[2])

greater efficiency in x-ray production. Less patient motion is likely as exposure times are shortened; additionally, there will be less interference from reciprocity law failure.

3. A lower x-ray dose to the patient.
4. Size—smaller components are required in building a machine; therefore the units can be compact and take up less space.

kVp Selection

The two methods by which x-rays are produced are the Compton effect (Fig. 5-9) and the photoelectric effect (Fig. 5-10). Screen-film mammography employs the photoelectric effect to produce its very special high-contrast x-ray spectrum.

The photoelectric effect depends on the atomic number of the substance (the target material) being bombarded. Elements with atomic numbers between 40 and 45 will give off characteristic radiation in the 15- to 30-kV range; the photoelectric effect predominates in this range. Molybdenum, with an atomic number of 42, produces characteristic peaks at 17.4 and 19.6 keV. In screen-film mammography, a 0.03-mm molybdenum filter is used with a molybdenum target to absorb anything produced below 17 keV or above 20 keV; thus a very narrow band of essentially monochromatic radiation is being utilized (Fig. 5-11).

The photoelectric effect deals with atomic numbers. In examining the composition of the breast, it can be seen that the atomic numbers of the two major components of breast tissue are closely grouped:

Three-quarters of the mass of adipose tissue is composed of carbon atoms (atomic number 6).

Three-quarters of the mass of glandular tissue is composed of nitrogen (atomic number 7) and oxygen (atomic number 8).

Approximately 40% of all breast cancers will appear as microcalcifications; calcium (atomic number 20) is also composed of phosphorus (atomic number 15).

The objective then, is to produce contrast that will distinguish between atomic numbers 6, 7, 8, 15, and

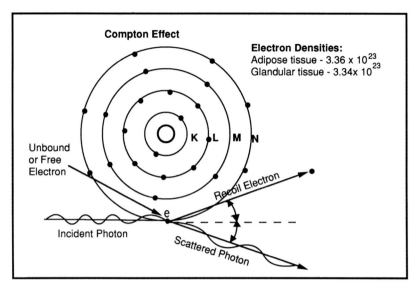

FIGURE 5-9   The Compton effect involves the release of an outer-shell electron. The radiation given off is the difference between the incoming x-ray photon's energy level and the amount of energy required to remove the loosely held outer-shell electron. Since only a portion of the incoming photon's energy is transferred in this interaction, the photon continues to travel, but with less energy. This photon may have more collisions and give up more of its energy, always at a different quality of radiation. (Adapted from Johns HE: *The Physics of Radiology.* Springfield, IL, Charles C Thomas, 1964.)

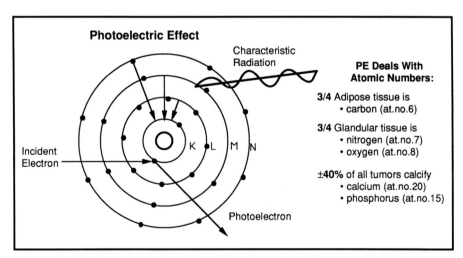

FIGURE 5-10   In the photoelectric effect, an electron from the cathode of the x-ray tube strikes the target and removes a tightly bound inner-shell electron, known as a photoelectron. The original x-ray photon then completely disappears because all of its energy was required in this action. The resulting hole created by the ejected photoelectron is then filled by an electron from an outer orbit. Characteristic radiation is emitted as the outer-shell electron gives up some of its energy in moving closer to the nucleus. (Adapted from Johns HE: *The Physics of Radiology.* Springfield, IL, Charles C Thomas, 1964.)

Mammographic X-ray Spectra
(Screen/Film Systems)

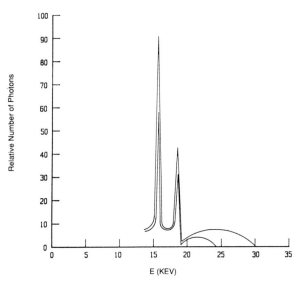

FIGURE 5-11   Typical x-ray emission spectra (normalized to unit area) used in screen-film mammography. A 0.03-mm molybdenum filter is used for the molybdenum target, and the spectra from 24 and 30 kV settings are shown. (Courtesy of Eureka X-ray Tube, Inc.)

20. This is quite a formidable task for any system to accomplish! This is why it is crucial to keep to a minimum the factors that will degrade contrast.

The Compton effect deals with electron densities. The electron density of fat is 3.36×10^{23} electrons/g whereas that of glandular tissue is 3.34×10^{23} electrons/g. There is virtually *no contrast differentiation* here; thus every effort should be made to avoid Compton scatter.

"According to Johns and Cunningham, in soft tissue at 20 keV there is a 70 percent likelihood of photoelectric absorption and a 30 percent chance of Compton interaction. . . . At 26 keV, there is an equal chance of either interaction."[3] As noted by Feig, "A low kV beam is essential to maximize the number of photoelectric interactions. Below 20 kV, the Photoelectric Effect predominate in all soft tissue. From 20 kV to 28 kV, most absorption in fat is due to the Photoelectric Effect, whereas most absorption in fibroglandular tissue results from the Compton Effect. Above 28 kV, Compton scattering accounts for most interactions within those tissues. These relationships occur because Photoelectric Effect increases more rapidly with a decrease in energy than does the Compton Effect. Therefore, contrast between fat and fibroglandular tissue increases with a reduction in kV. . . . To achieve the highest contrast practically attainable, settings of 25 kV to 27 kV should be used in screen/film mammography."[4] Settings of 26–27 kV may be useful when performing magnification or grid studies, and settings in the low 20s can be used with specimen radiography.[5]

Recently a tungsten target mammography unit has been designed that employs different K-edge filters. The kilovoltage and filter combinations can be varied to obtain an appropriate x-ray spectrum for each patient, according to the thickness of her breast and its ratio of adipose to glandular tissue. Clinical experience and time will tell if this type of unit will prove beneficial, particularly for thicker breasts. If so, the kVp settings employed will be far different from the 22–23 kVp utilized with the existing tungsten target systems.

Settings of 25 kV with a molybdenum target tube or 22 kV with a specially designed tungsten tube will create the highest possible contrast image while maintaining an acceptable radiation dose to the patient. If one is unable to use these low kV settings to produce a film with the proper density, the problem is generally not that a kilovoltage that low cannot penetrate the breast; rather the inability is inherent in the design of the x-ray machine or the recording system. Design features that make the use of low kilovoltage impossible include:

1. A limited generator output of the x-ray unit
2. Limited tube loading capability of the unit
3. A long SID used to compensate for a large focal spot or for the shallow angle of the target
4. A slow-speed recording system
5. Poor film processing conditions

Other factors that affect the ability to use low kVp settings are:

1. Use of a grid. Ideally, a grid study using 25-kV molybdenum or 22-kV tungsten would produce the highest contrast. However, when a grid is used, so much primary and secondary radiation is absorbed by the lead strips that increases in kilovoltage are sometimes unavoidable.
2. Reciprocity law failure.

Reciprocity Law Failure

The reciprocity law failure (RLF) of film used in conjunction with an intensifying screen states that as the length of time of exposure increases, there is *not* a linear increase in the density on the film. For example, if two identical films are exposed, one for a given length of time and the other for twice that long, the second would not be twice as dark in its density measurement as the first. Figure 5-12A illustrates this concept for two types of x-ray film. With these two types of film, RLF begins after 0.5 second of x-ray exposure. A divergence in the optical densities begins at approximately 1.25 seconds, with type B film providing significantly less density than does type A. Every recording system has a point at which it "dies." When figuring the differences in optical densities at

each half-second for the two sample films in Figure 5-12A, a reasonable estimate is that type A film would "die" at 3.0 seconds while type B would "die" at 2.5 seconds (Fig. 5-12B).

Imaging in mammography employs a series of trade-offs. Ideally, operation at 25 kV with a molybdenum target tube or 22 kV with a tungsten target tube for all patients will result in the most contrast possible while keeping the radiation dose to the patient at acceptable levels, yet the length of the exposure must be less than 0.5 second so that *no* RLF is encountered. However, since the majority of mammographers in the United States use grids routinely, and since grids absorb radiation, an increase in the technical factors used is often necessary to obtain an adequate density on the film. One must increase either the kilovoltage, the milliamperage, the time, or

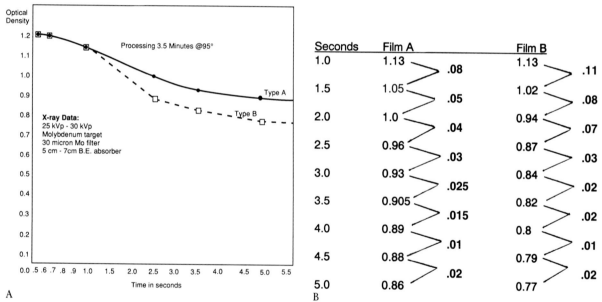

A

B

FIGURE 5-12   **A.** Comparison of the optical density of two types of film. The differences in the optical densities measured at each half-second show a dramatic decline in density between 2.5 and 3.0 seconds for type B film. Making exposures longer than 2.5 seconds will not result in this film becoming much darker. Hence, the useful life of the film exposure is over—it "dies." Estimating the time at which type A film "dies" is more difficult since there is no dramatic decline in density with longer film exposure. Yet experience indicates that other factors, such as patient discomfort and patient motion, must be taken into account. In our example, exposures that are longer than 3 seconds for type A film would risk an unsharp image because of these other factors, and without a significant gain in film density. (Courtesy of Transworld Radiographic X-Ray Systems.) **B.** The two columns in heavy print show the amount of density change between each half-second of exposure. In the column corresponding to film **B,** a dramatic decrease in density occurs between 2.5 and 3.0 seconds. Film **A** shows a gradual decrease in film density as the length of time of the exposure increases.

some combination of these factors to accommodate use of a grid. Because most mammography units have fixed milliamperage stations, the radiologic technologist is limited to altering kilovoltage and/or time. Time (length of the exposure) determines density (Fig. 5-13) while kilovoltage controls contrast (Fig. 5-14).

In order to use the optimal kilovoltage settings that will produce high contrast, as a compromise the length of the exposure should be increased up to the point at which RLF has a major effect. Exposures that continue beyond this point have adverse effects: they (1) invite patient motion, (2) increase the radiation dose to the patient, and (3) result in the capture

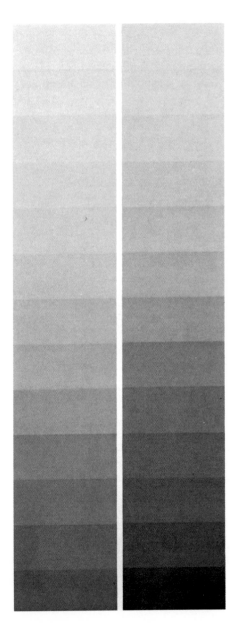

FIGURE 5-13 Two radiographs of an aluminum stepped wedge made with the same kilovoltage but with changes in milliamperage (one was exposed at 5 mAs, the other at 10 mAs). Note that density differences are apparent but the contrast is not appreciably altered. This is true of all small changes in milliamperage over a limited density range. (*The Fundamentals of Radiography*, ed 10. Rochester, NY, Eastman Kodak Co, 1960.)

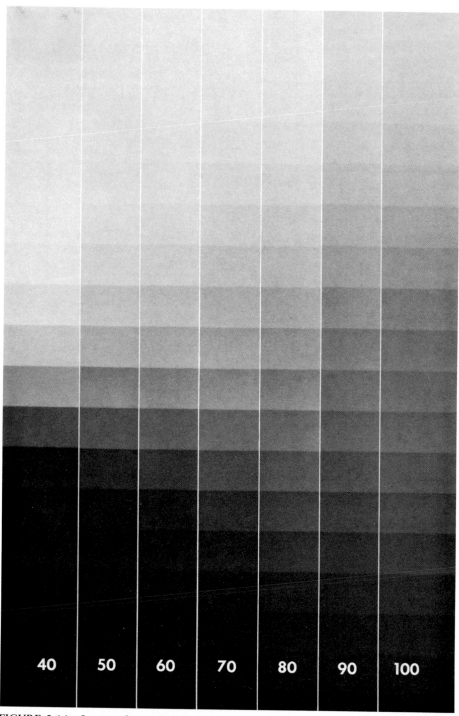

40 50 60 70 80 90 100

FIGURE 5-14   Seven radiographs of an aluminum stepped wedge made with kilovoltages ranging from 40 to 100, to demonstrate the effect of kilovoltage on subject contrast. Note that the lower kilovoltages produce high contrast (also called short-scale) and the high kilovoltage produces low contrast (called long-scale). The effect will be even more striking by turning the illustration sideways and selecting two densities in the high-contrast strip. Then note the number of intermediate tones made visible as the kilovoltage is increased. (*The Fundamentals of Radiography,* ed 10. Rochester, NY, Eastman Kodak Co, 1960.)

of excessive scattered radiation on the film. While scatter adds to the *density* of a film, it degrades the *contrast* of the image. Therefore, rather than make exposures longer than the time frame at which RLF has a major effect, at this point increasing the kVp setting to increase the density on the film would be the appropriate solution.

Grids

Contrast is of paramount importance in screen-film mammography. Anything that contributes to its degradation is undesirable and attempts should be made to avoid or reduce such contributing factors. Maintaining high contrast is difficult because the breast itself has very little inherent subject contrast; in addition, the "soft" x-ray spectrum utilized is easily attenuated.

Scatter production is by far the factor that causes the most degradation of contrast. Scatter adds to the overall density on the entire film, so it detracts from contrast (Fig. 5-15). Two methods used to combat scatter are (1) the use of specially constructed "soft" grids for mammography and (2) vigorous compression of the breast. The latter method is discussed in the next section of this chapter.

Grids improve contrast by allowing primary x-rays to pass through their interspace material while the lead strips absorb the secondary scatter (Fig. 5-16). The price paid for this increase in contrast is that the x-ray dose to the patient is increased to as much as three times that of a study performed without the use of a grid. A study by Sickles demonstrated that in virtually all mammograms use of a scatter-reduction grid improves image quality. However, the use of grids resulted in improved detection capability in only 37% of the patients. The images that benefited the most from use of the grid were of breasts that were greater than 6 cm when compressed or contained more than 50% radiographically dense tissue.[6]

Optimally, a reciprocating grid should be used; if using an older mammography unit in which moving grids cannot be retrofitted, the purchase of a stationary grid is recommended. These fine-line (up to 200 lines/inch, or 80 lines/cm) grids come in various sizes and focal spot–film distances (FFD). The FFD of the grid *must match* the SID of the unit. Because these

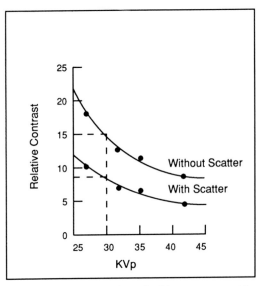

FIGURE 5-15   Variation of subject contrast with x-ray energy, with and without effect of scatter. Contrast increases dramatically as x-ray energy is decreased and scatter is eliminated. At 30 kVp, contrast is roughly doubled when scatter is eliminated. (From Zammenhof RG, Homer MJ: Mammography part 1. Physical principles. *Appl Radiol* 1984;13(5):86.)

stationary grids are focused, the center of the grid must align with the center of the central ray in order to minimize the grid lines. Offsetting of the grid will increase the shadowing of the lead lines on the radiograph (Fig. 5-17). Stationary grids, typically with a 3.5:1 grid ratio, are so thin (and therefore flexible) that aluminum interspace material is used to provide some rigidity. Since aluminum attenuates the x-ray beam to a greater extent than does the fibrous materials generally used with reciprocating grids, there is a slight increase in radiation dose with these grids over that of reciprocating grids.

Reciprocating grids for mammography have been in existence since 1978, when the Philips Company introduced the "soft" grid for mammography. Reciprocating grid ratios are generally 4:1 or 5:1, with some units having higher grid ratios. As the grid ratio increases, the clean-up of the scattered radiation will also increase, but a corresponding increase in radiation dose to the patient results as well. Various types of fibrous interspace material (carbon fiber, pressed cardboard, or wood) rather than aluminum interspace material (as is common with diagnostic x-ray

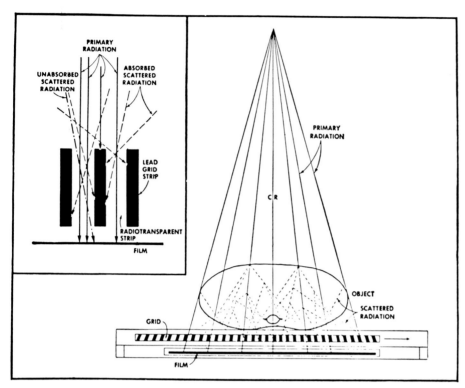

FIGURE 5-16   Location and function of a grid. (Inset: detail of a grid.) Note how a large portion of the scattered radiation is absorbed, but image-forming radiation passes through. (From Cahoon J: *Formulating X-ray Techniques.* Durham, NC, Duke University Press, 1974.)

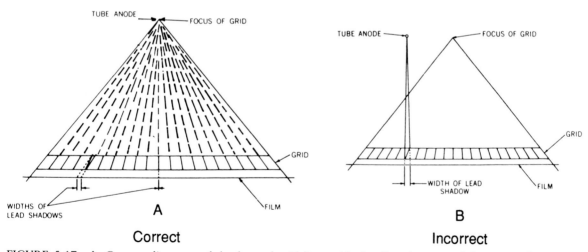

Correct   Incorrect

FIGURE 5-17   **A.** Correct alignment of the focused grid lines with the diverging rays of the x-ray tube. **B.** Incorrect alignment. Much of the primary radiation will be absorbed by the lead strips and the divergence of the x-ray beam will cause shadowing of the grid lines so they will be more apparent radiographically. (Adapted from Cahoon J: *Formulating X-ray Techniques.* Durham, NC, Duke University Press, 1974.)

grids) allow the Bucky factor to be kept low—between 2 and 2.5. The pressed carbon fiber surface of the Bucky device, which is separate from the actual grid, acts as a protective cover for this fragile grid, especially when the grid is subjected to the forces used in compressing the breast. Pressed carbon is very strong yet attenuates very little of the x-ray beam.

The mammography unit should have reciprocating grids in two sizes: 18 × 24 cm and 24 × 30 cm. A microswitch should prevent exposures from being made unless a cassette has been inserted; this is a fail-safe device. The grid should be free of artifacts. To check for artifacts, disconnect the grid from its electrical supply to prevent it from moving and make a light exposure on a film placed inside the grid tunnel. Reconnect the grid and insert a new film. Again make a light exposure. Compare the two radiographs to identify the artifacts that remain visable. Refer to Chapter 8 for a complete description.

When examining the reciprocating grid assembly, make sure the chest wall bend of the surface that covers and protects the grid is not too thick. The chest wall edge of the grid should be as close to the edge of the cover as possible. There should be just enough extra space so the grid can move freely. The important point is to minimize the "dead space"—any area of the receptor tray on which breast tissue rests but will not be visualized (Fig. 5-18). This area of nonvisualization affects all standard views.

In addition to minimizing the chest wall dead space, the area on either side of the cassestte must be kept as small as possible to avoid lateral edge dead space (Fig. 5-19). This area of nonvisualization af-

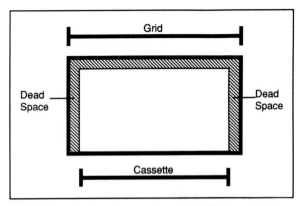

FIGURE 5-19   A reciprocating grid will always be larger than the film cassette. Lateral edge dead space must be kept to a minimum because breast tissue that rests atop this area will not be visualized on an oblique view.

fects any view in which the corner of the receptor tray is placed in the axilla. A certain amount of space on either side of the film cassette is necessary to allow the grid to reach operating speed before the x-ray exposure begins; the grid lines will then be blurred out during the exposure. Accommodating this space becomes critical when obtaining an oblique view, in which visualization of the upper portion of the tail of Spence is essential.

Compression and Compression Devices

Vigorous compression of the breast has an important role in screen-film mammography. Sickles[7] summary of Logan and Norlund's explanation[8] of the reasons for compression includes:

1. Decreased motion unsharpness (vigorous compression effectively immobilizes the breast, even for exposures as long as 3 to 4 seconds).
2. Decreased geometric unsharpness (compression brings intramammary abnormalities closer to the image receptor. . .).
3. Increased contrast (compression reduces the amount of scattered radiation by decreasing thickness).
4. Separation of superimposed areas of glandular tissue (vigorous compression spreads apart overlapping islands of dense breast tissue, thereby reducing confusion caused by superimposition shadows and facilitating the visualization of the borders of mass lesions).

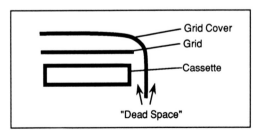

FIGURE 5-18   Side view of a Bucky device. The space between the chest wall edge of the cassette and the side of the grid that comes in contact with the patient's skin must be kept to a minimum. Breast tissue that rests atop this area will not be visualized.

5. Reduced radiation dose (by decreasing breast thickness, fewer photons are needed to expose the image receptor).
6. More uniform film density (vigorous compression flattens the base of the breast to the same degree as the more anterior regions, permitting optimal exposure of the entire breast in one image . . .).
7. More useful assessment of the apparent density of masses (cysts and benign glandular tissue usually are more easily flattened by vigorous compression than carcinomas, therefore appearing to be of lower density because size-for-size their decreased thickness stops fewer x-rays).

The only negative aspect of compression is the varying degree of discomfort which each patient will experience. Every woman will have her own level of tolerance for compression.

Figure 5-20 depicts how much compression can increase contrast on a film; examples of adequate versus inadequate compression in visualization of cancer in a glandular breast can be found in Chapter 12. While compression is a vital necessity, a statement concerning overcompression of the breast is warranted. "Compression forces in the range of 160–250 N [36–56 lbs.] should be obtainable. A minimum of 200 N should be generated by the compression systems in order to sufficiently compress large, dense breasts. Compression forces higher than 250 N may be harmful and should not be obtainable."[9] The maximum forces that are generated by four different mo-torized compression systems have been reported to be:[9]

Unit A: 70–160 N
Unit B: 70–235 N
Unit C: 200–485 N
Unit D: 120–180 N

This comparison illustrates that excessive compression certainly can occur, whether caused by the design of the equipment or by the hand of an overzealous technologist.

Compression Paddle Design

Manufacturers have dramatically improved the design of compression devices over that of earlier versions. The design and fabrication of the compression device is extremely important in allowing visualization of the posterior breast tissue and in maintaining contrast on the films. A compression device: (1) should be made of thin plastic; (2) must have a straight chest wall edge, meaning no "cut-out" for the ribs; (3) must have sufficient height and angulation of the chest wall edge; (4) must have a squared-off rather than a rounded chest wall edge; (5) must remain parallel to the receptor tray when compression is applied; (6) must have perfect vertical alignment between its chest wall edge and that of the receptor

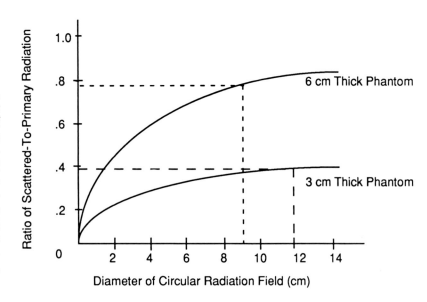

FIGURE 5-20 With a 6-cm thick, minimally compressed breast that measures 9 cm in diameter, 80% of the density of the film results from scatter. If that same breast were reduced to 3 cm in thickness with good compression, with an increase in diameter to 12 cm, scatter would contribute only 40% of the density. Thus a two-fold increase in contrast would be achieved. (Adapted from Barnes GT, Brezovich IA: Intensity of scattered radiation in mammography. *Radiology* 1978;126:243.)

tray; and (7) must be controlled by hand during final compression, although the initial positioning and compression should be aided by a motor-driven assembly.

Thin Plastic Composition   The use of non–fire-retardant Lexan plastic (the bulletproof plastic manufactured by General Electric) is recommended. This plastic will attenuate little of the x-ray beam as compared with Plexiglas, which is used by many manufacturers. The thicker the plastic the more rigid the compression device will be, but also the greater the attenuation factor. While the attenuation from the compression device will not cause one to miss a carcinoma, the role such a minor design feature has on the clinical image is not negligible (see "Image Contrast Summation Effects," later in this chapter). The use of 1.5-mm thick Lexan is preferred.

Straight Chest Wall Edge   The compression device should have a straight chest wall edge. Since 1987, all manufacturers have produced the straight-edge design. It is strongly recommended that a device that has a curve for accommodation of the ribcage be replaced or remade. Figure 5-21 illustrates compression of the breast in the oblique position using a straight-edge versus a curved compression device.

Height and Angulation of Chest Wall Edge   The chest wall edge of the compression device should extend upward approximately 2 inches in height and form an 85° angle with the horizontal (Figs. 5-22 and 5-23). The 2-inch height in this design will keep the axillary fold from superimposing itself over the posterolateral aspect of the breast; units that have short chest wall edges require the patient to sublux her shoulder and thereby pull some breast tissue off the film. Additionally, the 2-inch height will help avoid shearing fractures of a thin plastic compression device upon vigorous compression of the breast. With compression devices made of thinner plastic, an 85° angle will allow enough forward displacement of the plastic by the patient's ribcage as she leans into the machine while being positioned to avoid causing superimposition of the ribs and plastic over the central posterior aspect of the breast.

Squared-Off Chest Wall Edge   The chest wall edge or bend of the compression device should be squared off rather than rounded (Fig. 5-24). The sharper edge will allow the compression device to grip the tissue closer to the ribs than a curved edge would allow. Curved edges allow some of the breast tissue closest to the ribs to "roll" backward and not be compressed.

Parallel Alignment with Receptor Tray   The compression device should remain perfectly parallel to the receptor tray upon final compression of the breast.[1] The breast must be compressed to a flat, even thickness over its entire surface. Any inclination of the compression device will usually result in less compression of the thickest portion of the breast, exactly the area that requires the most. Figure 5-25 illustrates the correct and incorrect relationship of the compression device to the receptor tray.

Vertical Alignment with Receptor Tray   The chest wall edge of the receptor tray and the chest wall edge of the compression device need to be in perfect vertical alignment along the entire length of the tray. Figure 5-26A illustrates proper alignment while Figures 5-26B and C demonstrate two common incorrect design features found on many mammography units currently in use. Improper alignment will cause posterior breast tissue to be missed.

Controls of Compression   It is recommended that final compression be manually applied and controlled by the technologist utilizing a hand-controlled compression device for two reasons: (1) the patient needs reassurance that a *person*, not a machine, is in complete control of the amount of compression that is to be applied to her breast, and (2) the technologist can feel the resistance increase with each turn of the handwheel and receives direct feedback as to when the breast is adequately compressed. The foot on a pedal positioned on the floor cannot "feel" when enough is enough; the foot pedal simply stops when its preset limit in foot-pounds per square inch has been reached. Therefore, the amount of compression able to be exerted by the foot pedal device of a mammography machine should be minimal to avoid the possibility of overcompressing the breast.

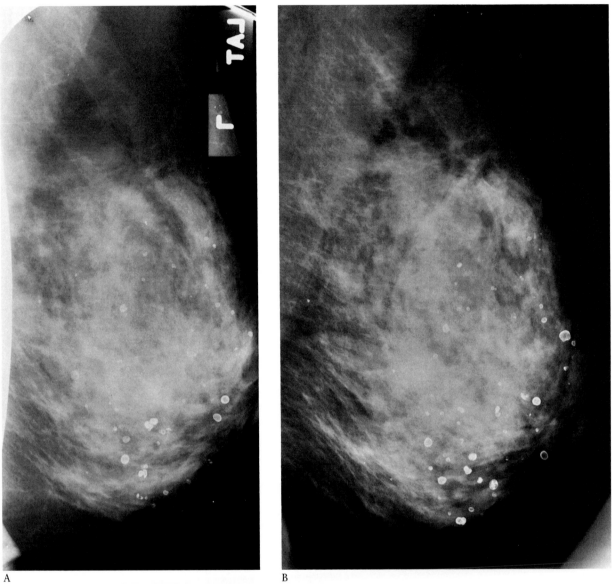

A   B

FIGURE 5-21   **A.** An oblique view mammogram performed with a curved compression device causes loss of visualization of tissue at the chest wall. **B.** An oblique view of the same patient performed with a straight-edged compression device visualizes much more posterior tissue.

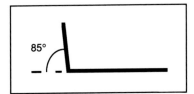

FIGURE 5-22   Side view of a compression device.

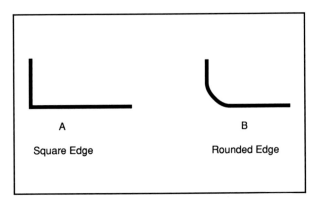

A	B
Square Edge	Rounded Edge

FIGURE 5-24   Side views of a square-edged versus a rounded-edged compression device.

Spot Compression Device and Quadrant Paddles

The "spot" or "coned-down" compression device supplied with many mammography units is typically very small, perhaps 2 inches in diameter. These small devices are adequate to use with patients who have a nonpalpable area in a very small breast or with any size breast containing a palpable lesion. However, they are of little value in attempting to obtain an extra view of a nonpalpable lesion in a large breast. If the technologist is unsuccessful in locating this suspicious-looking nonpalpable area during the first attempt with a 2-inch diameter device, the patient will typically allow a second try, albeit grudgingly. More attempts than this usually result in increased resistance from the patient. Unless the technologist is extremely adept in aligning this smaller compression device over a nonpalpable area in a large breast, it is suggested that a local plastics fabricating company be asked to make a larger spot device if the manufacturer of the equipment does not have a quadrant paddle available. Quadrant paddles are, on average 3–4-inches wide. This paddle usually allows the nipple to be visualized as a point of reference when performing special views of the breast.

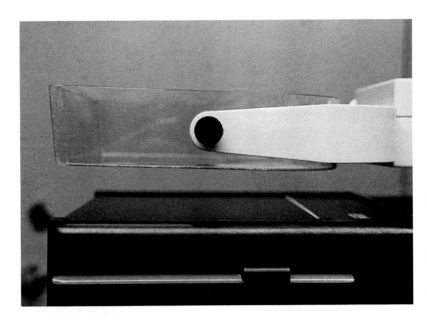

FIGURE 5-23   The chest wall edge of the compression device should extend upward approximately 2 inches and should angle slightly toward the patient. Note that the edge is squared rather than rounded at the chest wall. Also, the compression plate must be parallel with the film.

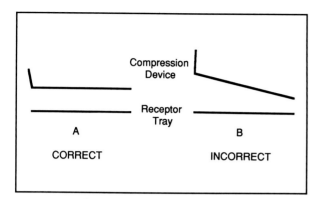

FIGURE 5-25 **A.** The correct relationship between the compression device and the receptor tray. **B.** Incorrect sloping of the compression device.

Magnification

The crucial question to ask of a unit that performs magnification is, "Can the unit truly produce the magnification factor specified; that is, are the images sharp and are they produced with an acceptable radiation dose?" The equipment should allow compression as well as collimation to just the portion of the breast that is of interest.

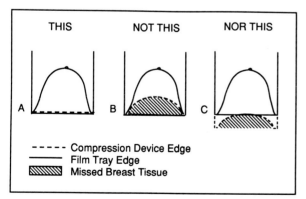

FIGURE 5-26 The chest wall edge of the compression device must have a straight edge. This straight edge must align perfectly with the chest wall edge of the film receptor tray, as shown in **A.** The design and alignment of the compression devices shown in **B** and **C**, respectively, will cause central and posterior tissue to be missed.

Magnification factors range from $1.3\times$ to $2\times$. The increase in radiation dose associated with magnification when compared to routine imaging of the breast will range from:

$1.3\times$	non-grid technique	$1.7\times$ increase in dose
mag	grid technique	$0.7\times$ increase in dose
$2.0\times$	non-grid technique	$4.0\times$ increase in dose
mag	grid technique	$1.7\times$ increase in dose

To maintain acceptable doses and exposure times, "grids are not recommended for use with magnification since both the air gap . . . and the small field size reduce scattered radiation. . . . The use of a grid increases patient exposure, increases tube loading and increases motion artifacts due to the prolonged exposure time."[10]

Aside from the increase in dose as the magnification factor increases, another problem is introduced—that of maintaining radiographic sharpness. In order to maintain a sharp image as the magnification factor increases, either the focal spot must become increasingly smaller (it cannot because this is an internal part of the equipment's design), or the thickness of the body part being radiographed must be decreased. "While some units are equipped to provide $2\times$ magnification geometry, most focal spots perform better at $1.5\times$ magnification. Images at lower magnification are usually sharper due to the finite size of the focal spot."[10] "For $1.5\times$ magnification, the optimal 'equivalent' focal spot size is about 0.2mm, while for $2\times$ magnification the optimal 'equivalent' focal spot is about 0.1mm."[11] A nominal focal spot measurement is not a reliable indicator of the resolving capability of a mammographic unit. The actual size of the focal spot is allowed to be ± 50%. The equivalent or measured focal spot provides specific data for the calculation of resolution in line pairs/mm.

Magnification Factor Versus Focal Spot Size

The manufacturers of films and screens continue to improve their products, with many systems now able to resolve approximately 20–22 line pairs/mm. To see how this improving imaging technology influences magnification, a brief discussion of some basic concepts in imaging is in order. Figure 5-27 compares mammographic x-ray unit geometric resolution (line pairs per millimeter) for two focal spot sizes. Note

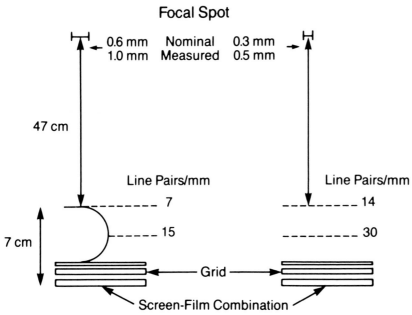

FIGURE 5-27 Example of the use of a grid in routine imaging of the breast. The distance from the top of the breast to the film measures 7 cm. The smaller of the two measured focal spots would therefore be required to obtain good resolution on the resulting radiograph. The very top of the breast induces a bit of geometric unsharpness (the 14 line pairs/mm produced by the equipment is worse than the 21 line pairs/mm current recording systems can visualize), but by the time mid-breast is reached the radiographic resolution is being limited by the recording system (the equipment is now able to produce 30 line pairs/mm although the recording system is unable to "see" anymore than 21 line pairs/mm). Remember—the part of the object closest to the film always has the best resolution while the part farthest from the film has the worst. With the larger of the two focal spots, only the bottom half of the breast, closest to the film, would have good resolution. (From Haus AG: Recent advances in screen/film mammography. *Radiol Clin North Am* 1987;25(5):913.)

the improved resolution when a smaller focal spot is used.

With magnification, regardless of the magnification factor, the recording system is still limited to resolving the current 20–22 line pairs/mm. With the parameters set in Figure 5-28 (unknown SID, unknown breast thickness, 0.15-mm measured focal spot), using a 1.5× magnification factor allows visualization of 13 line pairs/mm at midbreast, whereas with 2× magnification this is reduced to 7 line pairs/mm. Since the focal spot cannot be made smaller to give more line pairs of resolution, the thickness of the object being radiographed must be altered. Furthermore, the higher the magnification factor used the thinner the object must become. The numbers of line pairs per millimeter that can be resolved at various magnification factors and focal spot sizes are given in

Table 5-3. Chapter 12 provides a further description of positioning in relation to magnification.

X-Ray Tubes

The tube is the heart of the x-ray unit. On the outside the x-ray tube designed for mammography may look similar to other medical x-ray tubes, but the specialized interior design dramatically affects the operating characteristics and performance features necessary to produce a mammogram. A basic understanding of the problems screen-film mammography poses to x-ray tube engineers, and their solutions to these unique problems, will allow a more critical evaluation of a mammography machine.

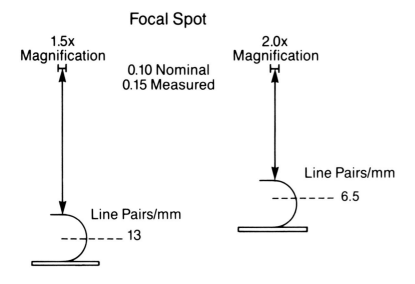

Focal Spot

1.5x Magnification

0.10 Nominal
0.15 Measured

2.0x Magnification

Line Pairs/mm
------ 6.5

Line Pairs/mm
------ 13

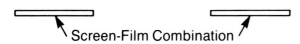

Screen-Film Combination

FIGURE 5-28   Diagram comparing mammographic x-ray unit geometric resolution (line pairs/millimeter) for 1.5 × and 2.0 × magnifications. (From Haus AG: Recent advances in screen/film mammography. *Radiol Clin North Am* 1987;25(5):913.)

TABLE 5-3   Line Pair Resolution in Magnification*·†

Focal Spot Size (mm)	Magnification Factor							
	1.5	*1.6*	*1.7*	*1.8*	*1.9*	*2.0*	*2.1*	*2.2*
10	20.00	16.67	14.29	12.50	11.11	10.00	9.09	8.33
11	18.18	15.15	12.99	11.36	10.10	9.09	8.26	7.58
12	16.67	13.89	11.90	10.42	9.26	8.33	7.58	6.94
13	15.38	12.82	10.99	9.62	8.55	7.69	6.99	6.41
14	14.29	11.90	10.20	8.93	7.94	7.14	6.49	5.95
15	13.33	11.11	9.52	8.33	7.41	6.67	6.06	5.56
16	12.50	10.42	8.93	7.81	6.94	6.25	5.68	5.21
17	11.76	9.80	8.40	7.35	6.54	5.88	5.35	4.90
18	11.11	9.26	7.94	6.94	6.17	5.56	5.05	4.63
19	10.23	8.77	7.52	6.58	5.85	5.26	4.78	4.39
20	10.00	8.33	7.14	6.25	5.56	5.00	4.55	4.17

*Courtesy of Transworld Radiographic X-Ray Systems.

†These numbers represent the resolving ability *at the surface the breast rests on* (the magnification tray). To figure the actual number of line pairs per millimeter (LP/mm), one would need to factor in how high above this surface the lesion lies in the breast using the following formula:

$$\text{LP/mm} = 1.1 \times \frac{\text{FOD}}{\text{FS}} \times \text{OFD}$$

where 1.1 is a constant, FOD is the focal spot–object distance (in centimeters), FS is the focal spot size (in millimeters), and OFD is the object-film distance (in centimeters).

Measured Output Rate

"Because of varying design characteristics of x-ray tubes, SID, window construction and ripple performance of different generators . . . specification of tube current can be misleading in predicting x-ray output. Measured output exposure data are much more useful."[10] With the recording instrument positioned 2 cm above the imaging plane, readings of at least 1000 mR/s at 25 kVp are desirable. Units recording lower x-ray output require longer exposure times or an increase in kVp settings to increase their output. Longer exposure times will induce reciprocity law failure and can result in patient motion. An increase in kilovoltage results in decreased contrast.

Filtration

Mammography x-ray tubes, whether they incorporate molybdenum in the target or consist of a specially designed tungsten tube, should have a beryllium window (1.0-mm aluminum equivalent or less filtration) rather than glass. Glass acts as a filter when dealing with this soft end of the x-ray spectrum, and it filters out photons that would provide contrast.

Tungsten tubes use 0.5 mm thick aluminum filters, although a recently designed mammographic unit uses one of three different filters, depending upon the kilovoltage selected. Molybdenum target tubes use molybdenum filters, usually 0.03 mm thick, to provide an almost monochromatic beam by filtering out the energy levels above 20 keV and below 17 keV. Do not substitute aluminum filtration for molybdenum filtration when using a molybdenum target tube; this will shorten the exposure time by severely compromising the contrast of the radiograph. If overfiltration of the x-ray beam occurs, a built-in microswitch should prohibit an exposure from being made.

Half-Value Layer

Half-value layer (HVL) affects radiographic contrast and dose. The half-value layer should be as close to 0.30 mm equivalence of aluminum at 30 kVp as possible. "At 28 kVp . . . the HVL should not exceed 0.37 mm AL."[10] "HVL should be >0.22 mm aluminum (AL) at 22 kVp and >0.25 mm AL at 25 kVp. Although dose decreases as HVL increases from the minimal allowable value, image quality deteriorates due to decreased contrast with increasing filtration."[9]

Stationary Versus Rotating Anodes

An advantage of the rotating anode is a higher tube loading capability; therefore the milliamperage can be higher thus exposure times can be reduced. The disadvantage is that there is more off-focus radiation produced with a rotating system. "This . . . may comprise from 5 to 25 percent of the total radiation output. Like scatter radiation, off-focus radiation adds an overall haze to the image, reducing the image contrast."[11] Much of this off-focus radiation can be removed by insertion of a diaphragm inside the tube housing; however, care must be taken to assure an unacceptable increase in the HVL has not occurred as a result. Stationary tubes produce less off-focus radiation but have lower tube rating capabilities.

Heel Effect and Anode Angle

Because the x-rays are actually produced 8 microns *inside* the target material, the angled target itself absorbs some of the x-rays it just produced—hence the heel effect (Fig. 5-29). Diagnostic x-ray tubes exhibit the heel effect in a left-to-right pattern; that is, the intensity of the x-rays is strongest at the cathode side of the tube and diminishes in strength toward the anode side. Mammography x-ray tubes exhibit the heel effect just as diagnostic tubes do, except the pattern is turned 90° so that the strongest x-rays are at the chest wall, diminishing outward toward the nipple (the cathode side of the tube will be closest to the patient's chest wall while the anode side of the tube will be toward the nipple).

The production of the x-ray beam requires a flow of electrons from the filament (cathode) of the tube to the surface of the anode. This electron stream is driven or forced to flow by the kilovoltage level, while the amount of electron flow is controlled by the milliamperage. Increasing the controlling factors (either kilovoltage or milliamperage) increases the heat to which the anode is subjected. To provide for better heat distribution, tube manufacturers angle the anode surface; thus a larger stream of electrons can be used to yield higher milliamperage values and the angle will also result in a smaller effective focal spot for better resolution. The negative trade-off is a more pronounced heel effect: a reduction in beam intensity

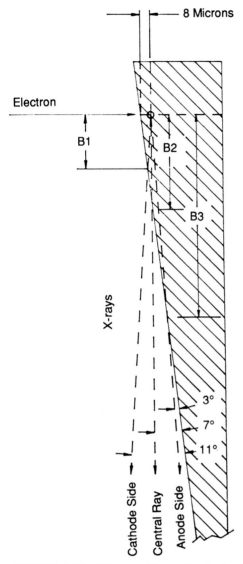

8 Microns

Electron

B1

B2

B3

X-rays

3°

7°

11°

Cathode Side

Central Ray

Anode Side

FIGURE 5-29 Diagram illustrating heel effect—self-absorption of x-rays in the upper target layer. X-ray production occurs 8 microns *inside* (at circle) the target (shaded area). Because the target is angled, the differences in exit lengths (B1 through B3) result in a falloff of radiation from chest wall (cathode side) to nipple (anode side). This is known as the heel effect. (Courtesy of Eureka X-ray Tube, Inc.)

as viewed from the chest wall to the nipple. Newer tube designs provide a balance between tube angle and focal spot size and the resulting optical density fall-off, or heel effect.

The heel effect, and therefore the optical density as well as the size of field coverage, is dependent upon the angle of the x-ray tube's target, the amount of tube tilt, and the SID (Fig. 5-30). Trade-offs in this facet of x-ray tube design are common because these three factors (heel effect, optical density, and field coverage) are closely interrelated. The steeper the anode angle (the closer to 0°) the more heat units the tube can withstand but the more pronounced the heel effect will be. The greater the heel effect the lower the intensity of the x-ray beam at the anode (nipple) side. The lower the x-ray intensity at the nipple side of the film the less field coverage there is available for the "24" dimension of a 24 × 30-cm film.

Effective focal spot sizes from many different mammography machines can be identical, regardless of the anode angle (Fig. 5-31). The factors that will be affected by the anode's angle are: (1) the actual focal spot size, (2) the amount of heat units the target can withstand, (3) the heel effect, and (4) variations in the flux rate (intensity of the x-rays). Since effective focal spots are sometimes measured at the half-angle axis, the longer the SID the smaller the half-angle, and hence the larger the actual focal spot will be. The positive effect of this design is that it would permit a higher milliamperage loading of the tube. However, there is an adverse effect with this design as well. The inverse square law states that the intensity of radiation varies inversely as the square of the distance; that is, as the tube is moved farther away from the film the x-ray intensity reaching the film diminishes. In practical terms, to go from a 60-cm SID to a 65-cm SID, the milliamperage seconds (mAs) must be increased by 20% to maintain the same density on the film. With a 10-cm increase in SID, a 36% increase in milliamperage seconds (mAs) is required.

Focal Spot Projection

Another factor relating to tube design is the projection of the focal spot as a function of the central ray. "It is extremely important that the unit be designed such that the central ray projects parallel to the chest wall. If the central ray from the tube (the ray that is perpendicular to the screen/film cassette) is toward the center of the image receptor . . . a few mm of tissue close to the chest wall is not imaged unless the compression device is moved in or out"[10] (Figs. 5-30 and 5-33).

The resolution toward the nipple edge of the film is twice as sharp as that at the chest wall edge of the

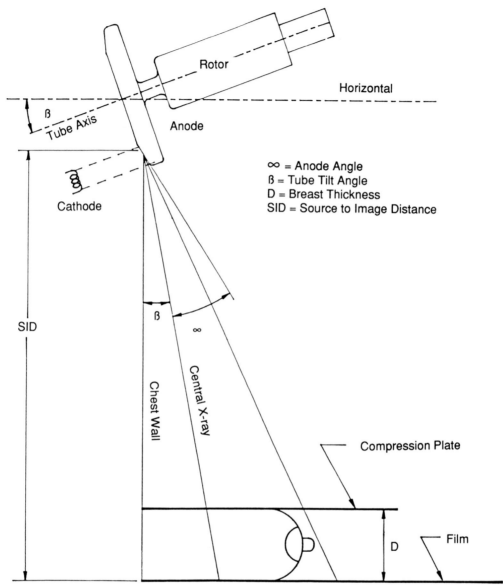

Horizontal

ß
Tube Axis

Rotor

Anode

∞ = Anode Angle
ß = Tube Tilt Angle
D = Breast Thickness
SID = Source to Image Distance

Cathode

SID

ß

∞

Chest Wall

Central X-ray

Compression Plate

Film

D

FIGURE 5-30 Tube angle relationships. X-ray tubes produce a diverging x-ray field. Mammography tubes utilize only one-half of this diverging beam—that from the chest wall out. If the other half were used, postero-superior tissue along the chest wall would not be visualized because of the divergence of the beam. The x-ray unit must be designed to provide the proper target angle plus tube tilt to assure a perpendicular ray through the chest wall and yet still provide coverage for the large film format (24 × 30 cm). This combined angle (target angle plus tube tilt) is a function of the SID of the machine. (Courtesy of Eureka X-ray Tube, Inc.)

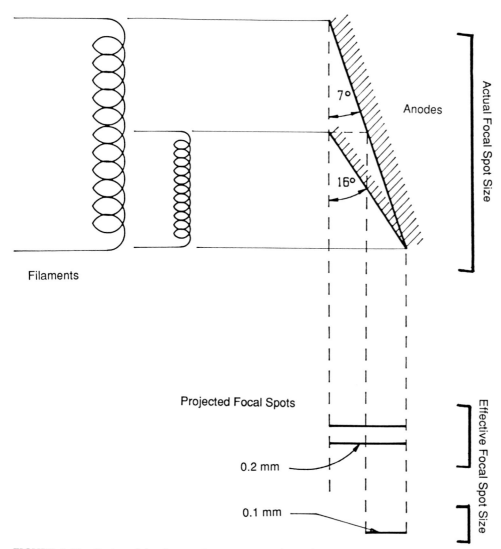

FIGURE 5-31 Projected focal spot sizes versus anode angle. Using a steeper anode angle with respect to the image plane (on this diagram it is the 7° angle), the actual focal spot (area on target's surface that the electrons strike) will be larger while the projected focal spot (effective focal spot at image plane) will be the *same size* as that produced by a more angled target (the 16° angle). The advantage of a 7° anode angle is that the system will be able to withstand more heat units because the target face is almost twice the length of that achieved with the other angle. This is known as the line focus principle. The disadvantages are that the heel effect on the 7° anode will be far greater, there will be a larger variation in the flux or photon energy (see Fig. 5-32), and size of field coverage will be less. (Courtesy of Eureka X-ray Tube, Inc.)

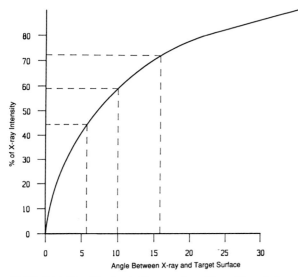

FIGURE 5-32   The heel effect produced by a 7° angled target will be greater than that from a 16° angled tube. The intensity of the x-rays provided by the steeper target (7°) will be 45% whereas that from the 16° target will be 72%. (Courtesy of Eureka X-ray Tube, Inc.)

film (Fig. 5-34). This factor becomes more critical when performing magnification views (Fig. 5-35). Utilizing the small 2-inch diameter spot compression device for magnification restricts imaging to the area that aligns at the chest wall edge (Fig. 5-36). Ideally, the area of the breast under clinical suspicion should be placed away from the chest wall edge of the machine and as far forward as possible on the receptor tray. Then the tissue will be under the portion of the x-ray tube that provides the best resolution.

The "Sweet Spot"

A mammographic unit that uses an x-ray tube with a biangulex design (large and small focal spots use separate areas on the target for production of x-rays) has a "sweet spot" that is approximately 4 cm out from the chest wall. With all other mammography x-ray tube configurations, this area of high resolution will be approximately 7 cm from the chest wall edge out toward the nipple edge. While the biangulex design has a decided advantage when performing magnification views, the current angle of the target produces

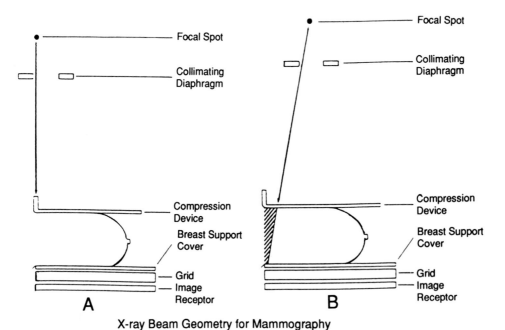

X-ray Beam Geometry for Mammography

FIGURE 5-33   A. The correct alignment of the focal spot over the chest wall edge of the receptor tray. There is no loss of posterior and/or superior breast tissue. B. Incorrect alignment causes a loss of tissue. (From Diagnostic X-ray Imaging Task Group No. 7.[10])

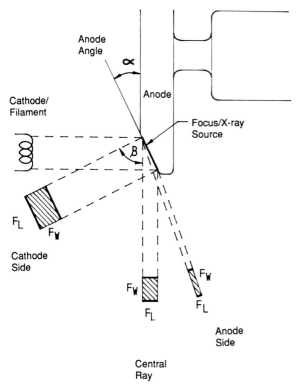

FIGURE 5-34 Projection of focal spot size as a function of the central ray. Resolution contains two dimensions: width and length. Only the length resolution (F_L) is two times worse at the chest wall; the width resolution (F_W) is unchanged. The apparent (effective) resolution is approximately the ratio of the orthogonal dimensions. (Courtesy of Eureka X-ray Tube, Inc.)

rather dramatic optical density fall-off because of its heel effect. It is hoped that advancements in x-ray tube design can maintain the ability to obtain excellent resolution for magnification views and eliminate some of the heel effect encountered in routine imaging.

Automatic Exposure Control (AEC)

"The discovery of AEC dates back to Russell H. Morgan in 1942. Morgan used a theory developed by Heinrich Franke, who recognized that on every radiograph there is a dominant area, the darkening of which is proportional to the average darkening and

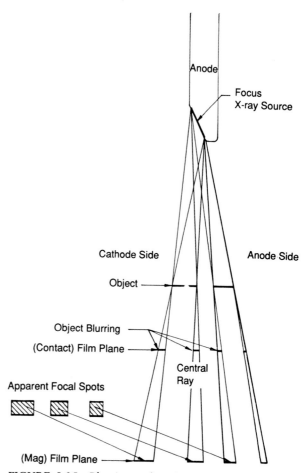

FIGURE 5-35 Blurring and projection of focal spot size as a function of the central ray. The resolution on the anode side of the tube (toward the nipple edge of the film) will be better than that at the chest wall. This holds true whether magnification or contact imaging is being performed. (Courtesy of Eureka X-ray Tube, Inc.)

general appearance of the entire image. This theory has formed the basis on which every AEC device operates. Radiation that is transmitted through an object is converted into an electronic signal, which terminates the exposure when the predetermined level of radiation has been reached."[12]

Phototimers have been a standard feature on most types of diagnostic equipment for many years but have been incorporated in mammography units only since the early 1970s. Only recently have phototimer designs been adapted effectively for mammography.

The unique problems associated with breast im-

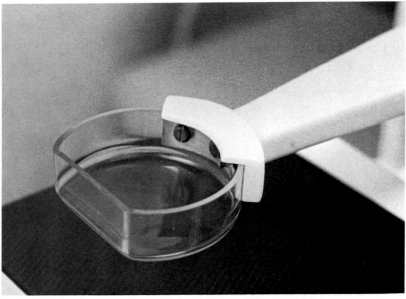

A

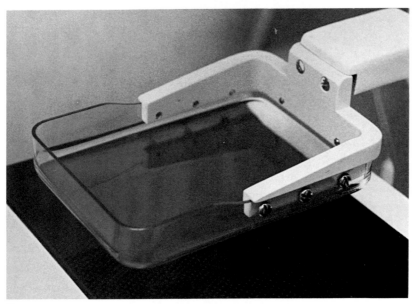

B

FIGURE 5-36 **A.** The 2-inch round spot compression device requires precision positioning and restricts the imaged area close to the chest wall edge of the film. **B.** The 4-inch rectangular spot compression device allows visualization of a larger area of breast tissue.

aging required waiting for the development of "smart" phototimers that rely on electronic high technology to reproduce accurate densities on the film. Prior to the development of the smart phototimer, most skilled technologists employed manual techniques.

In order to understand the unique phototiming problems the breast presents, we must first look at the anatomy of the breast (Fig. 5-37). The side view of the breast reveals the skin line at the outer edge, the subcutaneous fat layer immediately beneath the skin, the ductal structures and functional glandular tissue, the retromammary fatty tissue, the pectoral muscle to which the breast is attached and that extends down to the level of the nipple, and finally the ribcage. Breast cancers do not arise in the skin or in adipose tissue. Breast cancers arise from within the ductal structures or the functional glandular tissue. Therefore it is this tissue that must be adequately visualized.

Adipose tissue shows up dark on the film because the soft x-ray beam used for mammography is strong enough to penetrate the fatty component of the breast; therefore many photons will exit out the bottom of the breast and strike the film, causing the silver halide crystals to clump and remain on the film during processing. The glandular tissue, however, is very dense, resulting in greater absorption of the soft x-ray beam; therefore only a few exiting photons will strike the film, so that most of the silver is washed off inside the processor. Thus the denser glandular tissue appears white on the film.

Single Pickup Phototimers

The majority of dedicated mammographic units equip the phototimer with one detector. This single pickup can be moved only within a specific area of the receptor tray. It is confined to the center of the chest wall edge of the tray and can move from the chest wall toward the nipple for an average distance of approximately 3 inches.

Patient positioning and differing types of breast tissue will require variable placement of the phototimer pickup. If the breast being examined consists of homogeneous tissue (i.e., entirely glandular or entirely adipose tissue), the pickup could not be placed incorrectly, as long as the breast completely covers the detector. However, suppose the breast being imaged is an adipose-replaced breast that contains one fluid-filled cyst, and the pickup is unknowingly placed directly underneath this cyst. The phototimer responds only to the tissue sample that covers its detector. In this case the x-ray exposure will not terminate until the resulting radiograph has the "perfect" density for the cyst, at which point contrast will be lost in the rest of the overexposed breast tissue. The opposite result will occur if the pickup were to be placed under a single region of adipose tissue in an otherwise glandular breast. The radiograph will be correctly exposed for the small area of adipose tissue, but will be underexposed for the rest of the glandular tissue.

When working with a breast that has a mixture of adipose and glandular tissue, the pickup must be placed under the glandular component of the breast to obtain the proper film density. It is critical for the successful detection of lesions to achieve adequate x-ray penetration of the glandular tissue. When phototiming the breast that contains adipose and glandular components, the pickup often needs to be advanced to stay under the glandular tissue when changing from the craniocaudal to the oblique position (Fig. 5-38). If the pickup cannot move far enough to remain under the glandular tissue on the oblique view, the density setting of the phototimer must then be increased to compensate for the underexposure that would result from the pickup being positioned under adipose tissue.

Smart Phototimers

The smart phototimer has a series of photocells rather than a single pickup like its predecessors. A high-technology microprocessor chip allows the smart phototimer to average the multiple photocell readings. The extreme high and low scores are rejected while the rest of the readings are averaged. For example, when imaging a fatty-replaced breast containing a solitary cyst, one (or a few) of the photocells will be covered by this fluid-filled cyst while the rest of the photocells will be covered by the fatty-replaced tissue. The readings from the majority of the photocells would indicate that the readings from those few covered by the cyst are not consistent with the overall density of the breast tissue. The few "faulty" readings would be ignored by the microprocessor chip and the rest of the information would be averaged to result in

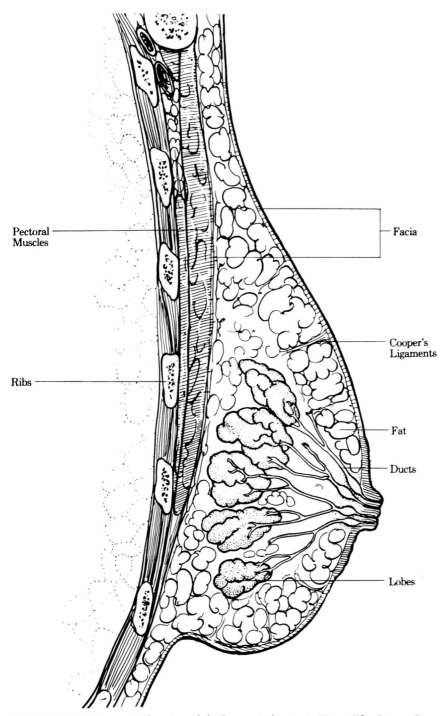

FIGURE 5-37   Anatomic drawing of the breast (side view). (From *The Breast Cancer Digest,* ed 2, National Institutes of Health Publication No. 84-1691. Washington, DC, Government Printing Office, 1984.)

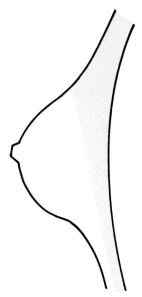

FIGURE 5-38   The shaded area comprises the pectoral muscle and retromammary fat stripe. This posterior breast tissue is not included on the craniocaudal view; however, it is visualized on the oblique view. (From Andersson I: Mammography in clinical practice. *Medical Radiography and Photography* 1986;62:2.)

the correct density. This is only one of the capabilities that make the newer phototimers more reliable.

Solid state technology allows the new phototimers to "remember" and to "repeat" kVp settings; thus they are able to respond to varying kVp settings. Earlier models were unable to maintain comparable film densities when changing from the most frequently used kVp setting to a different setting. When the kVp setting was changed, an adjustment had to be made to the density setting as well. Smart phototimers do not require additional adjustments in the density setting. Once the desired density level for the film is established and the "0" or "normal" density setting is programmed into the machine, the density setting will rarely need to be changed.

Smart phototimers also respond to varying thicknesses of breast tissue. Most breasts tend to be thicker in the oblique position than they are in the craniocaudal position. With single-pickup phototimers, an increase in the density setting often is required for the oblique position. Today's smart phototimers recognize and compensate for various thicknesses as positions are changed. These phototimers are also able to

compensate for reciprocity law failure. The phototimer should be able to:

1. Track (maintain the same optical densities) from one kVp setting to another.
2. Compensate for differences in breast thickness.
3. Obtain an adequate density for all of the varying densities in the breast.
4. Compensate for reciprocity law failure on the film.
5. Reproduce accurate densities on each film (reproducibility).
6. Provide an mAs readout after the exposure has been terminated.

With a smart AEC device it is virtually impossible to take a suboptimally exposed film. Figure 5-39 illustrates the wide range of technical factors required by varying tissue composition and thickness.

A "potential disadvantage of phototiming is that it might encourage a radiologist to employ an inexperienced technologist to do mammography, or assign infrequent mammography rotations to many technologists instead of forming a small cadre of highly skilled ones. It must be remembered that selection of exposure parameters is a relatively simple task whereas proper positioning and compression of the breast truly defines the success of the technologist, and thereby, of the images she produces. Phototiming must not serve as an excuse for slipshod technical performance; the result may well be correctly exposed yet poor quality mammograms."[7]

Automatic kVp Selection

An option available on many mammography units is AutokV. This system can be used only when the technologist has chosen to phototime the examination. During the exposure, the kVp will automatically be adjusted upward to prevent a long exposure time from occurring because of a low kVp/glandular breast mismatch.

Screens and Films

The contrast level exhibited by a radiograph depends upon the contrast of the film as well as that inherent

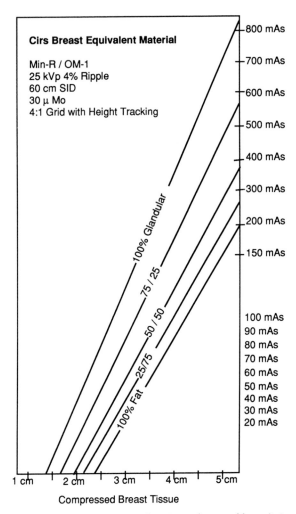

Cirs Breast Equivalent Material

Min-R / OM-1
25 kVp 4% Ripple
60 cm SID
30 μ Mo
4:1 Grid with Height Tracking

Compressed Breast Tissue

FIGURE 5-39 mAs as a function of type of breast tissue and thickness of breast with compression. The constant factor is the kVp setting. The variables include: (1) the ratio of adipose to glandular tissue (ranging from 100% glandular to 100% adipose tissue), and (2) the thickness of the breast, which ranges from 1.5 to 5 cm. A 4.5-cm thick, 100% glandular breast would require approximately a threefold increase in mAs to obtain an optical density equivalent to that of its 100% adipose counterpart. A 3.0-cm thick glandular breast would require only a twofold increase in mAs. (Courtesy of Transworld Radiographic X-Ray Systems.)

to the breast. Some breasts, just as some peoples' faces, are very "photogenic"; these breasts are high in subject contrast, which is the ratio of the intensity of the x-rays passing through the more radiolucent tissue to that passing through the more radiopaque tissue. The typical radiographic appearance of a photogenic breast is approximately 50% adipose tissue and 50% finely nodular glandular tissue, and the breast can be compressed to under 3 cm. However, the subject contrast of such a breast could be reduced or enhanced by the contrast level of the film being used. Film contrast determines how the intensity of the x-rays relates to the optical densities on the film.

Various types of films provide an array of contrast levels. For imaging the breast, which has little inherent contrast, a high-contrast film is desirable. Dedicated processing of single-emulsion film is highly desirable; without this, underdevelopment of the silver halide crystals occurs. Film companies are currently marketing single-emulsion films that are processed in standard 90 second processors but that are said to approach the results of films that have undergone extended processing. The fog level on the film will also adversely affect the contrast. Base fog should measure no more than 0.16–0.20.

There are many factors that affect image quality in mammography (Table 5-4). While discussing the design and performance of the components of a mammography unit, most of the radiographic sharpness factors affecting the mammographic image quality were described. Radiographic noise—the random variations in density perceived on an image—represents a second category of factors affecting mammographic image quality. While these two categories (radiographic sharpness and radiographic noise) can be independently defined and discussed, they are intimately related when looking at a radiograph.

Radiographic noise is caused by artifacts or by radiographic mottle. Radiographic mottle is caused by film graininess, which is related to the size of the individual grains of silver halide; by structure mottle—optical density fluctuation from non-uniformity within the phosphor layers of the screen; and by quantum mottle—the spatial distribution of the x-ray quanta. Quantum mottle is determined by the speed and the contrast of the film, the screen's absorption and conversion efficiency, the diffusion of light emitted from the screen (known as the line spread function), and the quality of the radiation that exits from the bottom of the breast.

Line spread function (LSF) exerts its effect when an x-ray photon strikes the intensifying screen; this occurs at varying depths within the screen, depending upon the energy level of the photon. The emitted light spreads out as it travels through the screen. This

TABLE 5-4   Factors Affecting Mammographic Image Quality*

		Radiographic Sharpness			Radiographic Noise	
Radiographic Contrast		Radiographic Blurring (Unsharpness)				
Subject Contrast	Receptor Contrast	Motion Blurring	Geometric Blurring	Receptor Blurring	Radiographic Mottle	Artifacts
Absorption differences in breast Thickness Density Atomic number Radiation quality Target material Kilovoltage Filtration Scattered radiation Beam limitation Compression Air gap Grid	Film type Processing Chemistry Temperature Time Agitation Photographic density Fog Storage Safelight Light leaks	Breast immobilization (compression) Exposure time	Focal spot size Focal spot–object distance Object–image receptor distance	Phosphor thickness Light absorbing dyes and pigments Phosphor particle size Screen-film contact	Quantum mottle Film speed Film contrast Screen absorption Screen conversion efficiency Light diffusion Radiation quality Structure mottle Receptor graininess	Handling Crimp marks Fingerprints Scratches Static Exposure fog Processing Streaks Spots Scratches Dirt Stains

*From Haus AG: Recent advances in screen/film mammography. *Radiol Clin North Am* 1987;25(5):914.

spreading of the light will produce an area of blur on the film, with the size of the blur being dependent upon the thickness of the screen (Fig. 5-40). LSF depends upon: (1) screen phosphor layer thickness, (2) screen phosphor particle size, (3) light absorbing dyes/pigments in the screen, and (4) screen-film contact. The thicker the screen the greater the blur, but the faster the screen will be; the faster the screen the lower the radiation dose to the patient.

Just as does increasing the speed of the screen, in-

creasing the speed of a film also results in a decrease in radiation dose but an increase in noise. When choosing a faster recording system, if the choice is between a faster screen and a faster film (whether this is achieved by the actual speed of the film being increased or by using dedicated processing to increase the film's speed), the faster screen will not cause as much of an increase in quantum mottle (noise).

An increase in the contrast of a film will reduce the recording latitude visible on the image; this affects the range of optical densities on the image. "For film, an optical density of 1.0–1.3 above base fog for the main parenchymal area of the breast should be achieved."[10] The range of optical densities should vary from approximately 1.2 in the parenchyma to maximum density (3.0 +) just outside the skin line.

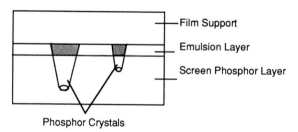

FIGURE 5-40   Line spread function. X-rays strike the phosphor crystals that comprise the intensifying screen and the crystals give off light in a diverging pattern. The farther away from the film the crystal lies, the greater the divergence. This divergence of the light beam will cause an area of blur on the film. (Adapted from Haus AG: Technical improvements in screen/film mammography. *Radiology* 1990;174(3):628.)

Effect of Emulsion on Radiographic Quality

The state-of-the-art recording system today consists of a single-emulsion orthochromatic x-ray film that provides high contrast and good resolution. This film is encased in a specially designed mammographic cassette that employs a single rare-earth intensifying screen and that will attenuate little of the x-ray beam as it exits the bottom of the breast. The screen is located in the bottom half of the cassette so that it will

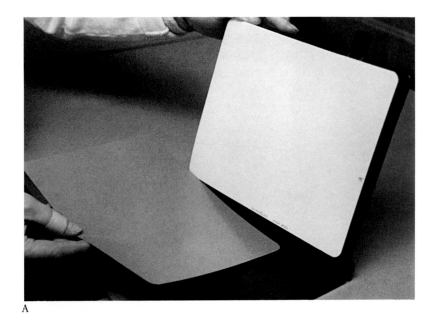

A

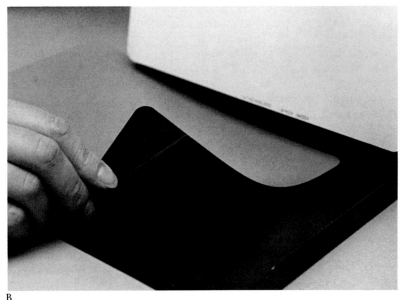

B

FIGURE 5-41 **A.** In a single-screen cassette the emulsion side of the film faces the screen. **B.** The nonemulsion, or shiny side, faces the plastic cover of the cassette.

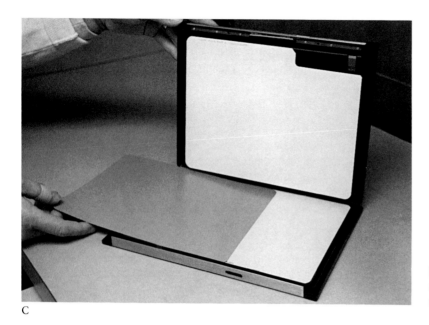

C

FIGURE 5-41 (*Continued*) C. The double-emulsion/double-screen imaging system.

not act as an attenuator of the x-ray beam (Fig. 5-41).

The nonemulsion, or "shiny," side of the film contains an antihalation coating. The purpose of this coating is to prevent the light from the intensifying screen, the inside of the cassette, or any other source of backscatter from the cassette from striking the film. Anyone who has ever loaded a cassette with the antihalation coating facing the light-emitting intensifying screen has seen how effective this coating is in performing its job!

Single-emulsion film contains a larger amount of silver halide and gelatin per emulsion layer than does double-emulsion film. For this reason the requirements for processing single-emulsion film will be far different than for double-emulsion film. Diffusion of the developer through the thickened emulsion layer requires a longer immersion time in the developer tank, an increase in the developer temperature, and movement of the film through the rollers in a serpentine pattern to bend and flex the film, thus giving the enhanced developer chemistry better access to the exposed silver halide crystals. Extended processing (see Chap. 6) does result in an increase in radiographic noise (Fig. 5-42). Film companies are currently marketing single-emulsion films that are processed in

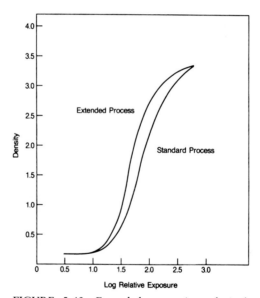

FIGURE 5-42 Extended processing of single-emulsion film will enhance contrast, increase the speed of the film so exposure times can be shortened, and increase the density on the film. (From Tabar I, Haus AG: Processing of mammographic films: Technical and clinical considerations. *Radiology* 1989;173:65.)

standard 90-second processors but that are said to approach the results of films that have undergone extended processing.

A double-emulsion film, Min-R T, has been introduced by the Eastman Kodak Company. While not in widespread use, this film certainly does serve a need in limited applications, such as:

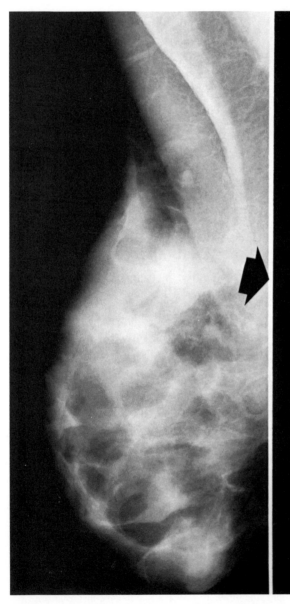

FIGURE 5-43   When the film extends beyond the screen inside the cassette, a narrow band of clear unexposed film will be seen (arrow).

1. Use with any low-generator-output mammographic unit.
2. Use with magnification.
3. Use with a grid when imaging a very thick, very glandular breast.
4. Use to reduce the radiation dose to young patients.

The double-emulsion/double-screen imaging system of today is said to exhibit zero percent crossover; compared to the earlier versions of this film, this was a needed improvement. Although the contrast inherent in this system is less than that of single-emulsion film, its real advantage is in its increased speed—it is 60% faster than Kodak's standard Min-RM film. A low-generator-output mammography unit requires increases in the kVp settings in order to obtain an adequate density on a film once the RLF of the film has been exceeded. Increasing the kilovoltage decreases contrast; however, if a 60% faster recording system can be employed in this instance, the required kVp increase would be reduced. The ability to limit the increase in kilovoltage would offset the slight loss of contrast inherent in the film. Double-emulsion film is also less susceptible to problems associated with processing conditions and to artifacts.

The "Racing Stripe" Effect

A common problem that occurs on many screen-film images is the white "racing stripe" effect that shows itself as a narrow band of unexposed film along the chest wall edge of the film (Fig. 5-43). The effect occurs when the intensifying screen shifts inside the cassette. As a result, a band of unexposed film several millimeters wide occurs. The screen must be remounted or a new cassette purchased.

Concluding Remarks

This chapter primarily examined the features of a dedicated screen-film mammography machine. The competent radiologic technologist must have a thorough understanding and mastery of the relationships and interdependence between the mammographic unit components, accessories, films, processing techniques, and patient positioning techniques.

Image Contrast Summation Effect

Many of the trade-offs encountered in screen-film mammography are made to obtain the best contrast at an acceptable radiation dose. Many elements of the imaging process will not, by themselves, cause a cancer to be missed on a film, but when added together they could compound the inherent problems in breast imaging and result in an image with very low contrast. This is the summation effect. It is possible to achieve high-contrast images produced with an acceptable radiation dose while reducing the summation effect by following the guidelines listed here:

The HVL of the mammography machine should be equivalent to 0.30 mm aluminum when measured at 30 kVp. Slight increases in HVL will result in *much lower contrast* because the unit is filtering out the soft energy required by screen-film mammography.

When performing screen-film mammography with a molybdenum target tube, the molybdenum filter should be used. Use of an aluminum filter should be prohibited.

The window of the x-ray tube should be made of beryllium, not glass. A glass window causes a threefold reduction in the skin dose, but it does this by filtering out the soft x-rays necessary for contrast.

The compression device should be made of a thin piece of Lexan plastic to reduce the attenuation of the x-ray beam while still providing a sturdy device for good compression.

The specially designed mammography film cassette should attenuate the x-ray beam as little as possible. If using a vacuum pack system, select the disposable polyethylene bag. *Do not use* the reusable polyvinyl chloride bags because chloride will attenuate the x-ray beam.

When using a molybdenum target x-ray tube, 25 kV will produce the highest contrast; with a specially designed tungsten target x-ray tube 23 kV will produce an acceptable film. Use as low a kVp as possible to maximize contrast yet minimize the effect of RLF. For specimen radiography, using a molybdenum tube below 25 kV is acceptable.

A variety of contrast levels are available from film manufacturers. Choose a high-contrast film that allows good resolution at an acceptable speed.

Rare-earth intensifying screens are excellent for imaging the breast.

Be sure the film and screen combination being used are compatible with one another as well as with the chemistry in the automatic film processor. If they are incompatible, a loss of contrast occurs.

Compression of the breast is a critical technique in producing useful mammographic images. The thinner the breast the lower the amount of scattered radiation. However, this is the only significant factor from this entire list that cannot be controlled by the radiologic technologist; the patient's cooperation is required.

Summary

This chapter presented:

The ergonomic features that make the equipment easier to use.

The electromechanical features of the machine that are critical to producing a clinically useful image of the breast on film.

The basic considerations and the underlying physics of screen-film mammography that are important in selecting and using equipment that will produce high-quality films.

The relationships between these design features and the peripheral equipment (i.e., grids, cassettes, film, and processing), all of which has an effect on the process of producing a good image.

While the trend in equipment design is to automate screen-film mammography with improved units and useful peripheral equipment, producing a good clinical image is still based on an understanding of how the equipment and film produce an image so that the best trade-offs can be made.

References

1. *Mammography—A User's Guide,* NCRP Report No. 85. Bethesda, MD, National Council on Radiation Protection and Measurements, 1986.
2. Weigl W: A new high-frequency controlled x-ray generator system with multi-pulse wave shape. *J Radiol Eng* 1983;1(1):7.
3. Radiologic Exchange. Eds. Stears JG, Gray JE, Frank ED: *Radiol Technol* 1990;61(3):221.

4. Feig S: Fundamental Considerations in Xeromammography and Screen/Film Mammography. Syllabus for the Categorical Course on Mammography, American College of Radiology, September 1984.

5. Tabar L, Dean P: Optimum mammography technique. *Administrative Radiology* May 1989; p. 54.

6. Sickles EA, Weber WN: High contrast mammography with a moving grid: Assessment of clinical utility. *AJR* 1986;146:1137.

7. Sickles EA: Dedicated equipment. Syllabus for the Categorical Course on Mammography, American College of Radiology, September 1984

8. Logan WW, Norlund, AW: Screen-film mammography technique: compression and other factors, in Logan WW, Muntz EP (eds): *Reduced Dose Mammography*. New York, Masson, 1979.

9. ECRI: Mammography units. *Health Devices* 1989; 18(1):41.

10. Diagnostic X-ray Imaging Task Group No. 7: *Equipment Requirements and Quality Control for Mammography*. American Institute of Physics, AAPM Report No. 29. 1990.

11. Ranallo FN: Physics of screen-film mammography. In: Peters ME, Voegeli DR, Scanlan KA, eds. *Handbook of Breast Imaging*. Churchill Livingstone 1989.

12. Sterling S: Automatic exposure control: A primer. *Radiol Technol* 1988;59(5):421.

6

Valerie Fink Andolina

Processing

A major factor in quality imaging that is often overlooked is processing. In mammography, where contrast is of the utmost importance and where artifacts could obscure a tiny cancer, better than adequate processing conditions are imperative. As is discussed in Chapter 7, processor and darkroom cleanliness, proper ventilation and chemicals, and routine maintenance all play vital roles in obtaining the best possible images. This chapter deals specifically with the different types of processing available for single emulsion films.

Many facilities are able to dedicate processors specifically for mammographic film. This enables them to obtain the best possible contrast, reduces the risk of processor-related artifacts, and in some instances reduce the patients' radiation dosage.

There are two types of processing generally used for mammographic films: standard and extended. Standard processing refers to the type used for general radiography. It is usually a faster cycle time (approximately 90 seconds with an immersion time in the developer of approximately 23 seconds), and can accommodate both single- and double-emulsion film types. Extended or "push" processing are the terms used for processors dedicated to single-emulsion

films in which the cycle has been prolonged or "extended," usually to approximately 3 minutes with immersion time in the developer of approximately 45 seconds, in an effort to "push" more contrast and speed from the film. *The difference between standard and extended processing is not the total cycle time, but the time that the film is immersed in the developer solution.*

To ensure the highest quality image, a mammographic film must be used that is compatible with the chemistry and timing of the processor. There are many films and screens being manufactured specifically for mammography; the type of processing available in a facility should be a major factor in deciding which combination will be used. Most processor and film manufacturers employ mammographic specialists; it is recommended that such a representative be consulted to aid in making this decision.

Standard Processing

Standard processing is employed in general radiography, and standard processors can be found in any multipurpose imaging department. These processors usually have a cycle time of approximately 90 seconds, although they can have a cycle time of up to 4 minutes. Regardless of the total cycle time, the film is immersed in the developer for a minimal time to achieve average contrast and speed. Standard processing can accommodate many film types, both single and double emulsion.

If the equipment is properly cleaned and maintained, standard processing is adequate for mammography when film for this type of processing is used. Facilities using film-screen mammography that utilize standard processing cite these reasons for their choice:

1. Less radiographic noise on the image. Radiographic noise can be caused by radiographic mottle, which is a combination of film graininess, quantum mottle, and object mottle (variations in thickness of screen phosphors). Increasing the speed or contrast of a film (see "Extended Processing") will increase its noise. Standard processing keeps noise to a minimum while allowing acceptable speed and contrast.
2. Dedicated processing is not available, or not practical for the facility's patient load.
3. A prolonged processing time is undesirable because it may decrease productivity.
4. The amount of image quality gained with extended processing is not significant enough to warrant the investment in both time and money that may be involved.

Extended Processing

Extended processing is a technique that was developed in an effort to achieve the best possible image quality on a mammographic film by enhancing its contrast. Until recently, extended processing has been experimental and was only available by making mechanical modifications to existing standard processors. Since it has proven its worth, manufacturers of processing equipment are now marketing dedicated extended processors for mammography.

This type of processing increases the amount of time the film is immersed in the developer, and in some instances also involves an increase in developer solution temperature over that of standard processing. As with standard processing, these units must be properly cleaned, maintained, and monitored for maximum performance. This is even more critical when developer temperatures are increased, because even slight upward variations in temperature may increase film fog or adversely affect developer stability.

With extended cycle processing, the speed and contrast of some single-emulsion films are increased. However, the speed and contrast of double-emulsion film has not been found to increase significantly with extended processing.

As the speed and contrast of single-emulsion films increases, so does radiographic noise. However, the desirable increase in contrast, combined with the increase in speed, results in approximately a 35% reduction in radiation dose as well. When choosing a processing system, each facility must decide for itself whether less noise or increased speed, contrast, and reduced dosage is most desirable.

Facilities that use extended processing cite reasons such as:

1. Improved image quality
2. Increased contrast
3. Reduced radiation dose
4. Increased tube life
5. Reduced reciprocity law failure

Conclusion

Regardless of which type of processing is utilized, steps must be taken to maintain the highest quality images possible from the system. Routine cleaning and maintenance of the processor, as well as a quality assurance program, are recommended. Chapters 7 and 8 discuss these procedures in greater detail.

Bibliography

Andersson I: Mammography in clinical practice. *Medical Radiography and Photography* 1986;62:2.

Eastman Kodak Co. Screen-film mammography: A team approach. *Medical Radiography and Photography* 1985; 61(4):10, 11.

ECRI: Mammography units. *Health Devices* 7010;19(5-6):153–173.

Equipment Requirements and Quality Control for Mammography, report no. 29. New York, American Association of Physicists in Medicine, 1990.

Haus A: Screen-film-processing systems and quality control in mammography. Presented at the Symposium on the Physics of Clinical Mammography, St. Louis, 1990.

Haus A: Technological improvements in screen-film mammography. *Radiology* 1990;174(3):628–637.

Homer M: Extended processing—who's using it, who isn't and why [survey]. Boston, MA, Society of Breast Imaging, 1990.

Kimme-Smith C, Rothschild P, et al: Mammographic film—processor temperature, development time, and chemistry: Effect on dose, contrast and noise. *AJR* 1989;152:35–40.

Law J, Kirkpatrick A: Film processing for mammography. *Br J Radiol* 1988;61:939–942.

Lillie R: *Push Processing for Mammography Films*, Technical Summary, Rochester, NY, Eastman Kodak Co, 1987.

Rothenberg L: Patient dose in mammography. *Radiographics* 1990;10(4):739–746.

Tabar L, Dean PB: Quality aspects in mammography. *Medicamundi* 1984;29:2.

7
Valerie Fink Andolina

The Darkroom

As with any type of radiographic examination, obtaining a quality image begins with setting high standards in the darkroom. The proper equipment and attention to its care are key ingredients in the outcome of the final product. Proper equipment includes not only the processor, but the safelights, air quality, and overall environment.

Safelights

Safelight filters that correspond with green light–sensitive films such as those used in mammography should be installed in lamps located at least 4 feet above the work area. The Kodak GBX-2 (Fig. 7-1) and Wratten 1 or 2 are a few examples of this type of filter. Be certain that the proper wattage light bulb is used in the fixture to prevent fogging: no more than a 15-W bulb in an overhead ceiling fixture, and no more than 7.5 W in closer fixtures. The light intensity from higher wattage bulbs may damage safelight filters because of the excessive heat produced. Filters must be installed properly, so that the printing on the face of the filter can be read when looking at the lamp. If installed improperly, heat buildup inside the lamp may cause the filter to crack, leaking "unsafe" light.

Most films have some sensitivity even to the light radiated through safelight filters. Exposed films should not be subjected to safelighting for extended periods of time, nor should unexposed films be left on the work counter; this could cause them to become fogged. Since radiographic film is more sensitive to light after it has been exposed to radiation, it is important to process these films promptly to avoid fogging.

Fog may not be distinguished on routine radiographs because of differing exposure factors and scatter radiation. Darkroom safelights should be tested periodically using the type of film that is processed routinely in that darkroom. This is essential to determine the amount of "safe" time available before noticeable fogging occurs on the film, and to determine if faulty filters or other white light leaks are present in the darkroom. (See Chapter 8 for a more detailed discussion of this test.)

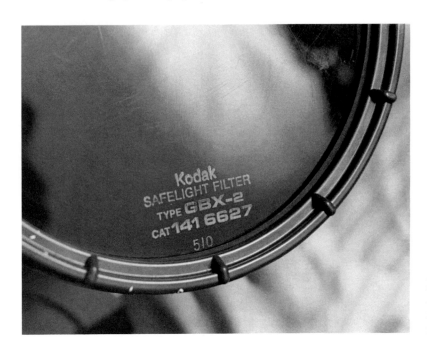

FIGURE 7-1   A safelight filter such as the Kodak GBX-2 is recommended for use with the green light–sensitive films used for mammography.

Other Sources of Fogged Film

Fog can sometimes arise from exposure to sources other than improper safelighting. Most commonly, white light leaks in around doors, through cracks in walls or ceilings (especially the suspended type), or where processor vibrations cause small openings in gaskets or covers. The afterglow from fluorescent lighting can cause fogging; incandescent lighting is recommended as a source of white light in the darkroom for maintenance and cleaning.

Film stored outside of the darkroom should be kept away from sources of radiation and developer chemical fumes to prevent fogging. Improper chemical replenishment or increased solution temperatures can also cause fogging of the image. These should be monitored in a quality assurance program, as discussed in greater detail in Chapter 8.

Air Quality

The atmospheric conditions, specifically temperature and humidity, and ventilation of the darkroom are often overlooked as contributors in obtaining a qual-

ity radiographic image, but they are major factors. A thermometer and hygrometer should be considered standard darkroom equipment, and measures should be taken to ensure a positive air flow to the processor.

Temperature and Humidity

The temperature of the darkroom should be kept at approximately 70 °F. This should be comfortable for the technologist and a benefit to image quality. When film is exposed to excessive heat, its emulsion becomes softer and more susceptible to scratching. A cooler temperature may cause the emulsion to crack and peel.

The humidity of the air in the darkroom should be kept at approximately 50–60% (K.B. Mathers, Eastman Kodak, personal communication). If the air becomes too dry (less than 50% humidity), static marks on the film may result (Fig. 7-2). This is especially frustrating in mammography because pathology can easily be obscured by such an artifact.

If the humidity of the darkroom air is allowed to rise over 60%, small droplets of water from the air may cling to the film and cause the emulsion to clump. The resulting image will look as if it has been misted with ink (Fig. 7-3). This clumping detracts

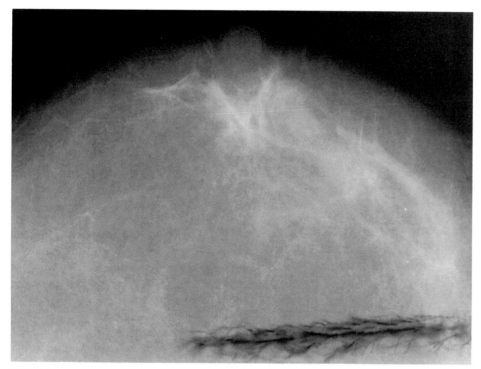

FIGURE 7-2   Dry air in the darkroom (humidity less than 50%) may cause static marks on the film that could obscure pathology.

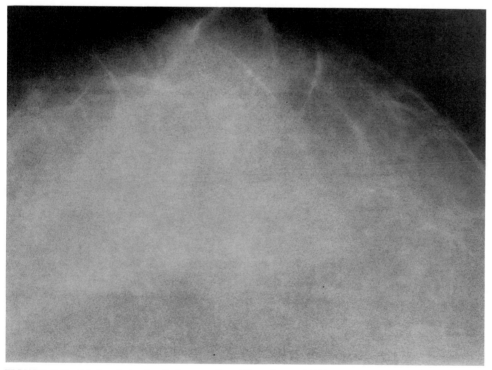

FIGURE 7-3   Moist air in the darkroom (humidity above 60%) may cause water droplets to cling to the films emulsion, causing artifacts that reduce resolution.

from the fine resolution of the film necessary to image microcalcifications and borders of lesions, and may cause a misdiagnosis.

To maintain the proper humidity in the darkroom, a room-size humidifier/dehumidifier may be used. By monitoring the hygrometer daily, the technologist will know which unit to operate. Temperature can be maintained by adjusting existing air conditioning, or by installing an additional unit if necessary.

Ventilation

Poor air flow to the processor can be detrimental to image quality, causing streaking and mottling of the emulsion. The blame for this type of artifact is usually placed on rollers that are worn and should be replaced, or on a poorly cleaned processor; ventilation problems are often overlooked.

The first step in checking for good air flow to the processor is to check the air flow *out* of the processor; the exhaust vent of the processor should be pushing air out. This can be felt by disconnecting the venting hose at the processor and placing one hand at the opening. If air is being pulled into the processor here, or no air is moving, there is a definite ventilation problem. If the air flow from the processor does not seem powerful, a representative from the manufacturer of the processor should be consulted. This person will be able to conduct testing of the air flow and determine if a problem exists.

Proper ventilation is necessary not only for image quality, but to ensure the health of the technologists and darkroom personnel. Poor exhaust ventilation may cause a buildup of chemical fumes in the darkroom that may lead to chronic headaches and nausea in persons who spend a great deal of time in this environment.

Processor Maintenance

There are many different makes and models of processors and different types of processing available. No matter which make or model of processor is used, whether it is standard or extended processing, two rules must always be applied in order to obtain maximum quality:

1. Install and operate the processor as the manufacturer suggests.
2. Clean, maintain, and monitor every processor on a routine basis.

When installed, a processor's developer and dryer temperatures should be set according to the manufacturer's recommendations. Any change of temperature in either component, even a slight change, will have an impact on the processed films. A 1°F change in temperature in the developer solution will change the overall film density by 5%. For example, if the developer solution is 2°F lower than the manufacturer suggests, films developed in this processor will be 10% lighter, as if the automatic exposure control density setting of the x-ray unit was set at −1. This would result in longer exposure times and unnecessary increased radiation dosage to the patient in order to create a film of the desired optical density.

A change from the suggested temperature in the dryer of a processor can result in streaking artifacts on the film if the temperature is set too high, or wet films if it is set too low.

To consistently obtain quality radiographs from any processor, a quality assurance program should be implemented. This type of program, once it has been established, will aid in diagnosing service problems, as well as determining whether the problem exists with the processor or with the x-ray unit. Chapter 8 discusses this type of program in greater detail.

Chemical replenishment should also be monitored in a quality assurance program, because improper replenishment can also be detrimental to film quality. Generally, replenishment is governed by the number of films processed, and by the length of time the processor is turned on. If the processor is left on but not used, replenishment rates will become inconsistent. It is best to turn the processor off if it will not be used for an unusually long period of time. Chemical tank levels should be checked periodically; if solution levels are allowed to become low, sediment from the tanks could enter the processor, causing artifacts. The processor's chemical tanks would then need to be emptied, cleaned, and refilled, and the transport roller racks cleaned.

All processors should be cleaned routinely in order to provide high-quality images (Fig. 7-4). Crossover racks should be cleaned at least once every day (Fig. 7-5), transport cleanup film should be processed

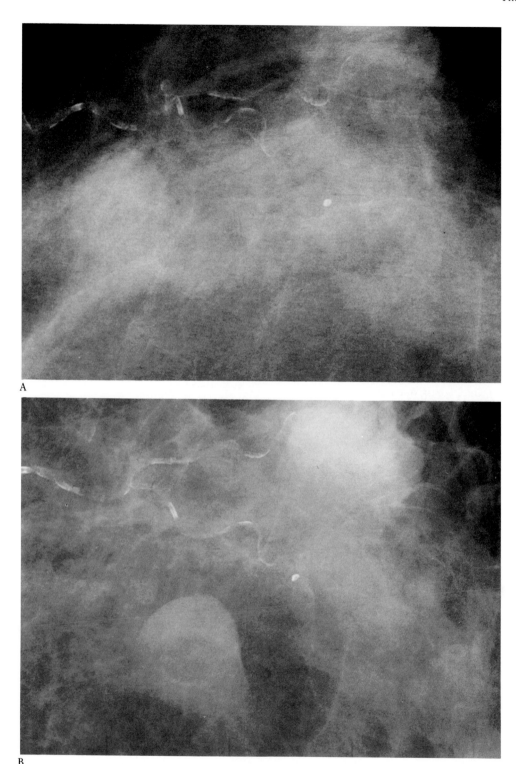

A

B

FIGURE 7-4   **A.** A processor that is not cleaned routinely or properly can cause streaking and mottling of the image, obscuring pathology—in this case, the borders of the lesion. **B.** A clean processor clearly shows the border of the lesion and an overall higher quality image.

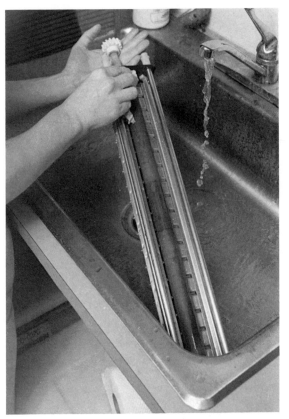

every morning and during the day as needed (Fig. 7-6), and the main racks should be cleaned once a week. Chemicals should be changed and tanks cleaned routinely, according to the type of processing used. Extended processing requires more frequent changes of chemicals than standard cycle processing because the films are immersed in the solutions for a longer period of time, depleting them more quickly.

The developer solution filter cartridge of the processor should be changed monthly. This helps prevent colloidal silver from the films' emulsion from settling on the rollers. If this type of buildup occurs, the silver can be deposited on films or can cause "wet pressure" artifacts. This is seen as a lowering of contrast and an increase in fog.

Even clean, well-maintained processors can cause artifacts on films. Any time that artifacts become a threat to the diagnostic quality of the films, a service representative should be contacted to remedy the situation. If unavailable, consult a representative from the processor or film manufacturer.

Dust Management

FIGURE 7-5   The crossover racks of the processor should be cleaned at least once each day to prevent crystallized chemicals on the rollers from being deposited on the films.

Dust is the greatest enemy of a darkroom, especially one that is used for mammography. Because single-

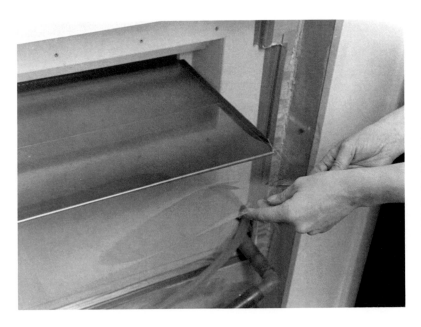

FIGURE 7-6   Processing of specially manufactured transport roller clean-up film should become a routine part of the start-up procedure of the processor. Dirt and sludge from the transport rollers will cling to the cleanup film, helping to keep the rollers free of dirt between routine cleanings. Cleanup film should also be used when the processor has been sitting for an extended period, or anytime dirt is noticed on patient films.

emulsion films and single-intensifying-screen systems are widely used, dust is visualized more easily as an artifact. Dust particles can obscure an area of minute calcifications or can mimic a carcinoma, causing a misdiagnosis. Steps should be taken to minimize the dust in the air of the darkroom.

Carpeting should never be installed in a darkroom, because it generates dust, nor should boxes or cartons be opened or stored here. Countertops should be wiped with a damp cloth daily, and floors should be vacuumed routinely. An air purifier with an electrostatic air precipitator is suggested to help eliminate airborne dust particles. The air purifier filter and air conditioner filters should be changed routinely. Air conditioning systems within the darkroom should be serviced at least yearly to avoid emission of precipitates from within the system. Dust can never be totally eliminated, but taking these steps will help keep the problem to a minimum.

Bibliography

Burkhart R: *A Basic Quality Assurance Program for Small Diagnostic Radiology Facilities,* US Dept of Health and Human Services publication No. (FDA) 83-8218. Washington, DC, Government Printing Office, 1983.

Equipment Requirements and Quality Control for Mammography, report No. 29. New York, American Association of Physicists in Medicine, 1990.

The Fundamentals of Radiography, ed 12. Rochester, NY, Eastman Kodak Co, 1980.

Mammography—A User's Guide, NCRP Report No. 85. Bethesda, MD, National Council on Radiation Protection and Measurements, 1986.

Quality Assurance Programs for Providers of Mammography Services, publication No. PH-7. Albany, NY, New York State Dept of Health, 1987.

Tabar L, Dean PB: Quality aspects in mammography. *Medicamundi* 1984;29:2.

8 Valerie Fink Andolina

Quality Assurance

To assure patients of receiving a high-quality mammographic study, many states are implementing new laws requiring adherence to mandatory quality assurance (QA) programs by mammography facilities. On the national level, The Mammography Quality Standards Act of 1992 and the Health Care Financing Administration (HCFA) both require that QA be performed in mammography facilities. The American College of Radiology (ACR) policy statement on mammography recommends QA programs to examine the equipment, film quality, and developing criteria. To enforce this statement, the ACR has made available an accreditation program to qualify institutions performing mammography through evaluation of staff, films, phantom images, and thermoluminescent dosimeter readings.* A listing of accredited institutions is made available to the public through the American Cancer Society.

*ACR accreditation information is available through:

Ms. Marie D. Zinninger
Mammography Accreditation Program
American College of Radiology
1891 Preston White Drive
Reston, VA 22091

This chapter discusses many of the types of testing performed by the technologist in a thorough QA program specifically designed for mammography, but does not exclude the quality assurance measures that might be performed for other types of studies as well. A very important aspect, but only briefly discussed, is testing performed on mammography equipment by a qualified radiation physicist.

The benefits of maintaining a QA program are twofold. The first is assurance to technologists, referring physicians, and patients that equipment and films are of consistent and excellent quality. Second, if an inconsistency does arise, records will help diagnose the cause of the trouble, enabling rectification of the situation before a major problem with the mammography unit or processor develops. Keeping precise records will also aid the service technician in pinning down a problem.

Mammography Checklist

Before beginning a QA program, it is important to establish that all components of the imaging system

87

TABLE 8-1 Mammography Quality Assurance Checklist†

	Screen-Film	Xeromammography
Type of x-ray equipment		
special-purpose	___	___
general-purpose	___ *	___
Target material		
tungsten (W)	___ *ᵃ	___
molybdenum (Mo)	___	___ ᵇ
W/Mo alloy	___	___ ᵇ
Minimum kVp setting		
28 or less	___	___ *
29–39	___ *	___ *
40 or more	___ *	___
Indicatedᶜ kVp for an "average breast"		
28 or less	___	___ *
28–34	___ *	___ *
35–50	___ *	___
Compression device		
none	___ *	___ *
balloon	___ *	___
curved or contoured (mild compression)	___ *	___
uniform thickness (vigorous compression)	___	___
Screens and films		

Screens and films for routine use should be specifically designed and specifically marketed for mammography. Direct exposure film or the use of mammography films without screens is not recommended.

*Checking one of these items may indicate that the mammographic system is inappropriate for the image receptor being used.
ᵃNote exceptions for special-purpose units.
ᵇAdded aluminum filtration should be used in place of molybdenum filtration for molybdenum and molybdenum/tungsten alloy targets.
ᶜInappropriate kV range can be identified from checklist. The actual value should be determined in the quality assurance program.
†From *Mammography—A User's Guide,* NCRP report No. 85. Bethesda, MD, National Council on Radiation Protection and Measurement, 1986.

are compatible. Table 8-1 is a sample checklist taken from the National Council on Radiation Protection and Measurement (NCRP) Report No. 85.[1] Completion of a checklist such as this will indicate if a part of your system is inappropriate for your image receptor. If such a condition does exist, optimum-quality radiographs will be impossible to obtain even with a thorough QA program.

Establishing a Quality Assurance Program

The Food and Drug Administration's (FDA's) National Center for Devices and Radiological Health suggests ten elements to be considered in establishing a QA program:

1. Assignment of Responsibility A QA committee must be established to determine who will perform each test, to whom these individuals will report, who will be responsible for maintaining the written records, and so forth. One person should be appointed as head of the committee, usually the radiologist, chief technologist or Radiation Safety Officer (RSO), to monitor the program as a whole and be responsible for calling service representatives.

2. Purchase Specifications The minimum technical specifications necessary for any x-ray unit to be placed within the facility should be recorded for use in considering future purchases. Also, the specifications of any units already in the facility should be recorded. These can then be compared to acceptance testing surveys at the time of purchase, or to semiannual testing results to ensure the unit is performing as expected.

3. Monitoring and Maintenance All pieces of equipment used to obtain and/or read the radiograph must be tested and maintained to ensure that they are performing optimally.

4. Standards for Image Quality The quality of the image produced at each facility will vary according to each site's equipment and processing conditions. Quality standards must be discussed and set by the committee for all aspects of image production: film type, screen type, processing, x-ray equipment, etc.

5. Technical Evaluation Procedures Once image quality standards have been delineated, testing must be performed periodically to ensure that the standards are maintained. All aspects of the system should be tested on a set schedule.

6. Record Keeping Paperwork is always a nuisance, but is necessary to determine if any component of the system is failing. A breakdown of one component could have disastrous consequences for the system as a whole.

7. Manuals A listing of test procedures and standards, as well as department policy, should be kept in the event that testing assignments change or questions of policy arise.

8. Training Policies and standards should be set for the training required for technologists who will be performing patient examinations. Training policies should also be set for committee members according to the testing assigned to the individual.

9. Communication Channels Policies should be set for each member of the committee, so that each will know to whom a discrepancy should be reported, and to ensure each will be prepared for any paperwork that must be filed.

10. Review For any QA program to work, it must be reviewed periodically to check its effectiveness against updated technology and to keep the entire committee apprised of any changes that may affect other areas of testing.

The staff of each individual facility must decide the extent to which each of these elements is addressed in their QA program. However, unless all are addressed to some extent, there may be no guarantee that measurements are performed properly and consistently, that their results are analyzed, or that proper corrective measures are taken.

Technical Testing

The technical areas that should be covered, recorded, and evaluated in a QA program are as follows:

1. **Mammography Unit**
   Compression device
       design
       alignment with film tray
       minimum and maximum pressure allowed
       accuracy of breast thickness indicator
   X-ray field alignment with edge of film tray
   Collimator light–x-ray field congruence
   Collimator luminance
   Source–image detector distance (SID)
       accuracy of indicators
   Tube
       focal spot sizes (actual measurements)
       type of target
       filtration
   Half-value layer
   Peak kilovoltage (kVp) accuracy and reproducibility
   Timer accuracy and reproducibility
   Milliamperage (mA) linearity and reproducibility
   Reproducibility of x-ray output
   Representative entrance surface exposure†
   Automatic exposure control (AEC) (phototiming)
       reproducibility
       kVp compensation
       backup timer accuracy
       minimum response time
       exposure switch
       interlocks
2. **Films/screens/cassettes**
   Type of mammography film and screens
       compatibility with each other
       compatibility with processing (standard or extended)
   Condition and cleanliness of screens
   Condition and cleanliness of cassettes
   Cassette identification for artifact control

---

†Using this, the average breast thickness, and the half-value layer measurement, the average glandular dose can be calculated. The average glandular dose measurement is more valuable than is a skin dose measurement, since glandular tissue is most sensitive to radiation and thus warrants greater concern about dosage.[2]

3. **Film processing**
   Speed index
   Contrast index
   Base plus fog
   Solution temperatures
   Replenishment rates
   Chemical changes
   Developer filter cartridge changes
   Processor cleanings and maintenance
4. **Darkroom**
   White light leak integrity
   Safelight conditions
   Cleanliness
   Air quality
   Ventilation
5. **View boxes**
   Consistency of light output each time
   Consistency of light output from one box to another
   Condition of viewing surface
   Ambient light control and image masking
6. **Entire system as a whole**
   Dose calculations
   Phantom imaging
   Repeat/reject rate analysis

Testing Schedule

Table 8-2 outlines the testing and routine maintenance suggested for a thorough QA program. The scheduling is based on the minimum frequencies recommended by the ACR in their accreditation program. However, it should be understood that if problems are detected or if equipment becomes unstable, it may be necessary to carry out some testing more frequently.

Most of the tests and maintenance can be performed by the technologist, but some tests, such as peak generating potential (kVp), half-value layer, focal spot size, and exposure calibration, must be performed by a qualified radiation physicist. In fact, the ACR requires that each facility in its accreditation program have an affiliated physicist. Protocols for QA testing of these parameters have been published by the American College of Radiology,[3] The American Association of Physicists in Medicine (AAPM),[4] and by the Center for Services and Radiological

TABLE 8-2 Testing Schedule

Frequency	Technologist	Physicist
Daily	Film processor Darkroom cleanliness	
Weekly	View box cleanliness Screen cleanliness	
Monthly	Replenishment rates Phantom imaging Visual checklist	
Quarterly	Light field–x-ray field alignment Fixer retention analysis Repeat/reject rate analysis	
Semiannually	Exposure switch Interlocks Darkroom fog test Lead aprons, gloves, and drapes View boxes Compression Film-screen contact	Timer accuracy kVp accuracy mA linearity Automatic exposure control Reproducibility of output (mAs) Mean glandular dose
Annually		Half-value layer Collimator luminance Focal spot measurements
At installation of new equipment		Radiation protection surveys Acceptance testing

Health.[5] The NCRP Report No. 66 discusses these measurements in more detail.[6]

From the technologists' point of view, it is important to know the reasons behind these tests. Chapter 5 offers a better understanding of the measurements taken on a machine, and what the acceptable limits are.

Daily QA Testing

Film Processor

QA testing of the processor must be performed daily in order to obtain an accurate assessment. Processor quality control testing is a very simple procedure that requires two separate pieces of equipment, a sensitometer and densitometer. The sensitometer, which is used in the darkroom, exposes a film with a gray scale of gradually increasing densities simulating a step wedge. The sensitometer produces a consistent exposure time, and is considered a constant; images of conventional step wedges are not acceptable because of the variable exposures of x-ray units. A single box of film is set aside for the specific purpose of quality control, and this film is used exclusively each day. In lieu of a sensitometer, presensitized strips of film may be purchased and processed on a daily basis. However, these images will degrade with time.

Once the film has been exposed by the sensitometer, it is developed in the processor. Whether using strips or film, processing should be done at approximately the same time every day—after the processor has been on for some time so the solutions are at their maximum temperatures. Next, the developer solution temperature is taken using a thermometer independent of the internal thermometer in the developer. A digital-type thermometer is best because this type is the most accurate. This thermometer should be used exclusively for quality control. Do *not* use a glass thermometer; if it breaks, the mercury will damage the processor.

The second piece of equipment used is a densitometer. Readings of the densities of specific areas of the film and the gray scale are recorded and then plotted on a graph to show changes in gross fog, contrast, and speed. Developer solution temperature is also plotted on the graph. Graph paper made specifically for processor QA testing is available through film or sensitometer manufacturers. Figure 8-1 shows an example of the graphs produced. Notice that changes of chemicals and processor maintenance are also recorded. By following this procedure daily, any unusual fluctuation in the curves will show a problem with the processor before it becomes severe.

Before beginning a processor QA program, it is advisable to contact local film and chemical sales representatives for guidance. Clean the processor's tanks and racks, start with fresh chemicals, and record the findings for 2 weeks in order to establish the normal range for that processor.

Procedure

1. Using a box of film that has been set aside specifically for quality assurance, expose one sheet with the sensitometer (Fig. 8-2). Check the owner's manual of the sensitometer for its proper use.

2. Develop the film in the normal manner through the processor being tested (Fig. 8-3). If the processor is dedicated for mammography, sensitometry should be performed with mammographic film.

3. Immediately after the film has been processed, record the temperature of the developer solution using a digital thermometer. Plot the temperature on a graph. This value should remain relatively constant, because even a slight variation in developer temperature can considerably degrade the image.

4. Mark the film with the date and temperature.

5. Using a densitometer, take a reading of the *base plus fog*. This will be any area on the film that has not been exposed by the sensitometer, and appears clear. Plot this reading on a graph.

6. Using a densitometer, select the step on the wedge with the density closest to 1.2; record this as the *speed index* (sometimes known as the mean density or MD) (Fig. 8-4). Note which step was used—this step will remain constant throughout the QA program. Every day this same step will be read for the speed index.

7. Using a densitometer, select and read the step with the density closest to 2.20. Next, select and read the step with the density closest to 0.45. Subtract the lower density value from the higher density value. The difference of those two density values is called the *contrast index* (sometimes known as the density difference, or DD). Record the contrast index on the graph. Again, note which steps were used; these same steps will be read each day with the densitometer.

Evaluation   After the temperature, fog, speed, and contrast are recorded on a graph, the findings should be evaluated. Tolerance limits set by the QA committee should be noted on the graph for each value. Recommended tolerances are ± 0.15 optical density units (OD) for speed and contrast and ± 0.03 OD for gross fog. Temperature variations should not exceed $\pm 2°F$. In Figure 8-1, note that both the temperature and the fog lines are relatively straight, whereas both the speed and contrast index vary slightly from day to day. If the variations begin to show a continuing trend in either direction, the pro-

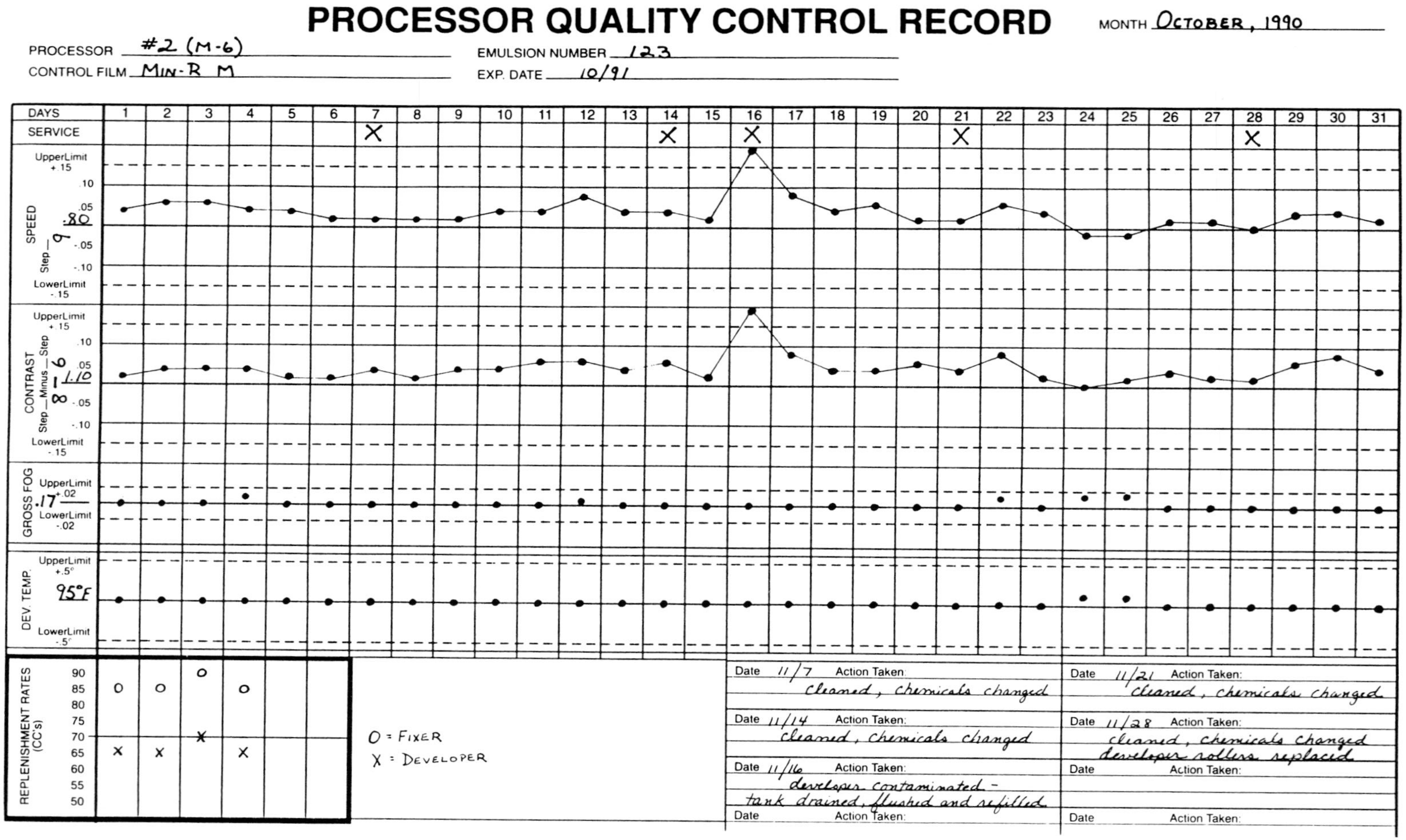

FIGURE 8-1 An example of sensitometric graph paper for processor quality assurance. Maintenance, cleaning, chemical changes, and replenishment rates are noted on this graph for quick correlation in the event of any variation in the curves.

92

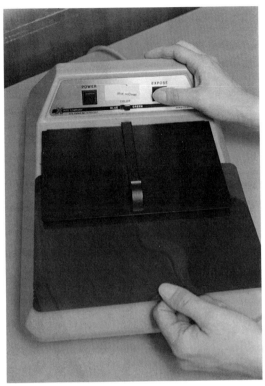

FIGURE 8-2   Each day, a single sheet of film must be exposed by a sensitometer and then processed.

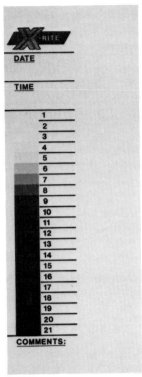

FIGURE 8-3   The processed sensitized film will reveal a graduated gray scale, simulating the image of a step wedge.

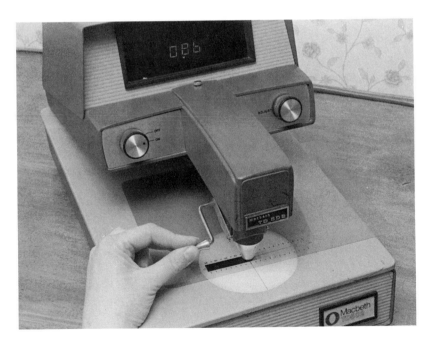

FIGURE 8-4   The optical densities of selected steps on the gray scale are read with a densitometer. The speed index and contrast index are determined by these values.

cessor service or maintenance representative should be consulted.

Monthly QA Testing

Replenishment Rates

Accurate replenishment of developer and fixer solutions is essential to proper processing of the film and to the long life of the processing solutions. If the solutions are not properly replenished the films may not dry or be transported correctly. An unusual trend in daily sensitometry may be correlated with improper replenishment.

Overreplenishment of the *developer* will result in lower contrast and lower maximum density. Slight underreplenishment results in a gain of speed and contrast, and severe underreplenishment results in a loss of both as well as failure of the film to transport correctly.

Overreplenishment of the *fixer* does not affect the transport of the film or its quality, but is wasteful. Underreplenishment of fixer results in poor fixation, insufficient hardening, inadequate washing and drying, and possible failure to transport in the fixer rack or at any point beyond. Poor fixation may cause image quality to be unstable, and staining may occur.

The replenishment rate is calculated by estimating the number of films processed and the number of hours processing occurs daily. The rate is then adjusted in the processor's replenishment pump. This usually can be done at the time the chemical tanks are cleaned. If the replenishment rate for the processor cannot be measured and adjusted by the technologist or a service and maintenance representative, the manufacturer of the processor should be consulted regarding the proper procedure, because it varies with each make and model.

Phantom Imaging

One of the most important aspects of a quality assurance program is phantom imaging. Evaluation of the images from a given unit over a period of time supplies a great deal of information about resolution, density changes, contrast, unit output discrepancies, and tube degeneration. The exact information obtained depends on which phantom is used, and how it is used.

Currently, the certification program sponsored by the ACR uses the RMI (Radiation Measurements, Inc.) 156 Mammographic Accreditation Phantom. Since this is the only nationwide accreditation program at this time to standardize and upgrade the quality of mammography, the 156 phantom is widely used in mammography facilities and is the one that is used in this testing procedure.

The Phantom   The RMI 156 Mammographic Accreditation Phantom (Fig. 8-5) is a square acrylic block with a wax insert containing simulated masses, fibrils, and calcium specks of varying specified sizes. The phantom itself approximates a breast of 4.5 cm thickness, considered to be the average size of a compressed breast.

Figure 8-6 shows a schematic view of the RMI 156 phantom giving the test objects sizes and approximate locations. The objects within the phantom range widely in size, from very minute objects undetectable on most mammography systems to objects that can be detected on even the poorest imaging system. In a QA program utilizing this phantom, nu-

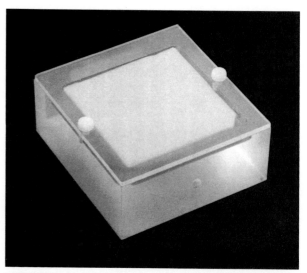

FIGURE 8-5   The RMI 156 Mammographic Phantom is currently used in the ACR accreditation program. Note the nipple indent marker, which should be positioned away from the chest wall edge of the film tray when being radiographed.

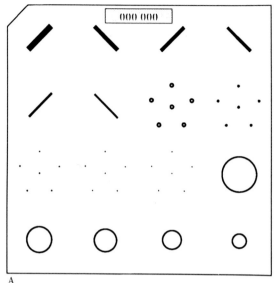

A

B

1 1.56 mm fiber **1**	2 1.12 mm fiber **1**	3 .89 mm fiber **3**	4 .75 mm fiber **5**
5 .54 mm fiber **9**	6 .40 mm fiber **10**	7 .54 mm al speck **1**	8 .40 mm al speck **1**
9 .32 mm al speck **6**	10 .24 mm al speck **7**	11 .16 mm al speck **10**	12 2 mm mass **1**
13 1 mm mass **1**	14 .75 mm mass **1**	15 .5 mm mass **7**	16 .25 mm mass **10**

C

FIGURE 8-6   **A.** Schematic view of the contents of the RMI 156 phantom. **B.** Radiographic image of the RMI 156 phantom. Most mammography units will not fully visualize all of the fibrils, specks, and masses contained in the phantom. **C.** Each object within the phantom is assigned a numerical value, which is the score awarded if the object is visualized on the radiographic image.

merical values are assigned to each position containing an object. A radiographic image of the phantom is obtained and that image is "scored" based on what is actually seen. The higher the phantom image score, the better the imaging system.

What The Image Monitors   Depending on the manner in which the phantom image is exposed, several factors concerning the x-ray unit can be monitored. However, it must be stressed that processing of the film must be consistent; therefore a good QA pro-

gram for film processing must be used in conjunction with phantom imaging.

Using Automatic Exposure Control (AEC) Many facilities now have mammography x-ray equipment with very reliable phototimers, and most, if not all, images in these facilities are obtained by using the AEC. Logically, then, the phantom images should be obtained the same way, using the same technique (density setting and kV) as would normally be used when imaging a 4.5-cm thick compressed breast.

When using the phantom this way, the consistency of the x-ray unit's AEC, as well as the quality and consistency of detail and resolution of the images, can be monitored. Charting the mAs readout on the unit each time a phantom image is made will evaluate the reproducibility of the mA stations. Density readings recorded from the same area of the image each time a phantom image is made will monitor the reproducibility of x-ray output. Monitoring these will help to determine if there has been any drift in the quality of the unit's performance, and will help the technologist determine if a change needs to be made in technique settings (e.g., the density setting can be increased until service can be obtained if the density and/or mAs readout is low). These charts will also help the service technician to determine the exact problem.

Manipulating the Technique Some facilities, even those in which phototiming is routinely used for patients, prefer to obtain phantom images using manual techniques, or by manipulating the AEC to ensure that each month the optical density of the image will be the same. The technique used to obtain the image may change each month in order to achieve this consistency. This will show the maximum imaging capability of the unit. However, it is important to realize that when phantom images are obtained in this manner, it proves only the ability of the unit to acquire good images. If the phantom images are not made with the techniques used for patients, there is no way to determine if good-quality mammograms are being obtained with this same x-ray unit.

Procedure

1. One phantom image should be made for each focal spot. When exposing the film using the large focal spot, use a grid under the phantom if a grid is normally used when imaging a 4.5-cm breast (Fig. 8-7). The phantom image of the small focal spot should be magnified if that is the general use of the small focal spot on the unit. The same cassette/screen should be used each month for the exposures, because screens can vary slightly in intensity, and this variability will show in the consistency of the readings.
2. The phantom should be situated on the film tray in the same area as a patient's breast would be, with the nipple indent marker of the phantom positioned away from the chest wall edge of the tray. The ACR requires that a 1cm-diameter, 4mm-

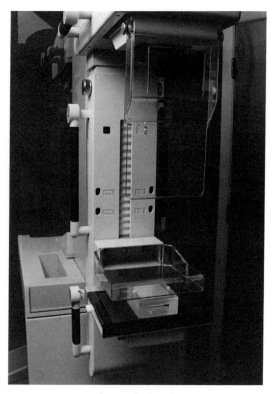

FIGURE 8-7   Radiograph the phantom in the same manner as a patient's breast would be radiographed. Use compression and a grid with the large focal spot if these are normally used when imaging a breast.

thick acrylic disc be placed on the phantom in the area of, but not overlapping, the fibrils in boxes 5 and 6 of Figure 8-6C. Place the disc in the same spot each time a phantom image is exposed. Lower the compression device to touch the phantom. If using AEC, position the detector under the center of the phantom.
3. Make exposures of the phantom using a technique that would normally be used for a 4.5-cm thick compressed breast with both focal spots. Process the films in the usual manner. The density of the resultant films should be one that the radiologist agrees visualizes the phantom best. Background density measured between blocks 11 and 15 of the RMI 156 phantom will usually be between 1.0 and 1.4 OD (Fig. 8-8). Once the technique and/or density has been established, it should remain consistent throughout the program. Record the optical density each month.

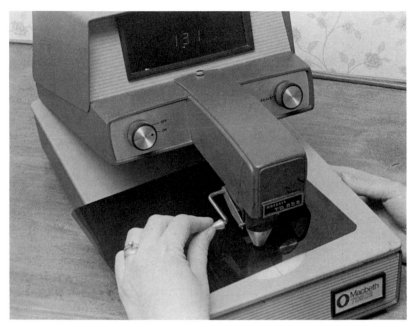

FIGURE 8-8   Measure the background density of the phantom image with a densitometer, taking care to not measure in the area of the structures within the phantom. The background density should measure between 1.0 and 1.4 OD.

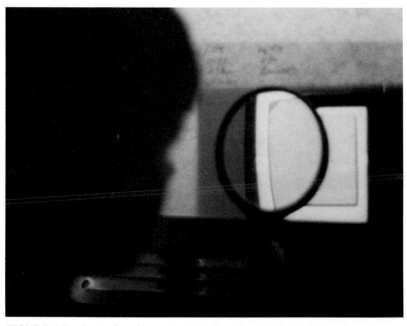

FIGURE 8-9   Score the phantom image by scanning the radiograph to determine which structures are visualized. Add up the assigned numerical values for each object seen to determine the total score.

Evaluation   Establish a consistent method for scoring the phantom images. Figure 8-6C shows the suggested scoring system recommended by RMI. The RMI scoring system recommends a minimum score of 10 for fibrils, 8 for specks, and 3 for masses, for a total of 21; the maximum score possible is 29 for fibrils, 25 for specks, and 20 for masses. Keep in mind that some states, such as New York, have scoring systems of their own. The ACR recommends scoring each structure seen as 1 point; 2 or 3 specks seen in the smallest visible speck group should be counted as ½ point, 4 or more as 1 point. The maximum total score for the ACR method is 16 points. The minimum passing score is a total of 10; 4 fibers, 3 speck groups, and 3 masses must be seen.

To score the phantom image, scan the radiograph to determine how many of the fibrils, masses, and calcium speck groups are visualized (Fig. 8-9). Add the assigned scores of each structure seen to determine the total score. By masking any extraneous light and using a magnifying glass, as with actual mammograms, additional structures may be seen.

With a densitometer, read the optical density (O.D.) of the image of the 4mm-thick acrylic disc between the fibrils and the O.D. of the background immediately to its left or right, but not over the fibrils. Subtract the O.D. of the disc from the O.D. of the background. This number is the density difference. The ACR recommends this number be approximately 0.40 O.D. when the image is exposed at 28 kVp. Phantoms exposed at a lower kVp will have more contrast, and the density difference number will be higher than 0.40, demonstrating the increased contrast. Graph the density difference for each phantom image taken. A discrepancy or trend to this graph may indicate possible kVp drift, exposure, or AEC problems.

For consistency, it is best to have one person assigned to score the image each month and chart the readings. However, these images should also be scored and checked routinely by other members of the QA committee, and by the radiologist. Each time this is done, it should be documented and initialed by the individual with his or her comments.

In the event there is a major discrepancy in scores from one month to the next, or if there is a downward trend in the score, the reason must be determined. Evaluate the techniques and focal spot size with your service representative.

TABLE 8-3   Visual Checklist for Mammographic Rooms*

C-Arm
  SID indicator clearly marked (especially on units with variable SID)
  Angulation indicator working
  Locks all working
  Field light working
  High tension cable/other cables—not frayed, not in field, not restricting motion of C-arm
  Smoothness of motion
Cassette holder
  Cassette lock (should hold cassette securely)
  Compression device in alignment with cassette
  Compression scale (cm) in working condition, clearly marked
  Amount of compression pressure adequate but not overtight
  Grid (alignment, smoothness of motion, correct focal SID)
Control booth
  Hand switch placement behind shield (technologist should not be able to step beyond shield with a hand on exposure switch)
  Ability to see patient (should not be impaired)
  Panel switches/lights/meters in working order
  Technique charts available
Other
  Gonadal shields/aprons/gloves available
  Corresponding cones, diaphragms, and compression devices available
  Cleaning solution available for patient surfaces
  Lead markers (left and right) and lead BBs available

*Adapted from Committee on Quality Assurance in Mammography: *Mammography Quality Control for Radiologic Technologists.* Reston, VA, American College of Radiologists, 1990.

Visual Checklist

In addition to components of the mammography system that require testing, there are elements just as crucial to unit operation for which testing is not necessary. Nonetheless, these items should be monitored and evaluated periodically to assure they are in correct working order. Table 8-3 lists some of these items, expanding upon those necessary for ACR approval.

Quarterly QA Tests

Light Field–X-Ray Field Alignment

Alignment of the light field and the x-ray field must be tested to ensure that the light field seen on the film is indeed the area that is being irradiated. If a breast is positioned within the light field but the x-ray beam does not cover the entire field, tissue may be inadvertently coned off, necessitating a repeat of the exposure. Areas being irradiated posterior to the chest wall or beyond the film tray subject the patient to unnecessary radiation. In some units, this might also indicate a problem with the alignment of the x-ray tube's central beam to the edge of the film tray. The ACR requires the physicist to perform this test at least annually to check that the beam is within the limits of the light field and film receptor and does not exceed more than 1% of the SID into the chest wall area. But it is simple for technologists to perform if there is a question of shifting of the field-to-beam alignment.

Procedure

1. Place a cassette on the film tray of the mammographic x-ray unit being tested so that it slightly overhangs the front edge of the film tray, where the patient would stand.
2. Turn the field light on and collimate or use a diaphragm that exposes an area smaller than the size of the film.
3. Place radiopaque objects such as coins or paper clips intermittently within the border of the light field, along its perimeter (Fig. 8-10). Also, note the location of the light field with respect to the front edge of the film tray; note whether the light goes beyond or is short of meeting the edge.
4. Expose and develop the film.

Evaluation   If the border of the x-ray field does not align with the border of the field light and the difference is more than 2% of the unit's SID (e.g., 50-cm SID = 1.0-cm tolerable difference), alignment adjustment may be necessary. Call the service representative.

Fixer Retention Analysis

The quantity of fixer (or hypo) retained in any processed film is an indicator of the length of time the film will keep its image quality. Excess residual fixer can degrade the stability of the image, and may indicate insufficient washing within the processor. Residual hypo test solution is available through film manufacturers.

Procedure

1. Process one unexposed sheet of film through each processor being tested.

2. Place one drop of residual hypo test solution on each processed film. For single-emulsion films, place the drop on the emulsion side. Double-emulsion films should be tested separately on both sides.
3. Allow the solution to stand on the film for 2 minutes.
4. Blot off the excess solution.
5. Place a sheet of white paper beneath each film and compare the color of the stain with the hypo estimator included with the hypo test solution. This provides an estimate of the amount of residual hypo in the film. The estimated amount should be 0.05 g/m² or less. If the stain indicates more than this, repeat the test.

If an excess amount of hypo is retained on the films, processor wash tanks and wash water flow should be checked by a service representative to determine adequacy. Fixer replenishment rates should also be checked to ascertain that the recommended rates are being used.

Repeat/Reject Rate Analysis

A repeat/reject rate analysis will provide information concerning the aspects of imaging in a department that might need more attention, and enable correction of a problem that might otherwise go unnoticed. If the department will be beginning a QA program in the near future, an analysis of rejected films obtained prior to starting will give an idea of the impact of the program's efforts.

Procedure   Before beginning the analysis, all bins containing rejected films throughout the department must be emptied. On the same day, establish a method to determine accurately the amount of raw film consumed.

1. After about a week, or the time it takes to use approximately 1,000 sheets of film, collect all of the rejected radiographs and determine the actual number of sheets of film consumed.
2. Analyze all of the rejected films to determine the reason for their rejection. If feasible, a log book near the rejection bin will help speed this step. If a log book is not kept, it may be impossible to determine if a light or dark film is due to improper processing or poor technique.
3. Tally the number of films rejected according to cri-

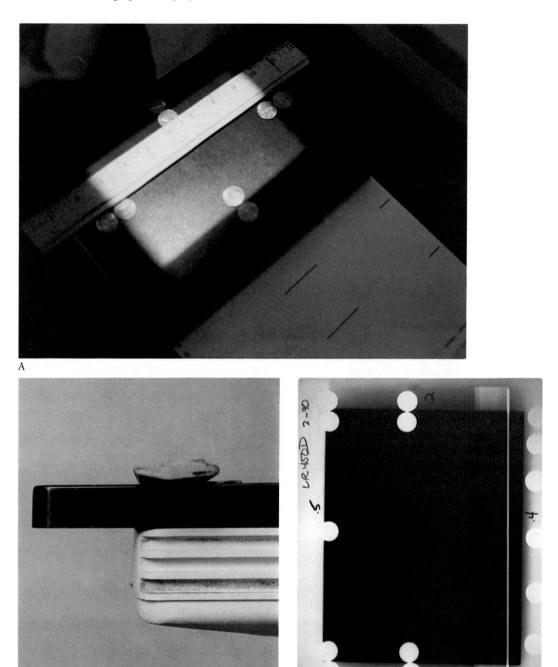

FIGURE 8-10   **A.** To determine if the light field and x-ray field are in alignment, a radiograph is taken using coins to mark the borders of the light field. **B.** A ruler with a metal edge is used to mark the chest wall edge of the film tray. **C.** The resulting radiograph clearly shows any misalignment of the light field with respect to the actual area being irradiated.

teria such as "poor positioning," "processor problem," "too light," or "too dark."

4. Determine the overall percentage of rejected films:

$$\frac{\text{number of rejected films}}{\text{total number of films used}} \times \frac{100}{1}$$

5. Determine the percentage of rejected films from each category:

$$\frac{\text{number of films from rejected category}}{\text{total number of rejected films}} \times \frac{100}{1}$$

Evaluation Analyze the rejection percentages and take corrective steps if necessary. For mammography, the ACR recommends that the standard rate not exceed 5%; the ideal rate is less than 2%.

Semiannual QA Tests

Exposure Switch

The switch must be able to terminate the exposure if manual pressure is removed. Choose an exposure time greater than 1.0 second to test the switch.

Interlocks

Interlocks should forbid exposure when in the open position. Any interlocks on the machine should be checked by attempting exposure while they are in the open position.

Darkroom Fog Test

The darkroom fog test is done to assure that fogging of the film is not occurring as a result of cracks in safelights or other sources of leaked-in white light. Most film manufacturers have easy-to-use darkroom fog test kits available through their technical sales representatives (Fig. 8-11). However, the procedure is also easy to do without a kit as explained below.

Procedure Before beginning the test, the person performing it should turn off all safelights and other lights in the darkroom and allow his or her eyes to adapt to the darkness (5–15 minutes). After this any sources of light leaking into the darkroom should be sought. Pay special attention to the seals around processors, passboxes, doors, and the like and to ceilings (particularly the suspended types, which can leak

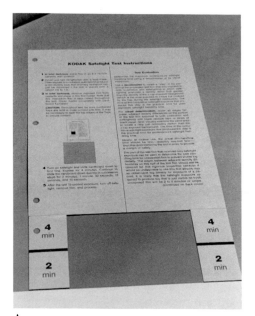

A

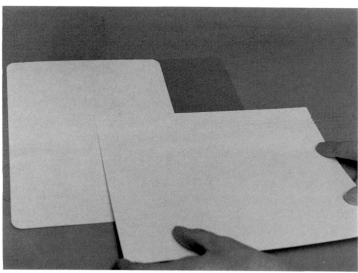

B

FIGURE 8-11 **A.** Darkroom safelight fog test kits are available through many film manufacturers, with detailed instructions included. **B.** If unable to obtain a commercial safelight test, the procedure is easy to perform using readily available equipment.

light from adjacent rooms). If any light leakage is noted, measures should be taken to eliminate it. Cover any machinery indicator lights or luminous clock dials before beginning the test.

1. In *total darkness,* open a new box of film. Load a film into each of two cassettes. Store the remaining film in the film bin. Take the cassettes from the darkroom to the x-ray unit.
2. Lightly expose one of the films to x-rays. The exposed film should have a density reading of approximately 1.0. To be certain of the technique, develop the first film and check its exposure immediately. If the density of the exposure reads approximately 1.0 on the densitometer, continue the test by exposing the second film using the same technique; if not, adjust the technique appropriately and then expose the second film. If the x-ray unit used shows a heel effect, position the film so that the effect will show at the 8-inch end of an 8 × 10 film.
3. In the darkroom, in *total darkness,* place the second film on the counter where cassettes are normally loaded and unloaded; if using single-emulsion film, the emulsion side must face up. Cover one half of the film lengthwise with a cardboard sheet (i.e., cover a 4 × 10 area of an 8 × 10 film). Keep this half covered throughout the remainder of the test.
4. Cover all but the upper one quarter of the remaining visible film with a second piece of cardboard. Turn on the safelights and machinery indicator lamps, and expose this portion to the safelights for *2 minutes.* At the end of 2 minutes, shift the cardboard so that one half of this side of the film is uncovered. Expose for *1 minute.* Shift the cardboard again so that three quarters of this side of the film is uncovered and expose for *1 minute.* The film now has exposures of 4, 2, and 1 minutes in the three exposed areas.
5. Process the film in the usual manner.
6. Determine the density differences of the various areas of the film with a densitometer, and record these values. If there is a difference between two adjacent exposure time areas of more than 0.05 OD, a problem may exist. Reexamine the darkroom for light leaks, the safelight filters for cracks, and the safelight bulbs for correct wattage. Note also the difference between the safelight exposed areas and the side of the film that was cov-

ered during the test. This will give an indication of how long a film is "safe" in the darkroom.

The ACR recommends a fog test that involves covering half of a sensitometric strip and allowing the uncovered half to be exposed to safelighting for 2 minutes (Fig. 8-12). The recommended difference in optical density between adjacent areas should be no more than 0.02 OD. This test is much less time consuming but not as accurate; some sensitometers will differ in optical density between the right and left sides of each step on the imaged wedge.

Lead Aprons, Gloves, and Drapes

Lead aprons, gloves, and drapes should not have tears that prohibit their usefulness as radiation protection garments. The easiest way to check this equipment is to use a fluorographic unit to visualize any "cracks" in the lead.

View Boxes

An evaluation of illuminators will help to maintain uniformity among all illuminators in the department, as well as assuring maximum perceptibility and optimum contrast and density ranges in the films. The most important areas that should be checked when examining the view boxes are the color or color "temperature" of the light, and the light intensity, as well as the cleanliness of the cover panel.

The *color or color temperature* used should be that which is most pleasing to the eye of the viewer or person reading the films. All fluorescent tubes within the illuminators of a department should be of the same type and brand to help ensure consistency in the color. A change in color temperature between illuminators can result in apparent changes in image contrast, leading to nonuniform exposure techniques.

The *intensity of illuminator lights* themselves is extremely important. A dim illuminator will reduce the visibility of detail by simulating increased density on the film; technologists may underexpose films to compensate. Underexposure records information on the lower contrast portion of a film's H and D curve, thus reducing detail further.

The balance between room light and illuminator light is important for minimizing glare to provide proper viewing conditions. Excessive glare will cause a loss of perception and will increase eye fatigue. A

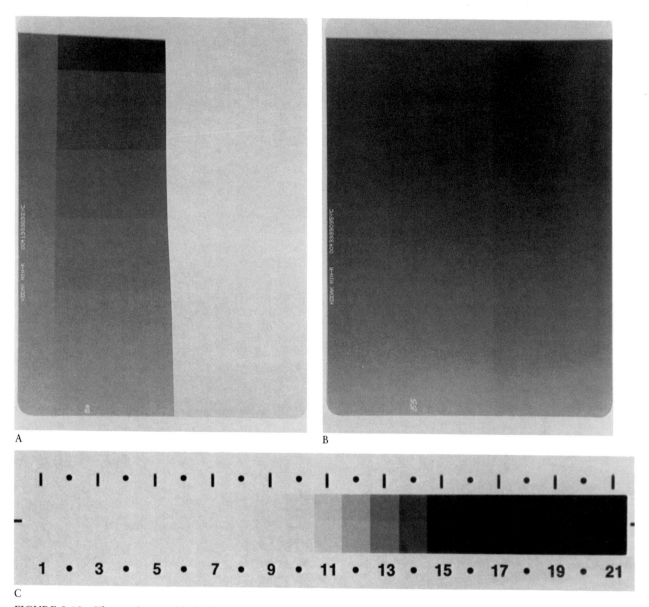

FIGURE 8-12   The resulting safelight fog test images from: **A.** the Kodak safelight test; **B.** the "do-it-yourself" safelight test, detailed in this chapter; and **C.** the ACR sensitometric safelight test.

ratio of approximately 10:1 is recommended between illuminator intensity and ambient room light intensity.

Both illuminator light and ambient room light can be measured with light meters. Specially made meters such as the GE type 214 read directly in foot-candles (ft-c). Photographic light meters can also be used by setting the ASA (speed) at 64. The denominator of the shutter speed at f8 is the light intensity in ft-c (e.g., with ASA 64 and a shutter speed of 1/400th second at f8, the light intensity level is 400 ft-c).

Ambient room light should measure approximately 30 ft-c. To measure the intensity of illuminator lights, take a reading with the meter very close to or in contact with the view box. Pass the light meter over the entire illuminator surface and record maximum and minimum intensities; calculate the average. Illuminators should average 500 ± 100 ft-c.

Viewboxes used for mammography should provide a higher luminance level than those used for general radiography. General use viewboxes have a luminance level of approximately 1500 nit (candela/m²). The ACR suggests that mammographic viewboxes should have an output of at least 3500 nit. This specification of the viewbox should be available from the manufacturer.

Many radiologists also appreciate a masking system to reduce glare when reading mammography images, because the films are odd sizes in relationship to standard view box sizes and allow a great deal of harsh light to filter around the image. This glare makes it more difficult for the eye to distinguish the contrast differences so vital in mammography. There are special viewing systems available for mammography with shutters to mask excess light. Pieces of cardboard or exposed and processed film can also be used to block the glare.

All illuminator bulbs within a department should be replaced periodically and the inside of the viewbox should be cleaned every six months. Viewing surfaces should be cleaned weekly.

Compression

The pressure applied by the compression device must be adequate to thoroughly separate the glandular tissue. However, compression should not be allowed to exceed the point at which it could cause injury to patients, or damage to the compression device and its components.

Adequate compression force should range from 25 to 40 lb in both automatic and manual modes. If maximum compression exceeds 45 lb, adjustments are necessary. Some units allow the technologist to adjust the compression rate, while others must be adjusted by a service engineer.

A flat bathroom scale, placed between towels to protect the cassette holder and compression device, can be used to measure the amount of pressure obtainable. The maximum amount of compression should be measured separately for both automatic and manual compression.

Film-Screen Contact

All cassettes should be checked with a film-screen contact mesh to determine clarity of the image. Finer meshes with 40 wires per inch are now being manufactured specifically for testing mammography screens. The image of the mesh taken with each cassette will show any areas that are out of focus because of poor film-screen contact.

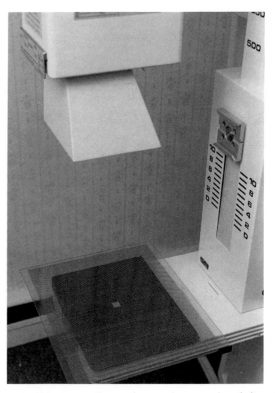

FIGURE 8-13   The mesh test object is placed directly on the cassette to be tested. Use of a grid will detract from the image of the mesh.

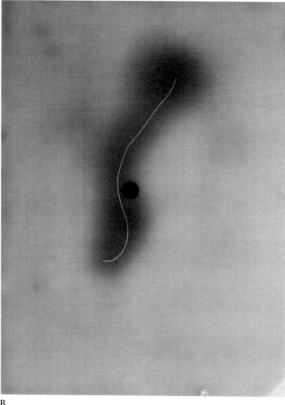

A   B

FIGURE 8-14   **A.** Radiographic image of a mesh with acceptable darkened areas of reduced sharpness. **B.** Radiographic image of a mesh showing reduced sharpness caused by an artifact within the cassette.

When imaging the mesh, be sure to allow the cassette to sit at least as long as it would between normal uses. The sponge backings on some screens need approximately 15 minutes to totally expand and allow entrapped air to escape for maximum film-screen contact.

Procedure

1. Place a filled cassette in the film holder of the x-ray unit or above the grid location. *Do not use the grid,* because this may detract from the image of the mesh.
2. Place the mesh directly on the cassette, so that the mesh is centered with the cutout toward the chest wall edge of the film (Fig. 8-13), if it has a cutout. Newer mesh tools do not have cut-outs.
3. It may be necessary to use an acrylic block to obtain the required film density. If so, place an acrylic block approximately 4 cm thick on the compression device, and raise it as close to the port of the x-ray tube as possible.

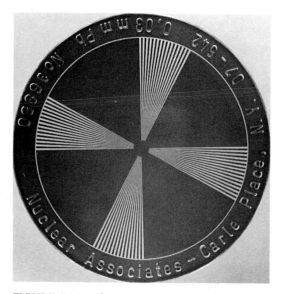

FIGURE 8-15   The star pattern testing device used to assess the focal spot size of the tube.

4. Expose the film at 28 kVp to yield a measurement of 0.70–0.80 OD at the chest wall edge of the radiograph, or as the background density.
5. Place the film on a view box and step to the side and back about 6 ft to examine it (Fig. 8-14). Areas of decreased film-screen contact will appear darker and less sharp. Cassettes with large areas (greater than 1 cm) of poor film-screen contact should be removed from service.

Focal Spot Size Assessment

The actual size of a focal spot should be measured by a physicist using the slit camera technique.[7] However, a technologist may use the star pattern test as a subjective way of assessing focal spot size by evaluating the resolution visualized by the tube (Fig. 8-15). It must be remembered that the star pattern is not an accurate measurement of the size of the focal spot, but if performed in the same manner each time it can serve to inform of any *change* in the size or shape of the focal spot. If star patterns are to be part of a mammographic QA program, a 1° or smaller pattern is necessary to detect the fine resolution obtainable with the smaller focal spots used.

Procedure The pattern is placed close to the port of the x-ray tube (Fig. 8-16). The image obtained on the film will be magnified, enabling the fine line res-

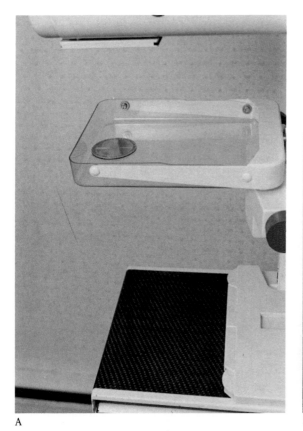
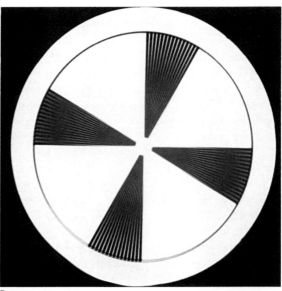

A
B

FIGURE 8-16 **A.** The star pattern testing device is placed close to the port of the x-ray tube. The resulting radiographic image will be magnified, allowing clearer visualization of the fine line resolution. **B.** The radiographic image of the star pattern is scanned to find the outermost areas of blurring, known as the zero contrast regions.

olution to be seen more clearly. As the image of the pattern is scanned from its periphery toward its center, areas of blurring can be seen. The outermost blurred areas are known as the *zero contrast regions*. The diameters of these regions are measured, and the focal spot size is determined by calculations using these measurements. The formulas for these calculations differ with the size (in degrees) of the pattern used, and are included in the instruction manual of each pattern.

Summary

This chapter has outlined much of the testing that is recommended for mammographic quality assurance. The importance of examining the results of these tests, and of reviewing the entire quality assurance program routinely, cannot be understated; the performance of any testing is insignificant if discrepancies are not acted upon.

References

1. *Mammography—A User's Guide*, NCRP report No. 85. Bethesda, MD, National Council on Radiation Protection and Measurement, 1986.
2. Haus AG: Physical Principles and Radiation Dose in Mammography, in Feig SA, McLelland R (eds): *Breast Carcinoma—Current Diagnosis and Treatment*. New York, Masson, 1983.
3. Committee on Quality Assurance in Mammography: Quality Control for Medical Physicists. Reston, VA, American College of Radiology, 1990.
4. Equipment Requirements and Quality Control for Mammography, report No. 29. New York, American Association of Physicists in Medicine, 1990.
5. Hendee W, Rossi R: Quality Assurance for Radiographic X-Ray Units and Associated Equipment, HEW Publication (FDA) 79-8094. Washington, D.C. Government Printing Office, 1979.
6. NCRP report No. 66. Bethesda, MD, National Council on Radiation Protection and Measurement, 1980.
7. *Quality Assurance for Diagnostic Imaging Equipment*, NCRP report No. 99. Bethesda, MD, National Council on Radiation Protection and Measurement, 1988.

Bibliography

Bureau of Environmental Radiation Protection: *Guide for Radiation Safety/Quality Assurance Programs*. Albany, New York State Department of Health, 1985.

Burkhart R: *A Basic Quality Assurance Program for Small Diagnostic Radiology Facilities*, US Dept of Health and Human Services publication, No. (FDA) 83-8218. Washington, DC, Government Printing Office, 1983.

Committee on Quality Assurance in Mammography: *Mammography Quality Control for Radiologic Technologists*. Reston, VA, American College of Radiology, 1992.

Diagnostic Quality Assurance Plan. Rochester, NY, Upstate Medical Physics, Inc., 1987.

ECRI: Mammography units. *Health Devices* 1990;19(5–6):153–173.

Equipment Requirements and Quality Control for Mammography, report No. 29. New York, American Association of Physicists in Medicine, 1990.

Gray J: *ACR Program on Mammography Control for Radiologists, Medical Physicists, and Technologists*. Reston, VA, ACR, 1990.

Haus AG: Screen-film processing systems and quality control in mammography. Presented at the Symposium on the Physics of Clinical Mammography, St. Louis, 1990.

LaBella J: Complete Breast Imaging Seminar—Quality Assurance, Rochester, NY, 1990.

Logan-Young, WW: Quality Assurance Booklet for the Search for Breast Cancer Seminar, Rochester, NY, 1990.

Mammographic Accreditation Phantom Model 156 Instruction Manual. Middleton, WI, Radiation Measurements, Inc, 1990.

Mount CJ, Gray JE: Improved tool for testing screen-film contact in mammography. *RadioGraphics* 1990;10(6): 1049–1054.

Process Control Procedure for Radiographic Processors. Rochester, NY, Eastman Kodak Co, 1988.

Quality Assurance for Mammography. Wilmington, DE, E.I. Dupont, 1988.

Quality Assurance Programs for Providers of Mammography Services, publication No. PH-7. Albany, NY, New York State Department of Health, 1987.

Star X-Ray Test Patterns Instruction Manual. Carle Place, NY, Nuclear Associates, 1989.

X-Omatic Processor School, Reference Manual 7476T. Rochester, NY, Eastman Kodak Co, 1986.

The Transition from Xeroradiography to Screen-Film Imaging

The technologist with experience in xeroradiography will find the transition to screen-film imaging more difficult than if she were a novice learning breast imaging. Radiologic technologists who have made the transition have indicated that it is difficult to change work habits that have become ingrained during years of repetition. While both imaging systems involve x-raying the breast, this is where the similarities end.

The Major and Minor Differences

There are three major differences between xeroradiography and screen-film imaging: (1) the x-ray equipment and recording systems, (2) the technical factors and radiographic physics employed, and (3) patient positioning and radiographic landmarks. Various chapters in this textbook present information in each of these major categories as they apply to screen-film mammography. This chapter deals with the minor differences that often confuse technologists when making this imaging transition (Table 9-1). The author assumes the reader is experienced in xerora-

diography and is familiar with its radiographic principles.

Nipple in Profile

A basic protocol of xeroradiography is that the nipple must always be imaged in profile. In most women, the nipple will be centrally located on the breast; therefore the nipple will be in profile or nearly in profile upon final compression of the breast. However, this is not the case in some women. These women will either be very full inferiorly (the bottom half of the breast), with little tissue in the superior aspect, or the opposite. When positioning these women, it would be necessary to pull posteroinferior or posterosuperior tissue, respectively, *off the receptor tray* in order to image the nipple in profile. "The nipple should, whenever possible, be projected tangentially. However, it is not always possible to observe this rule and at the same time include a maximal portion of the breast. In general, it is more important to visualize the posterior portion of the breast. It is

TABLE 9-1 Comparisons between Mammographic Systems

Xeroradiography	Screen-Film Imaging
Major Differences	
Existing x-ray system (dedicated or overhead)	Dedicated mammographic unit
Tungsten target tube	Molybdenum target tube
Selenium plate	Screen-film recording system
Specialized processing for selenium plates	Screen-film darkroom techniques
Blue-and-white images (on paper)	Black-and-white images (on film)
Curved compression device	Straight-edge compression device
kVp settings >35	kVp settings <28
Minor differences	
Nipple always in profile	Not required
Visualization of ribs	Not required
True lateral position	Oblique position
Visualization of skin line	Not required
Use of sponges	Not required
No deodorant/powder	Not required
Breath holding	Not required

usually not difficult to identify the nipple even if it is projected over breast tissue in one of the views."[1] Radiologic technologists work diligently to capture all of the breast tissue on the film, and strict adherence to the protocol of imaging the nipple in profile would be counterproductive and nullify their hard work.

Many think the nipple must be in profile for preoperative localization of a lesion. Craniocaudal views indicate whether the lesion lies in the medial half of the breast or the lateral half relative to the nipple. A nipple rolled into the breast tissue will still provide this same information. Lateral views give superior or inferior location of a lesion with regard to the nipple. Again, the nipple need not be perfectly in profile to ascertain this.

If a lump or lesion is suspected in the nipple area on a patient whose nipples do not fall in profile, an additional film is required. The routine films should demonstrate as much breast tissue as possible, while the extra film visualizes just the anterior portion of the breast, with the nipple in profile. If possible, use magnification for the second image. The information obtained from a magnification view of the nipple and retroareolar region will be far greater than that from the standard image.

Visualization of the Ribs

It is disconcerting to the technologist in transition from xeromammography to screen-film mammography to exclude the ribs from the study. However, every position in which a patient can be placed results in specific areas of the breast that cannot be visualized—whether the imaging method is xeroradiography or screen-film imaging and whether or not the ribs are included. The reason for this is that the breasts are attached to the ribcage, which is a curvilinear structure. Technical differences between xeromammography and screen-film mammography made it necessary to modify positioning as well as technique to meet the specific requirements of each modality.

Xeromammography demonstrates the retromammary fat space and the ribs in the true lateral projection. It was believed that imaging these structures meant that all the breast tissue was visualized; however this created a false sense of security. In some cases the retromammary fat space visualized is only that portion tangential to the x-ray beam and, in fact, posterior breast tissue is not included. Xeromammography compensates for the nonvisualization of posterolateral breast tissue in the lateral view by requiring its inclusion on the laterally exaggerated craniocaudal view (Fig. 9-1A).

Xeroradiography receptors have the latitude to demonstrate the breast, from ribs to nipple, utilizing a curved compression device to allow visualization of the ribs. Screen-film systems do not offer this wide latitude, therefore an evenly compressed breast is required. Because the ribs will not be included on a screen-film image, a change in positioning (from true lateral to the new oblique position) was required.

Screen-film mammography has strengths as well as weaknesses (Fig. 9-1B). Visualization of one portion of the breast will be "sacrificed" in each standard position in order to completely capture other areas (Fig. 9-2).

No single radiograph can ever display all the structures contained within a three-dimensional object,

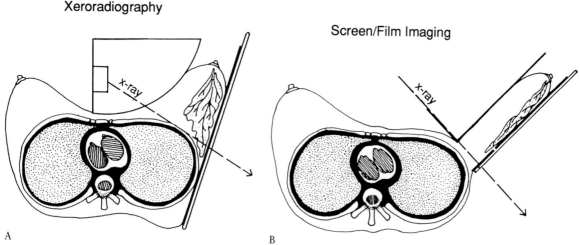

Xeroradiography

Screen/Film Imaging

A   B

FIGURE 9-1   **A.** In xeromammography the central ray is directed tangentially across the ribcage. Because of the curve of the compression device and the need to visualize into the lung field, the breast cannot be pulled away and kept away from the ribs as compression is applied. Thus posterolateral tissue is not visualized; however, the craniocaudal view will be laterally oriented to include this area. Medial tissue is also not included because of the divergence of the x-ray beam. **B.** In screen-film imaging, the chest wall edge of the cassette is placed along the midaxillary line. The posterolateral portion of the breast is captured on the film because the edge of the cassette has "gone around the corner" of the ribcage. By going this far around the curve of the ribcage, medial tissue will be missed when applying compression. Thus visualization of the medial portion of the breast is required on the craniocaudal view. (From NCRP report No. 85.[2])

however, it is the technologist's responsibility to visualize as much tissue as possible.

Lateral Versus Oblique Positioning

Prior to the design of the dedicated mammographic unit, mammography was performed on an x-ray table utilizing a ceiling-mounted x-ray tube. With this equipment, patients could be positioned so as to obtain craniocaudal, lateral, and axillary views. Versatility in positioning was made possible by the 1965 development of the C-arm design of the dedicated mammographic unit. By the mid-1970s, mammographers in the United States heard reports from their Scandanavian peers about the advantages of a new position—the oblique position.

The breast is situated anterior to the pectoral muscle, an obliquely running muscle. With the evolution of screen-film imaging, the C-arm design of the dedicated mammographic unit provided the opportunity to obtain an oblique view of the breast as opposed to the standard lateral view. Positioning for the lateral view required the compression device to "fight" against the direction of the muscular attachment of the breast to the body. Now that the force of the compression could coincide with the attachment of the breast to the body, more posterior tissue could be included on the oblique film than was possible to include with a true lateral. The lateral position is now relegated to the role of preoperative localization and is used as a supplementary view.

Visualization of the Skin Line

Breast cancers do not arise in the skin, nor do they arise from adipose tissue. "The primary focus of a breast cancer is rarely located in the subcutaneous fat zone. Thus, tumors with their epicenter in the subcutaneous tissue are, in all likelihood, benign, and are usually inflammatory processes or hematomas. It

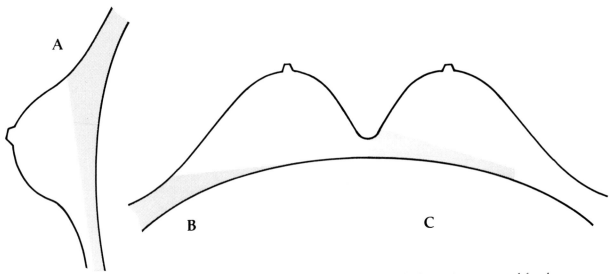

FIGURE 9-2   The "blind" areas of the standard mammography views. When the breast is compressed for the craniocaudal view, the superior posterior portion of the breast is not imaged (shaded area in **A**). Furthermore, either a posteromedial or a posterolateral portion is not included, depending on how the patient is rotated (shaded areas in **B** and **C**). In the lateral view the posterolateral portion tends not to be imaged (**B**), whereas in the oblique view the posteromedial portion of the breast tends not to be imaged (**C**). The craniocaudal projection can be either laterally or medially oriented. Usually it is obtained so that the lateral posterior portion is included rather than the medial posterior portion. This is logical only if two views are used, and the other view is the lateral, which tends to omit the posterior lateral portion. If, on the other hand, the oblique view is used together with the cranio-caudal view as a two-view standard, it might be wise to obtain the craniocaudal in a more medially oriented fashion. This is recommended since the oblique projection tends to miss the juxtathoracic medial portion of the breast. (From Andersson.[1])

should be noted that metastasis from cancers other than breast cancer may be located in the subcutaneous tissue."[1]

In high-contrast screen-film imaging, the skin line as well as the subcutaneous fat layer will be considerably darker than the parenchyma of the breast in all cases except in that of breasts that compress to approximately 1 cm or less and are composed primarily of adipose tissue. In direct opposition, xeroradiography utilizes low-contrast technique to allow for even densities on the resulting image of structures as radiolucent as the skin to structures as radiopaque as the ribs. It is this lack of contrast and density differentiation that has trained xeroradiographers to look at the "halo" just outside the skin line to ascertain whether or not their radiograph is properly exposed. For xeroradiography, visualization of the skin line is very important; with screen-film mammography, it is not.

In the early days of film mammography, when the ability to find a nonpalpable/minimal breast cancer was virtually nonexistant, the cancers that were confirmed by x-ray were already clinically evident; in fact, a pre-requisite for having a mammogram in those days was a palpable mass. By the time a breast cancer had grown to an advanced stage at which the person became symptomatic, secondary signs such as skin thickening, skin dimpling, and nipple retraction were often present. "The mass . . . has an irregular margin. In addition, there are spicules around its periphery, representing retraction of tissue strands towards the tumor. It is often referred to as scirrhous carcinoma. Microscopically, this type of cancer is characterized by retractive fibrosis. Thus, much of each tissue strand surrounding such a tumor represents thickened normal structures of the breast. The central lesion and the strands surrounding it undergo shortening (retraction), which is the basis for the skin dimpling and nipple retraction which is sometimes seen with these tumors. The skin is usually thickened in the area of retraction. *This type of breast cancer usually feels larger than its radiographic size*"[1] (Le-Borgne Principle) (emphasis added).

Minimal breast cancers, which are unexpected clinically but which have the best prognosis, will not exhibit the secondary signs of more advanced tumors. Diagnosis then rests primarily on evaluation of the mammogram. "*Retraction and thickening of the skin are secondary signs* of cancer which may be helpful radiographically. Besides being non-specific, *these signs are often not evident, or completely absent, with small tumors.* For the detection of small tumors, the demonstration of the mass and its primary characteristics on high quality mammograms are crucial"[1] (emphasis added).

As noted by Moskowitz, secondary signs also appear to be of little help in screening for breast cancer. "*We found vein dilatation, skin thickening, nipple retraction, and duct dilatation to be essentially of no help in screening.* When nipple retraction was present and a palpable mass was found, the lesion was very far advanced at detection.... If one eliminated all biopsies suggested for mass questionable, vein dilatation, skin thickening, nipple retraction, and duct dilatation approximately 204 biopsies could be eliminated with virtually *no* loss of minimal cancers"[3] (emphasis added).

With recent technical improvements in screen-film mammography, cancers of minimal size (not clinically evident) can be detected. It is necessary to image the breast with high-contrast methods to detect these lesions within the glandular tissue. This usually means overexposing the skin line and subcutaneous fat. It is necessary in most cases to "bright light" the skin.

Use of Sponges

Sponges are used as a positioning aid in xeroradiography when the ribs are to be included on the image. This is necessary to (1) support the breast to match the thickness of the ribs so that the tissue will not "disappear" around the curvature of the ribs as the woman lies on her side, and (2) help make the breast into a relatively flat surface over which compression

can be distributed evenly. The ribs are not included on screen-film mammograms, therefore sponges should not be used.

When viewing a mammogram, it is microcalcifications or the irregular border of a mass that must be visualized. By inserting a sponge between the breast and receptor tray, the body part being imaged is now moved away from the recording system—and unsharpness will result. In screen-film imaging, the breast will always be in direct contact with the film tray; as a result geometric resolution is improved. Additionally, sponges may contain artifacts that imitate or obscure pathology.

Use of Deodorants and Powders

Two substances common to deodorant are aluminum and zinc. If clumped together, these metallic specs could mimic microcalcifications. However, they will be found in the apex of the axilla, where there are no ductal structures or glandular tissue, only lymph nodes (refer to Fig. 5-37). "Approximately 30 to 50% of primary breast cancers have mammographically detectable calcifications. These calcifications may be the only radiographic finding that suggest malignancy. When such neoplasms metastasize to axillary lymph nodes, the nodes may appear dense but usually lack mammographically detectable calcifications or other abnormalities. Reports of calcified metastatic neoplasm in axillary nodes draining a primary breast cancer are rare.... Mammographically detectable calcifications in axillary lymph nodes usually are caused by previous inflammatory disease. Very rarely they may be associated with metastatic breast carcinoma, especially in advanced cases. A recent report even suggests that punctate axillary nodal calcifications are more often indicative of intranodal gold deposits (in patients treated for rheumatoid arthritis) than metastases."[4]

Talcum powder, which contains aluminum and calcium particles, often is applied over the entire surface of the breast but will tend to clump along the inframammary crease, where the bottom of the breast and the abdominal wall meet. This deposition of powder may be visualized on the mammogram because efforts are made to include this area on the craniocaudal view. Talcum powder can be distin-

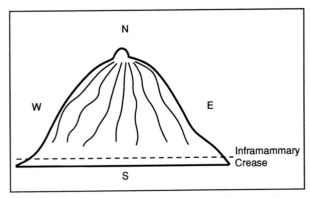

FIGURE 9-3   The ductal structures in the breast follow a "north-to-south" direction; the inframammary crease runs "east to west."

guished from tumors when looking at the craniocaudal film on the viewbox because the inframammary crease runs "east to west," whereas the ductal structures in which tumors would be found run "north to south" (Fig. 9-3).

The use of deodorants and powders should not interfere with the interpretation of a screen-film mammogram. Nevertheless, if a woman appearing for her mammogram has applied liberal amounts of powder or deodorant that have clumped in visible deposits along the moisture-prone inframammary crease or in the axilla, she should be asked to wash before the mammogram is performed. In contrast, patients should be advised to avoid these products if having a xeromammogram. The metallic specs that may be present would cause "toner-robbing" from adjacent areas (possibly obscuring a minimal cancer) because of the edge enhancement effect of xeroradiography.

Breath Holding

When the ribs and lung field are included on a xeromammogram, which uses considerably less compres-

sion than screen-film imaging, it is necessary to suspend respiration. Since screen-film imaging does not include the ribs or lungs and since one of the objectives of compression is to effectively immobilize the breast, the suspension of respiration is unnecessary except when: (1) the patient will not allow adequate compression of the breast, (2) imaging a woman who has implants, and (3) dealing with a patient who has emphysema or some other respiratory problem. Inadequate compression of the breast or excessive movement of the thorax invite motion; thus some patients may need to suspend respiration.

It is better to advise the patient to "stop breathing" rather than to hold her breath. When advised to "hold your breath," a person tends to inhale a large volume of air to last for the duration of the x-ray exposure. Inflating the lungs causes the ribcage to expand and the pectoral muscle to contract. Expansion of the ribs can result in the loss of some breast tissue on the mammogram because this bony structure now offers serious opposition to the compression device. Contraction of the pectoral muscle results in the breast being held more tightly to the body; in turn the compression will be more uncomfortable for the patient and the breast cannot easily be pulled away from the ribs. Instead, ask the patient to exhale and to "slump" as the compression is applied. Exhalation will result in the collapse of the ribcage (this positioning tip is especially helpful when dealing with thin women with prominent ribs). "Slumping" will loosen the muscle that attaches the breast to the body.

Summary

The transition from xeroradiography to screen-film imaging will require, first, an understanding of the differences and the rationale behind these differences and, second, conscientious effort, patience, and time to trade old habits for new.

References

1. Andersson I: Mammography in clinical practice. *Medical Radiography and Photography* 1986;62:2.
2. *Mammography—A User's Guide,* NCRP Report No. 85. Bethesda, MD, National Council on Radiation Protection and Measurement, 1986.
3. Moskowitz M: The predictive value of certain mammographic signs in screening for breast cancer. *Cancer* 1983;51:1007.
4. Helvie M, Rebner M, Sickles E, Oberman H: Calcifications in metastatic breast cancer in axillary lymph nodes. *AJR* 1988;151:921.

III

The Mammogram

10 Kathleen M. Willison

Breast Anatomy and Physiology

Anatomy of the Breast

The breast is a well-differentiated apocrine sweat gland of the same type found in the axilla and elsewhere in the body. These glands have evolved into an organ whose purpose is to produce and secrete milk during lactation.

External Appearance

Breast size and shape vary individually. The skin covering the breast is at its thickest at the base of the breast (about 2 mm thick)[1,2] and becomes thinner as it approaches the nipple (0.5 mm). The nipple-areola complex measures 4–5 mm (Fig. 10-1). As is the skin of the body, the skin of the breast is filled with sweat glands, sebaceous (oil) glands, and hair follicles that open to form the skin pores.[1] (The skin pores are sometimes evident mammographically as multiple tiny lucencies across the mammogram.) Of particular note are the sebaceous glands, which can become infected and imitate carcinoma radiographically (see Chapter 11).

At the breast's most distal point is the areola and nipple (Fig. 10-1). The placement of the areola and nipple on the breast again varies individually, but the nipple is considered the center point, and all things are described in reference to it. The areola is a smooth, circular darkening surrounding the nipple. Occasionally evident, especially during pregnancy and lactation, are many small protrusions on the surface of the areola. These are the Montgomery glands, a specialized sebaceous type named for the doctor who first described them. The nipple is a raised, darkened, circular extension with multiple crevices. Within these crevices are 15–20 orifices (collecting ducts)[3] that transfer milk from the lactiferous ducts.[4] Most often the nipple protrudes from the breast but occasionally it can be inverted; sometimes this occurs bilaterally. Sudden inversion or flattening of the nipple can indicate underlying malignancy. The breast usually has only one nipple, but one or more accessory nipples can occur. These accessory nipples can appear mammographically.

Internal Anatomy

The breast is enveloped between the posterior and the anterior superficial fascia of the skin.

119

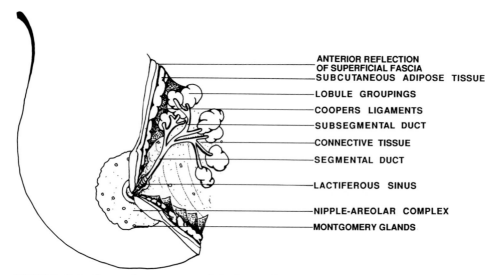

FIGURE 10-1   External appearance of the breast demonstrating nipple and areola placement. The cutaway exhibits the breast structures and shows the skin thinning as it approaches the nipple.

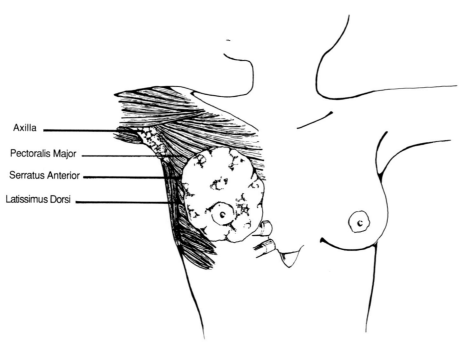

FIGURE 10-2   The breast lies anterior to and courses along the pectoral muscle. Its margins can reach the clavicle, superiorly, the latissimus dorsi laterally, and the sternum medially and can extend into the axilla.

The anatomic extent of the breast tissue should be kept in mind when considering mammographic positioning. This tissue covers a wide area (Fig. 10–2), sometimes reaching as far superiorly as the clavicle (level of the second or third rib), inferiorly to meet the abdominal wall at the level of the six or seventh rib (called the inframammary crease), laterally to the edge of the latissimus dorsi muscle, and medially to midsternum.[5] The organ also reaches into the axilla (this area is sometimes called the tail or the tail of Spence).[1,3,6] The breast lies anterior to the pectoralis major muscle, which runs in an oblique line from the humerus to the mid-sternum (Fig. 10-2). Separating the breast from the pectoral muscle is a layer of adipose tissue and connective fascia referred to as the retromammary fat space (Fig. 10-3).

The breast is made up of a varying mixture of fatty tissue, glandular components (Fig. 10-3), lymphatics, and blood vessels.

Distribution of Glandular Tissue   The pattern and distribution of the glandular tissue is essentially the same bilaterally. This is seen on the mammogram as a "mirror image." The majority of this tissue is dispersed centrally and laterally within the breast, and this distribution is recognizable mammographically (Fig. 10-4). Since breast cancer arises from the glandular tissue, it follows that the majority of cancers occur in these same areas (Fig. 10-5). The total amount of glandular tissue increases and decreases with hormonal fluctuation, administration of synthetic hormones (Fig. 10-6), pregnancy (Fig. 10-7), lactation, and menopause and subsequently atrophies with age (Fig. 10-8). Atrophy of glandular tissue be-

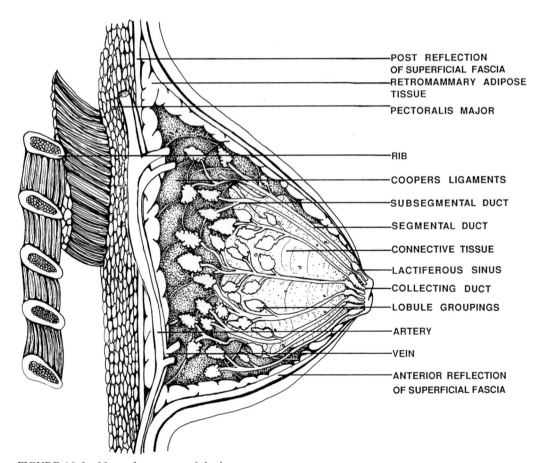

POST REFLECTION OF SUPERFICIAL FASCIA
RETROMAMMARY ADIPOSE TISSUE
PECTORALIS MAJOR
RIB
COOPERS LIGAMENTS
SUBSEGMENTAL DUCT
SEGMENTAL DUCT
CONNECTIVE TISSUE
LACTIFEROUS SINUS
COLLECTING DUCT
LOBULE GROUPINGS
ARTERY
VEIN
ANTERIOR REFLECTION OF SUPERFICIAL FASCIA

FIGURE 10-3   Normal anatomy of the breast.

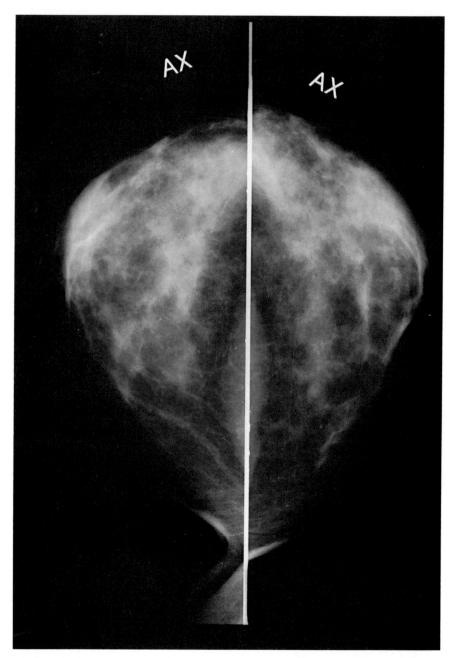

FIGURE 10-4   Bilateral craniocaudad mammograms demonstrating the pattern of centrally and laterally dispersed glandular tissue.

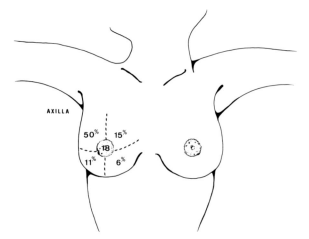

FIGURE 10-5   Distribution of breast carcinomas by quadrants. The majority of cancers arise in the upper outer quadrant of the breast, corresponding to glandular distribution.

gins medially and posteriorly, working its way to the nipple. This is an important point when interpreting the mammogram, because "new" tissue or growth of tissue in these areas in an aging woman can signal the presence of malignancy. "The ratio of glandular tissue to total breast tissue also depends upon each woman's genetic predisposition and her ratio of total body adipose tissue to total body weight [Fig. 10-9]. Therefore, it is not unusual to encounter young women whose breasts consist primarily of adipose tissue, or elderly women with extremely dense glandular tissue."[7]

The glandular tissue or "parenchyma" consists of 15–20 lobes that contain the ductal structures and the connective and supportive stroma (Fig. 10-3). The lobes are arranged in a radial pattern around the nipple.

The Lobes   Each of the 15–20 lobes contains a tree-like pattern of ductal structures (Fig. 10-10). From the nipple orifice extends a collecting duct that immediately widens into the lactiferous sinus (ampulla), a pouch-like structure that narrows and becomes the segmental duct. The larger main segmental duct branches into medium-sized subsegmental ducts. These subsegmental ducts branch into smaller ducts, branching further and decreasing in di-

ameter until coming to the lobule. The lobule is the very tiny (1–2-mm) portion of the duct that holds the milk-producing elements of the breast. A single lobe contains many lobule groupings.

The lobule is a structure loosely supported by a specialized connective tissue. The small duct just outside and leading to the lobule is the extralobular terminal duct. Once inside the lobule this duct becomes and further divides into the intralobular terminal ducts, which end at the terminal ductules, numbering anywhere from 10 to 100 in any lobule. The terminal ductule is a blind ending to the ductal pattern corresponding to what has been called the acinus, the sac-like, functional, milk-producing unit of the breast. It is believed by most authorities that acini are only truly formed during pregnancy, come to full maturity during lactation, and disappear at its completion.

The part of the ductal structure starting at the extralobular terminal duct and ending at the terminal ductules is termed the *terminal duct lobular unit* (TDLU) (Fig. 10-11). Many pathologies arise in the TDLU (see Chapter 11).

Connective and Supportive Stroma   The tissue that gives the breast its support can be divided into the extralobular and intralobular stroma. The latter is a specialized tissue that gives the lobule its shape and definition[3] (Fig. 10-11). It has an extensive capillary network allowing exchange of hormones into and secretions out of the lobule. The extralobular stroma holds the larger ductal structures.

The supportive structure of the breast are Cooper's ligaments,[8] which are of particular significance because of their notable effect on the glandular tissue mammographically (see "Mammographic anatomy," below). Cooper's ligaments are fibrous membranes that incompletely sheath the lobes of the breast, starting at the most posterior portion (the base) of the breast, extending outward, and attaching to the anterior superficial fascia of the skin. Figure 10-12 illustrates these structures and their dispersement throughout the breast.

Ductal Structures   The ductal structures are lined with two layers of epithelial cells[3] of many differing types (Fig. 10-13). Beneath these is a layer of myoepithelium, a form of smooth muscle whose purpose is to contract the acini and ducts, emptying milk dur-

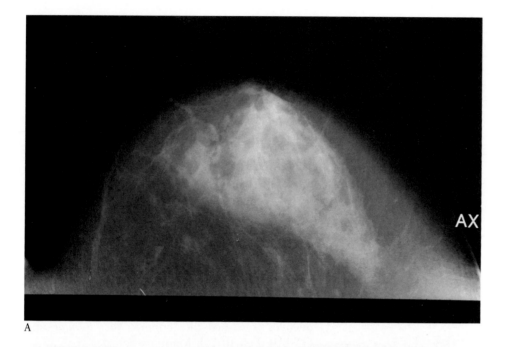

A

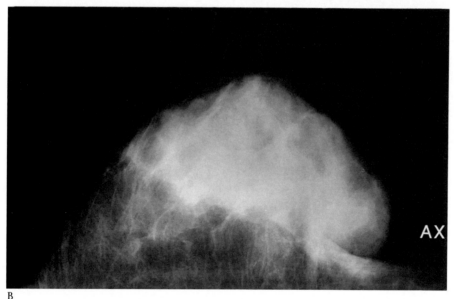

B

FIGURE 10-6   Effects of synthetic hormones on the amount of glandular tissue in the breast. **A.** Craniocaudad mammogram of a patient prior to synthetic hormones. **B.** Same patient 1 year after starting hormone therapy.

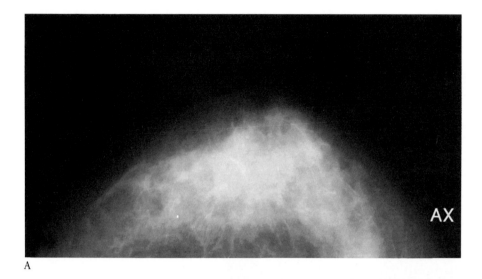

A

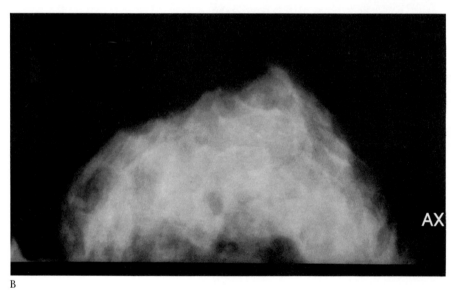

B

FIGURE 10-7   The amount of glandular tissue (**A**) increases with pregnancy (**B**).

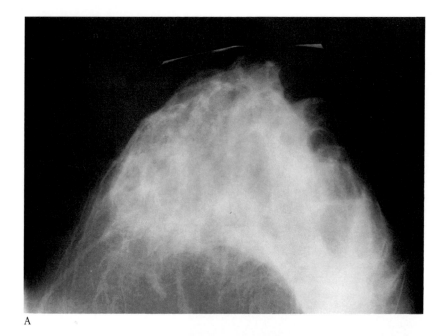

A

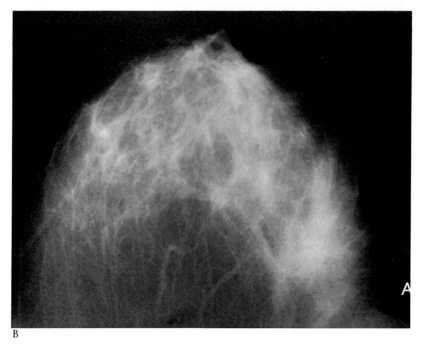

B

FIGURE 10-8 **A.** Craniocaudad mammogram of a woman prior to onset of menopause. **B.** Craniocaudad mammogram of same woman showing atrophy of menopause.

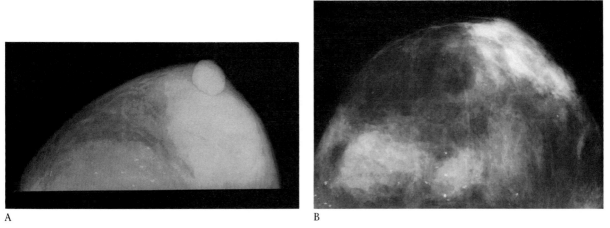

A   B

FIGURE 10-9   A dramatic example of how weight gain or loss affects the proportion of glandular to fatty tissue in the breast. **A.** Craniocaudad mammogram of a woman with anorexia nervosa. **B.** Craniocaudad mammogram of same woman after weight gain and recovery.

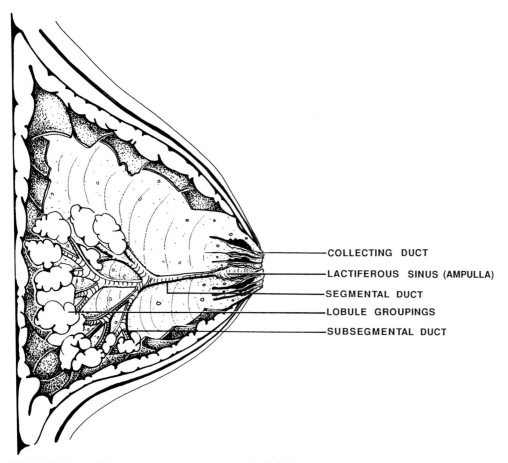

—COLLECTING DUCT

—LACTIFEROUS SINUS (AMPULLA)

—SEGMENTAL DUCT

—LOBULE GROUPINGS

—SUBSEGMENTAL DUCT

FIGURE 10-10   The anatomic structures of a single lobe.

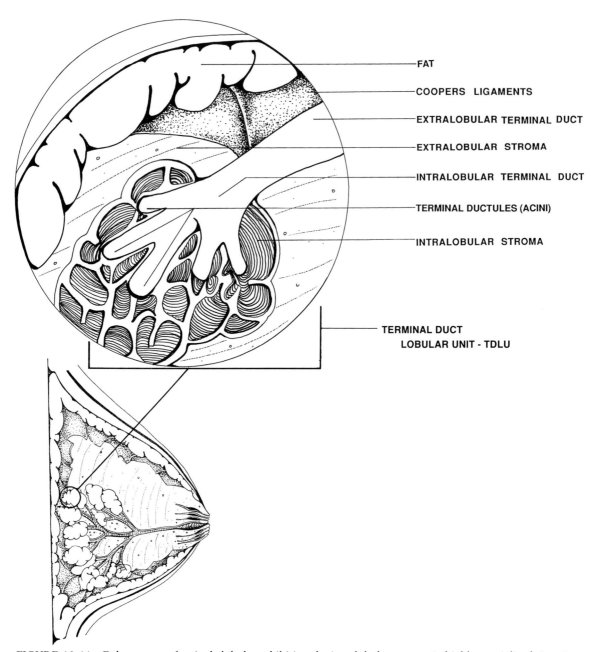

FAT

COOPERS LIGAMENTS

EXTRALOBULAR TERMINAL DUCT

EXTRALOBULAR STROMA

INTRALOBULAR TERMINAL DUCT

TERMINAL DUCTULES (ACINI)

INTRALOBULAR STROMA

TERMINAL DUCT
LOBULAR UNIT - TDLU

FIGURE 10-11   Enlargement of a single lobule, exhibiting the intralobular stroma (a highly specialized tissue) and other structures. The terminal duct lobular unit (TDLU) begins at the extralobular terminal duct and ends at the terminal ductules.

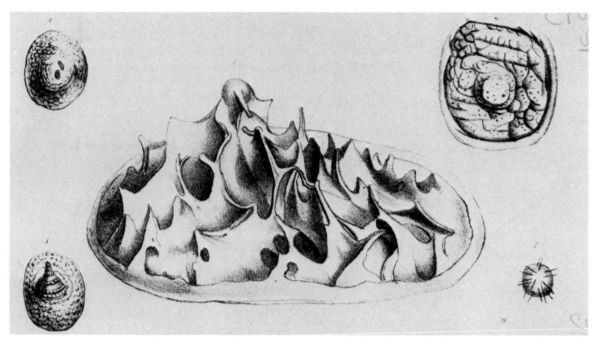

FIGURE 10-12   Drawing of Cooper's ligaments. Notice the outward projection from the base of the breast. (Drawing from Cooper.[8])

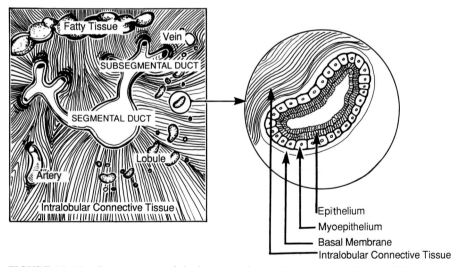

FIGURE 10-13   Cross-section of the breast with an enlargement to show cellular makeup of ductal walls.

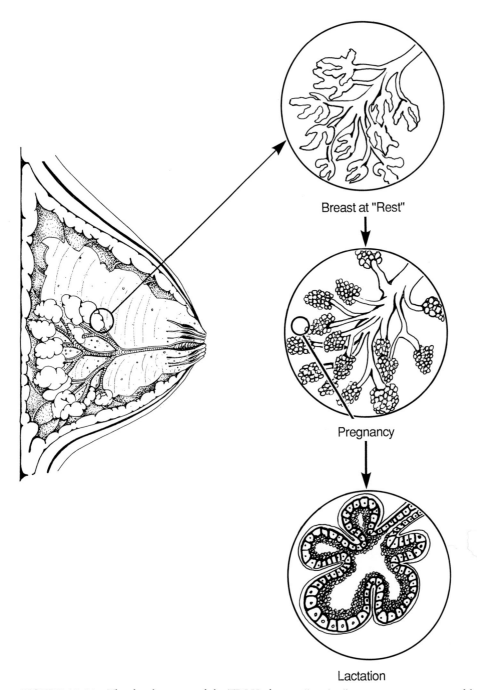

Breast at "Rest"

Pregnancy

Lactation

FIGURE 10-14   The development of the TDLUs from a "resting" state to pregnancy and lactation.

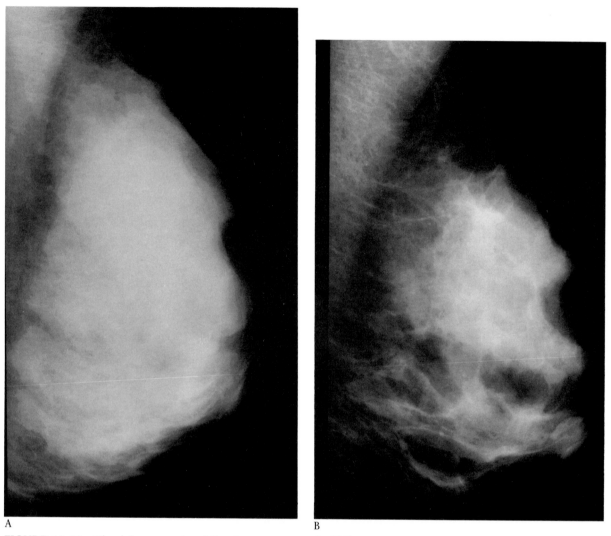

A   B

FIGURE 10-15   Glandular regression following pregnancy. **A.** Oblique mammogram prior to pregnancy. **B.** Same patient showing regression of glandular tissue 18 months after pregnancy and lactation.

ing lactation. This lies on a basement membrane. For the most part the changes that take place in the breast occur within the epithelial cells; however, the myoepithelium and the basal membrane do respond to hormonal changes. These occur in the normal expected physiologic conditions as well as in pathologic situations.

Physiology of the Breast

In order to discuss physiology of the breast it is first necessary to define the "resting breast." In this case "resting" means that there is no pregnancy or lactation. However, it should be made clear that the breast is never truly resting. It is in a constant state of change as a result of the menstrual cycle as well as changes that take place over a woman's lifetime. These range from proliferation of cells or ductal structures to involution, regression, and atrophy of these same structures. In addition, many of these structures fail to completely regress or involute, or there can be early atrophy. This wide variation in duct appearance at any given time causes difficulty for pathologists attempting to define "normal" breast anatomy especially when interpreting cytologic findings in fine-needle aspiration studies.

Hormonal Influences during the Life Cycle

At about the age of 17 years the ductal structures, including the lobule, have fully formed within the breast in response to earlier hormonal stimuli.

The normal physiologic changes that take place in the breast are related to hormonal secretions in the woman's body. The two most prominent hormones active in breast physiology are estrogen (responsible for ductal proliferation) and progesterone (responsible for lobular proliferation and growth). Prolactin is another prominent hormone but is present only during initial growth, pregnancy, and lactation. Other hormones also influence the breast tissue but are not discussed here.

Abnormal growth and change in the breast are related to the over- or underproduction of hormones, and also to inconsistencies in levels from one menstrual cycle to another.

Menstrual Cycle Changes   During the first part of the menstrual cycle, estrogen stimulates epithelial proliferation and enlargement within the *larger* ductal structures. During ovulation, epithelial cells proliferate in the lobule in response to progesterone,[1] forming new TDLUs in which the lobules enlarge and the terminal ductules become more apparent. Additionally, increase in blood flow and interstitial fluid retention leads to the lumpiness and tenderness felt by women a few days before the menstrual cycle begins. At the onset of menstruation, estrogenic influences cause involution and regression of the terminal ductal lobular unit and the lobules.[3] This regression can take several weeks,[9] and not all the lobules regress or involute, so some fully formed lobules are left behind.

Pregnancy and Lactation   Changes within the breast can be noted within several weeks of conception as a result of the increase in estrogen, progesterone, and prolactin production in the body.[5] At this time, the epithelial cells again proliferate, increasing the size and number of TDLUs (Fig. 10-14). The lobules enlarge and the acini become fully formed, readying for the production of milk (Fig. 10-7). After birth, the acinar epithelia undergo secretory changes as a result of the hormonal influence of prolactin, and secretion in the form of milk is produced. In addition, milk production causes ductal dilations.

After lactation ends, the structures begin to involute and regress. Hoeffken and Lanyi stated that "the degree of involution following lactation is variable. It can be quite extensive with almost total replacement of stromal and parenchymal tissue by fat with only fibrous septa, ducts and vessels remaining. In spite of this, however, the breast retains its ability to redevelop parenchyma and secrete milk during any subsequent pregnancy"[1] (Fig. 10-15).

Menopause   Atrophy of mammary structures commences at menopause and ceases 3–5 years later. This takes place beginning medially and posteriorly, then laterally, working its way to the nipple. In addition, atrophy can be spotty within one breast—one lobule may disappear while an adjacent one does not. Menopausal atrophy can be asymmetric from one breast to another. The involuting breast will lose its supportive tissue to fat, producing a smaller breast or a larger, more pendulous breast. This replacement by fat can occasionally give rise to a lump, physically imitating carcinoma; mammography is especially useful in these cases. The epithelial cells of the lobules will flatten and the basement membrane will become indistinguishable from the atrophied specialized connective tissue. Once this occurs the lobule loses its definition and eventually disappears completely. The smaller ducts involute; however, the larger ducts are not always affected (Fig. 10-8).

The above descriptions are an oversimplification of breast physiology and further reading is encouraged. The texts by Azzopardi[4] and Haagensen[5] are two good sources of information on the physiology of the breast.

Mammographic Anatomy

Normal Anatomy

Although some of the structures of the breast will be visualized on the mammogram, others will only be recognized by the effect or pattern they form (Fig. 10-16).

The nipple and its surrounding areola can be recognized as an increase in radiodensity along the skin line, if imaged in profile (Fig. 10-17A). If not imaged in profile, the nipple can be appreciated as a well-circumscribed radiopaque density (Fig. 10-17B), sometimes mistaken for a mass. Adipose tissue (fat) will appear as radiolucent areas (black, grayer, less dense areas) on the mammogram. The glandular tissue appears as a radiopaque "sheet" (the white or "denser" areas). This glandular "sheet" consists of the blood vessels, the lymphatics, the supportive and connective tissue (stroma), and the various ductal structures that were discussed earlier. The ductal structures are not appreciated as a single entity, but are recognized as a pattern of radial lines extending from the nipple. Specific ductal patterns are recognizable with ductography (Fig. 10-18). Blood vessels can often be noted as separate structures, especially when arteries calcify characteristically (Fig. 10-19). Occasional filling of a lymphatic channel can be seen during ductography, but is not usually recognized as such on the plain mammogram. Lymph nodes, in contrast, are well vis-

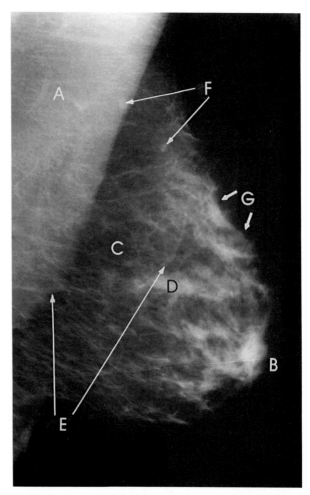

FIGURE 10-16   A 45° oblique mammographic projection demonstrating anatomic structures that are visualized with mammography: **A.** Pectoral muscle; **B.** nipple; **C.** fat; **D.** glandular tissue; **E.** blood vessel; **F.** lymph nodes; **G.** Cooper's ligaments.

ualized both in the axilla and often within the breast (Fig. 10-20). The connective stroma cannot be individually appreciated on the mammogram except for Cooper's ligaments, which can be seen as thin lines to the skin in the subcutaneous adipose tissue (Fig. 10-16).

Mammographic Changes

Pregnancy and Lactation   The appearance of the breast during pregnancy and lactation is one of in-

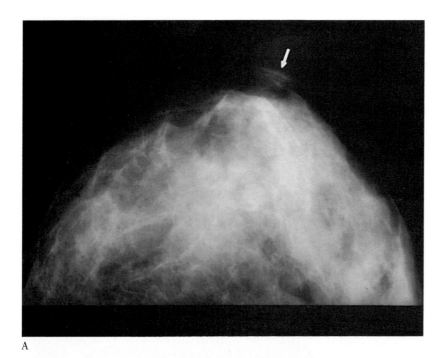

A

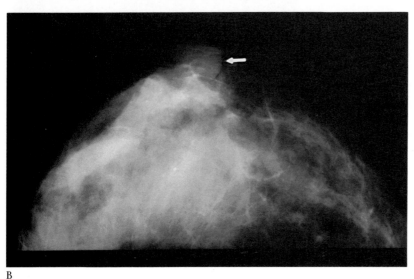

B

FIGURE 10-17   The nipple (arrows) shown in profile as an increase in density along the skin line (**A**) and demonstrating a well-circumscribed density when not shown in profile (**B**).

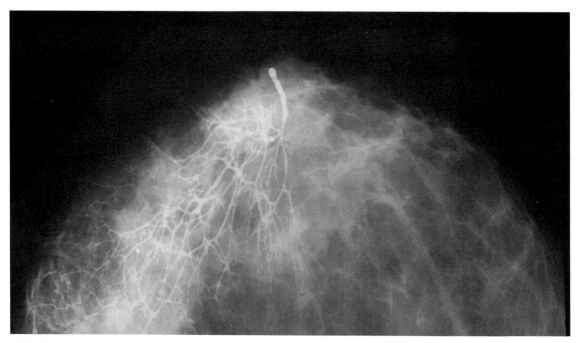

FIGURE 10-18   Craniocaudad ductogram showing the radial pattern of the ductal structures.

creased density, on the mammogram as a result of the changes already outlined but also because of the milk production and increased blood supply (Fig. 10-7). Mammography during this time is usually reserved for the symptomatic patient. In the case of lactation, the woman is asked to bring her baby with her and to nurse just prior to the mammogram being done. This removal of the superimposed milk increases visualization of the breast tissue.

Menstruation   Mammographically, an increase in overall density of the breast tissue during menstruation is usually not seen. (However, Haagensen described difficulty and discrepancies in physical exam during the premenstrual phase.[5]) Tolerating the vigorous compression necessary for mammography, during the premenstrual period will be more difficult for some women, and in fact the woman who has ex-

treme tenderness may tolerate only minimal compression. With this in mind, it would seem that the best time to perform mammography is during the week after the menses has ended. In large-scale screening programs this type of scheduling is extremely difficult; however, the patient can make an informed decision about scheduling if she has a regular menstrual cycle. Advising patients to decrease caffeine 2 weeks prior to the mammogram (since caffeine adds to the hormone effect) (see Chapter 3) may help prevent extreme discomfort during the compression of mammography.

Menopausal Changes   The menopausal breast will most often be of a greater fatty content on the mammogram (Fig. 10-8). The sometimes asymmetric appearance of the tissue is due to uneven atrophy.

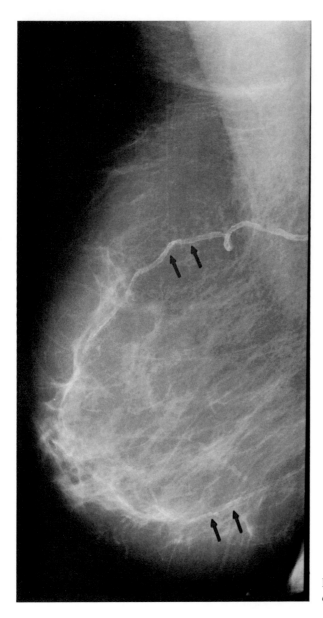

FIGURE 10-19 Oblique mammogram demonstrating characteristic calcification of an artery (arrows).

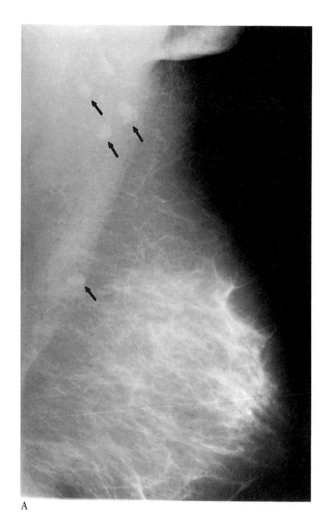

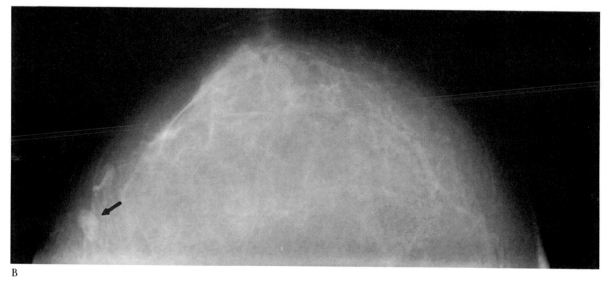

FIGURE 10-20   **A.** A 45° oblique mammogram showing lymph nodes in the axilla and trailing into breast (arrows). **B.** A craniocaudad mammogram demonstrating an intra-mammary lymph node (arrow).

References

1. Hoeffken W, Lanyi M: *Mammography*. Philadelphia, WB Saunders Company, 1977.
2. Shaw-de Parades E: *Atlas of Film-Screen Mammography*. Baltimore, Urban & Schwarzenberg, 1989.
3. Page DL, Anderson TJ: *Diagnostic Histopathology of the Breast*. Edinburgh, Churchill Livingstone, 1987.
4. Azzopardi JG: *Problems in Breast Pathology*. London, WB Saunders, 1979.
5. Haagensen CC: *Disease of the Breast*. Philadelphia, WB Saunders Company, 1986.
6. Egan RL, McSweeney MB: The normal breast, in Harper P (ed): *Ultrasound, Mammography*. Baltimore, University Park Press, 1985.
7. *Mammography—A Users Guide*, NCRP report No. 85. Bethesda, MD, National Council on Radiation Protection and Measurements, 1986.
8. Cooper Sir Astley: *Anatomy and Diseases of the Breast*. Philadelphia, Lea and Blanchard, 1845.
9. Gallager HS: Pathology of benign breast disease, in Harper P (ed): *Ultrasound mammography*. Baltimore, University Park Press, 1985.

Bibliography

Egan RL: *Breast Imaging Diagnosis and Morphology of Breast Diseases*. Philadelphia, WB Saunders Company, 1988.
Tábar L, Dean PB: *Teaching Atlas of Mammography*, ed 2. New York, Thieme Inc, 1985.
Wolfe JN: *Xeroradiography of the Breast*. Springfield, IL, Charles C Thomas, 1972.

11
Kathleen M. Willison

Mammographic Pathology

The description of mammographic pathology in this chapter is by no means all encompassing; rather, it is an introduction to pathologic patterns. Tábar and Dean[1], Shaw-de Paredes[2], Kopans[3], and Wolfe[4] (although Xerox mammographically oriented) give excellent descriptions in their atlases concerning mammographic findings. Page and Anderson[5], Azzopardi[6], Wellings et al.[7], Haagensen[8], and Layni[9] are good sources of information concerning etiology, development, and histologic changes of breast disease. While knowledge of this latter topic is not truly necessary for the technologist to be able to perform the study, it solves some of the mystery surrounding the disease.

The more versed the technologist is in pathologic patterns, the more adept he or she will be at imaging them. It is helpful for the technologist to become familiar with physical as well as mammographic patterns of pathology. Study the authors cited above in order to learn these pathologic patterns. The technologist will also gain more applicable information for day-to-day work by learning what the supervising radiologist recognizes as worrisome and in need of further study. This has been accomplished in a number of ways:

1. Working side-by-side with the radiologist when working up a patient is an excellent method of learning patterns of pathology.
2. In many clinics, the radiologist includes the technologist in the reading of the mammogram, indicating not only pathology but contrary findings that would indicate to the radiologist the necessity of an extra view. At many of these clinics the radiologist depends on the technologist for correlative physical findings and patient information.
3. In-service programs and inclusion of the technologist in tumor board meetings are useful methods of teaching pathology.

Mammography and the Breast

The breast is in a constant state of change as a result of cyclic monthly as well as life cycle changes. It is important to distinguish what is normal, benign, premalignant, and malignant among these changes. This is critical not only for the diagnosis, but also for patient prognosis and treatment.[5] While this can only be done with certainty by the histopathologist, mammography as a tool of detection certainly plays a role in this process:

The mammogram recognizes very early changes in a disease process, enabling the histopathologist to have more information regarding etiology of breast disease.

The mammogram "shows" processes that would otherwise remain hidden, thus adding more information about the breast and its metabolic processes.

The mammogram presses the histopathologist to further delineate breast changes in order that the mammographer can make a more exact diagnosis.[5]

Diseases of the Breast

The majority of breast diseases occur in the terminal duct lobular units (TDLUs) and arise predominantly from the epithelial cells; however, the fibrous or connective tissue can also be involved. Other lesions occur in the larger ducts. Figure 11-1 shows a breakdown of various breast diseases and their common site of origin.

Malignant Disease

The majority of cancers are thought to arise in the TDLUs. The extralobular terminal duct is thought to be the site of ductal carcinoma and the lobule the site of lobular carcinomas. However, the terms "ductal" and "lobular" are more often used to describe a cell type rather than a site of origin. There is much discussion regarding the potential for confusion because of this variance in terminology.

It is thought by most experts that malignant disease develops through a process that starts with epithelial hyperplasia (sometimes referred to as epitheliosis or papillomatosis), wherein the epithelial cells increase in number. There are three grades of epithelial hyperplasia: mild, moderate, and florid. Epithelial hyperplasia can progress to atypical hyperplasia, in which the epithelial cells increase in number and also change in a way that is not normal for these cells. At this stage, the process is believed to be reversible. The next step is carcinoma-in-situ, where there is no

invasion of the cell outside of the duct. At this stage the process is considered irreversible, and at some time the condition will progress. The next stage is infiltrating or invasive carcinoma, in which the cancer cells break out of the ductal walls and invade stromal tissue and lymph channels.

Both categories of carcinoma, ductal and lobular, are further divided into cancer types by changes that occur in the epithelial cells as well as other characteristics (Table 11-1). In addition, other types of cancers, although a small number, will arise from the stromal tissue and at the site of the nipple, as in the case of Paget's disease.

Benign Diseases

The majority of benign lesions are discussed in the "Masses" section of this chapter. This section is devoted to the various diseases that occur in the breast that are covered by the umbrella term "fibrocystic disease." Histologically, this phrase is falling by the wayside as histopathologists are trying to be more specific in their description of these benign processes, determining their subsequent likelihood of becoming cancerous and the degree to which they indicate increased risk. Some of these processes are adenosis, sclerosing adenosis, fibrosis, cysts, apocrine metaplasia, radial scar, epithelial hyperplasia, and duct ectasia.

These lesions may be evident physically and/or mammographically; however, some are only evident histopathologically as part of a disease process and are discovered as an incidental finding upon biopsy. These changes can give rise to masses, calcifications, or prominent ductal patterns which can be seen on the mammogram. Occasionally each lesion is found in isolation, but more often they are seen in conjunction with one another.

Adenosis   Adenosis is the enlargement and/or development of new lobular units. It can be considered "normal" change, as with the "adenosis of pregnancy," or pathologic when involved with other processes. Adenosis is not considered premalignant.

Sclerosing Adenosis   Adenosis with sclerosing of the intralobular stroma can present as calcifications or masses and is considered benign and not a premalignant condition.

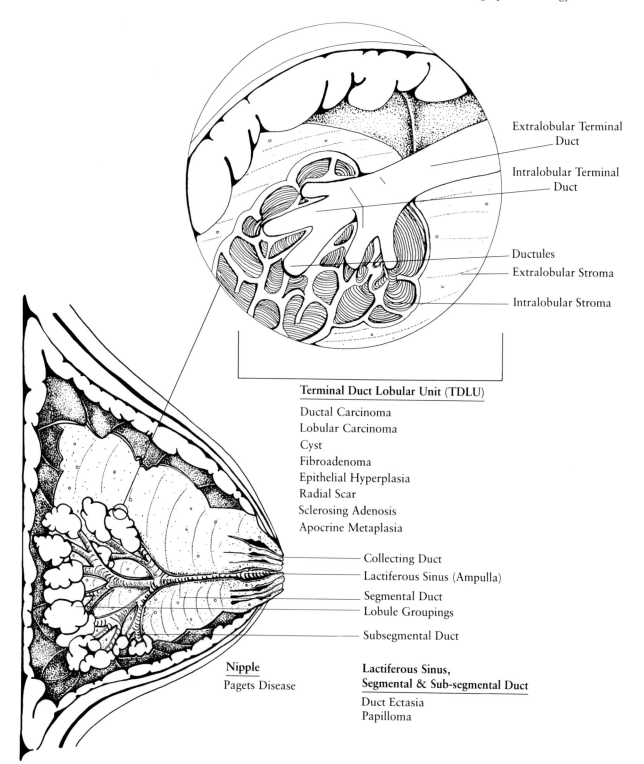

FIGURE 11-1   Various breast diseases and their most **common** site of origin.

TABLE 11-1   Cancer Types in Ductal and Lobular Carcinoma

Ductal	Lobular
Intraductal	In situ
Invasive	Invasive
Comedo	
Inflammatory	
Medullary	
Mucincus	
Papillary	
Scirrhous	
Tubular	

Fibrosis   Fibrosis is the formation of fibrous tissue stemming from the connective and supportive stroma. It is a benign condition.

Cysts   A cyst occurs in the TDLU when the extralobular terminal duct becomes blocked. The normal ductal secretions are not reabsorbed quickly enough and fluid begins to accumulate. When enough fluid accumulates the resulting pressure causes the TDLU to lose its shape and the cyst is formed. Occasionally, papillomas and carcinomas can arise in the wall of a cyst. According to Wellings et al.[7] there are three types of cyst, categorized by the cell type found in the lining: epithelial cyst, lined by epithelial cells; stromal cyst, an epithelial cyst that has lost its epithelial component; and apocrine cyst, in which the epithelial cells display apocrine metaplasia. The presence of cysts alone does not increase the risk of subsequent carcinoma; however, rarely an intracystic carcinoma or papilloma can arise from the epithelium of the wall of a cyst.

Apocrine Metaplasia (Apocrine Change)   Apocrine metaplasia is a change occurring in the epithelial cells whereupon they exhibit characteristics of apocrine sweat glands. Apocrine metaplasia alone does not increase the risk of breast cancer, but can occur with other more worrisome processes.

Radial Scar   The radial scar (also known as infiltrating epitheliosis, black hole, etc.) has a "central fibrous core"[5] with radiating arms made up of benign epithelial growth and sclerosis. It can mimic cancer both mammographically and histologically. It is not clear whether the radial scar signals premalignancy

or the likelihood of the breast tissue to develop carcinoma subsequently.

Epithelial Hyperplasia   Epithelial hyperplasia is the increase in number, over the normal amount, of epithelial cells lining the duct. Epithelial hyperplasia can be mild, moderate, or florid and can progress to atypical hyperplasia. Certain degrees of epithelial hyperplasia can be considered premalignant.

Duct Ectasia   A benign process consisting of widened ducts, containing thickened material. Inflammation surrounds the ducts. Its cause is unknown.

Physical Presentation of Pathology

The radiologist will depend in part on clinical and physical information to make a diagnosis (and/or recommendation for biopsy). Physical signs can often indicate whether a disease process is benign or malignant. The diagnostic use of some of these signs is summarized in this section.

Skin Changes

Redness   Infection, abscess, and inflammatory carcinoma most usually are associated with redness of the skin. However, redness is occasionally seen with other types of carcinoma and with benign diseases.

Edema (Skin Thickening)   These conditions can be associated with both infection and carcinoma, especially inflammatory carcinoma, in which the skin has the appearance of an orange peel ("peau d'orange").

Nipple Changes

Inversion   An inverted nipple(s) can be a part of normal development; however, inversion can also be associated with carcinoma.

Eczematous Changes   Reddening, flaking, and crusting of the nipple can be associated with Paget's disease of the nipple, a carcinoma that usually is seen in conjunction with an underlying intraductal carcinoma of the breast. This type of carcinoma constitutes just 2–5% of all breast carcinomas. Eczematous changes can also be due to a benign condition such as an allergy.

Discharges   Spontaneous, unilateral discharge is usually due to a benign condition such as duct ectasia, but can also be caused by a papilloma (benign tumor of epithelial cells) or carcinoma. Bilateral discharge or expressed discharge is usually hormonally related or of benign origin. Discharges can vary in color from clear to green to rusty or bloody. Carcinoma is usually associated with a bloody or watery discharge but exceptions can occur.

Contour Change

The radiologist will compare the shape of both breasts looking for asymmetry. This occurs as bulging of the skin, which can be associated with an underlying mass, benign or malignant, and as dimpling or

retraction of the skin, which can be associated with carcinoma.

Difference in Movement

When the arms are slowly raised the breasts should move symmetrically. Differences can indicate underlying pathologic processes, including carcinoma.

Difference in Size

Most often a difference in size of the breasts is associated with normal development; however, a shrinking or enlargement unilaterally can indicate underlying carcinoma.

Lump

An asymmetric palpable mass can be associated with carcinoma as well as benign disease. Carcinoma in its very early stages can have benign characteristics; that

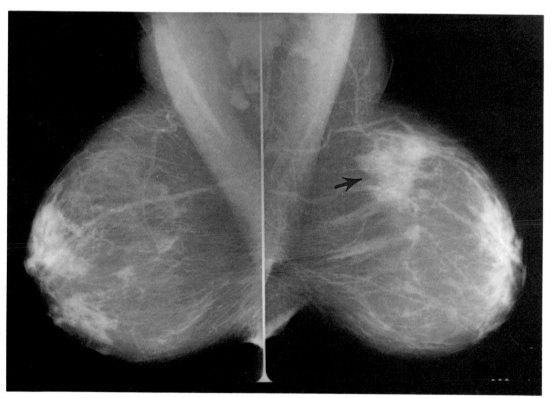

FIGURE 11-2   This asymmetric area (arrow) is a normal variant of development.

is, it can feel smooth and soft and can move freely rather than being fixed to the skin or underlying tissue. In addition, some benign lesions can feel very much like an advanced carcinoma—hard, irregular in outline, and fixed to the skin.

Pain

When a patient indicates pain bilaterally it is usually due to hormonal fluctuations or other body functions. Pain is unusual with carcinoma, but not unheard of.

Nodularity

Nodularity occurring bilaterally is usually associated with benign conditions.

Mammographic Presentation of Pathology

Pathology occurs mammographically as: (1) a mass, (2) calcifications, or (3) diffuse accentuation of the glandular tissue. However, these may only be made apparent by asymmetry, architectural distortion, and/or changes in contour of the parenchyma. Other mammographic signs of disease, although secondary, are dilated ducts, dilated veins, and skin thickening.

Asymmetry

The breasts are mirror images; therefore, mammographically the distribution of the glandular tissue should appear the same, with only slight variation from one breast to the other. If one breast is larger physically than the other the glandular components can be expected to be larger in that breast on the mammogram. However, a disproportionate amount of tissue in one area of one breast needs to be evaluated with further x-ray views.

Often asymmetry is a result of anatomic variations due to uneven development or prior surgery (Fig. 11-2). Asymmetry is the radiologist's greatest aid in determining abnormalities both benign and malignant.

Architectural Distortion

The ductal structures of the breast are seen mammographically as a pattern of radial lines that converge at the nipple. This is known as the normal architecture of the breast. Interruption of this pattern (i.e., lines that *oppose* this natural flow towards the nipple) is termed "architectural distortion" (Fig. 11-3). It occurs with both benign and malignant disease processes. Architectural distortion can occur with a

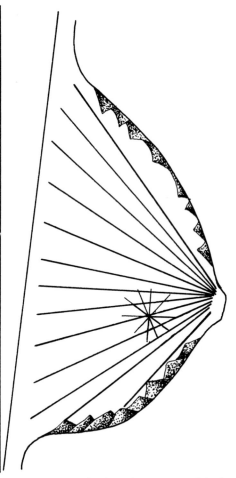

FIGURE 11-3 The ductal structures of the breast are seen as a pattern of radial lines that converge at the nipple. This is understood as the normal architecture. When lines appear that oppose this natural flow, it is termed "architectural distortion."

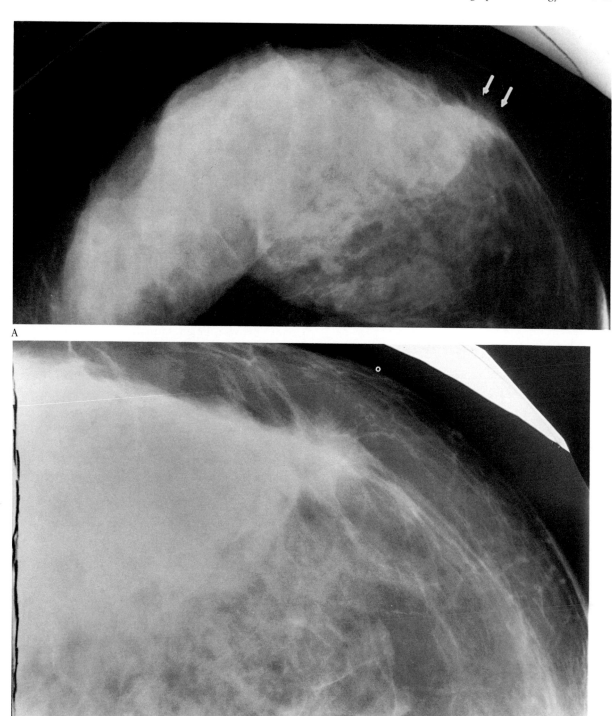

A

B

FIGURE 11-4   **A.** Architectural distortion—interruption of the normal flow of ductal structures to the nipple—is evident on this craniocaudad mammogram (arrows). **B.** With a special view the architectural distortion is more apparent.

mass and in fact may be the only indication that a mass is present.

Architectural distortion is a strong indicator of malignancy (Fig. 11-4). However, there are structures in the breast that can imitate architectural distortion. Blood vessels and Cooper's are often perpendicular to the duct lines radiating toward the nipple. These can contribute to a "pseudo (false) carcinoma effect," as can overlapped ductal structures. Surgical changes, resolving hematoma, and injury can also produce architectural distortion.

Change in Contour

The parenchyma of both breasts should be similarly smooth in outline. Asymmetric bulging or indenting of the skin can be caused by malignancy but can also be caused by prior surgery.

Masses

Mass densities that occur mammographically in the breast can be either benign or malignant. The radiologist will consider certain mammographic characteristics of a mass *in conjunction with* clinical and historical information to determine whether a mass should be biopsied. These characteristics include the border, density, and tissue makeup of the mass as well as the presence or absence of a capsule, a halo, or the silhouette sign.

Mammographic Characteristics

Border   A stellate border is a strong indicator of carcinoma, but can also occur with benign conditions such as hematoma and tension cyst. A smooth (or well-circumscribed) border is a strong indicator of a benign lesion, but a malignant mass can have a smooth border as well.

Density   Most malignant masses will be denser than surrounding glandular tissue; however, low-density carcinomas do rarely occur.

Makeup   The tissue composition of a mass indicates whether it is benign or malignant:

Fatty—always benign
Fatty and glandular mix—usually benign
Glandular or fibrous—benign or malignant

Capsule   A capsule is a thin radiopaque line surrounding a mass on the mammogram.[1] A mass that is encapsulated is most often benign; rarely this can occur with malignancy.

Halo   A halo is a thin, radiolucent curved line on the mammogram that is caused by the edge of the mass compressing surrounding fatty tissue[4] (see Fig. 11-6). A halo sign usually occurs with benign lesions but can occur rarely with a malignant mass.

Silhouette Sign   The silhouette sign can help the radiologist discern whether a lesion truly has a stellate border. If a mass is truly stellate, the lines radiating toward it will disappear in the middle of the lesion. Otherwise the lines are overlapped, rather than being connected to the lesion (Fig. 11-5 and 11-6).

Malignant Masses

Malignant masses are usually denser than surrounding glandular tissue and have a stellate border (Fig. 11-7). However, a malignant mass can be smoothly outlined or of a low density.

Benign Masses

There are a number of benign masses that occur in the breast. They are listed below with their etiology and mammographic characteristics.

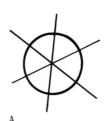 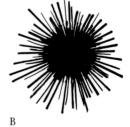
A   B

FIGURE 11-5   A "silhouette sign" (**A**) occurs when lines are able to be followed into and out of a mass. A true stellate mass (**B**) will have lines that disappear into the center of the lesion.

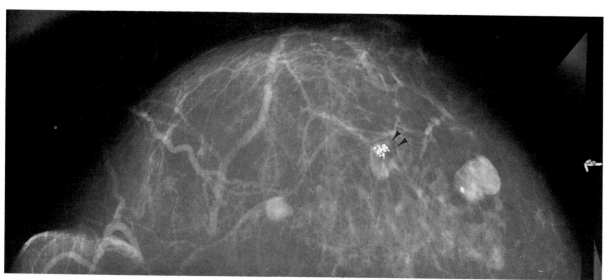

FIGURE 11-6   A thin radiolucent line, known as a "halo sign" (arrowheads), surrounds this fibroadenoma. Notice that one can see through these lesions and that lines that appear to extend from the borders of these three masses can actually be followed into and out of the lesions. This is the silhouette sign. Both the halo and the silhouette signs are indicators of benign disease.

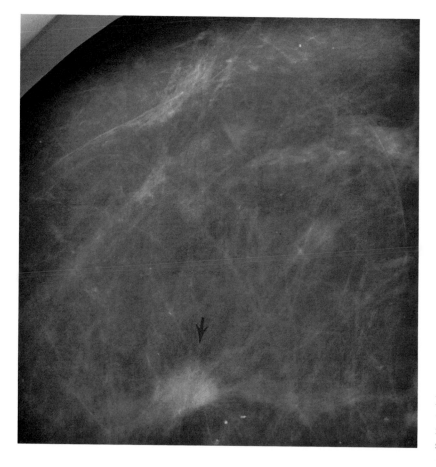

FIGURE 11-7   A malignant mass (arrow) is normally denser than surrounding glandular tissue and has stellate borders.

Lipoma   A lipoma presents mammographically as a benign-appearing, radiolucent, well-circumscribed, encapsulated lesion (Fig. 11-8). This is a fatty tumor with no epithelial component. A lipoma can feel soft and easily movable, but occasionally can have the physical attributes of a carcinoma.

Hamartoma   A hamartoma presents mammographically as a benign-appearing, well-encapsulated, smoothly outlined mass. A hamartoma is an island of glandular tissue separated from the normal ductal structures. Some experts believe that this is a variant of development. Hamartomas are sometimes mistaken for a new mass as they have become more visible with the technical improvements of the mammogram. They are separated into two categories:

Fibroadenolipomas—smoothly outlined, well-encapsulated *mixtures* of fatty and glandular components (Fig. 11-9). They are soft upon palpation. The fatty component will increase and decrease with weight fluctuations.

Fibrous hamartomas—smoothly outlined, well-encapsulated masses of varying density, but containing very little fat. They are soft upon palpation (Fig. 11-10).

Hamartomas can be quite large and sometimes respond to hormonal changes in the body.

Fibroadenoma   A fibroadenoma presents mammographically as a benign-appearing, oval, well-circumscribed mass (Fig. 11-11). Its density is normally that of surrounding glandular tissue. A fibroadenoma can also be lobulated and may exhibit a halo sign (Fig. 11-6), because it displaces surrounding structures. This lesion is a benign overgrowth of the fibrous tissue of the lobule. It contains epithelial tissue as well, responds to cyclical hormonal changes, and can characteristically calcify.

Cyst   A cyst presents mammographically as a benign-appearing, well-circumscribed mass (Fig. 11-12). Its density is usually that of surrounding glandular tissue; however, it can also appear more dense. When a cyst is under a great deal of pressure (termed a "tension cyst") its borders can look ragged, similar to a carcinoma (Fig. 11-13). A cyst can also demonstrate a halo sign because it compresses structures around it. While mammography can be suggestive of a cyst, only ultrasonography needle aspiration or biopsy can diagnose it.

Papilloma   A papilloma is an epithelial growth attached to the wall of larger ducts with a connective tissue stalk. Most papillomas are too small to be seen with the plain mammogram. Those that grow large enough to be visible are seen as a smoothly outlined,

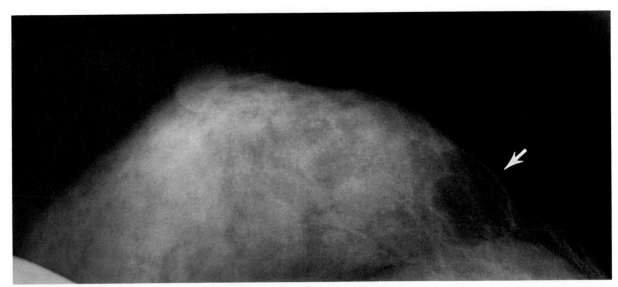

FIGURE 11-8   An example of a well-encapsulated fatty tumor known as a lipoma (arrow).

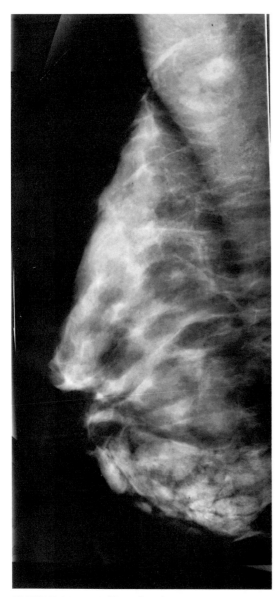

FIGURE 11-9   A fibroadenolipoma is a hamartoma containing both fatty and glandular components.

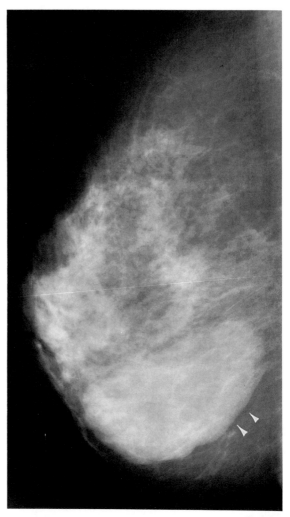

FIGURE 11-10   This large fibrous hamartoma (arrowheads) has been stable for 8 years.

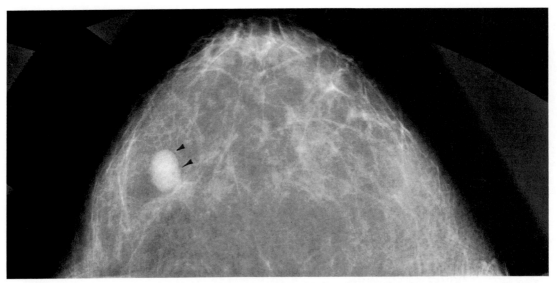

FIGURE 11-11   Smoothly outlined fibroadenoma, oval in shape, with a well-defined border (arrowheads).

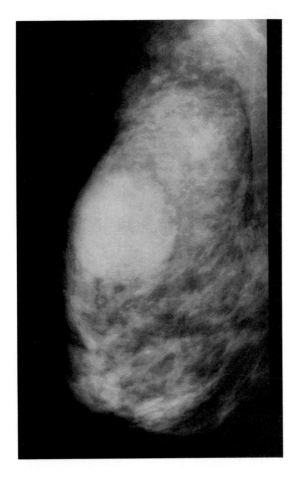

FIGURE 11-12 Large, smoothly outlined mass that was proved to be a fluid-filled cyst with ultrasonography.

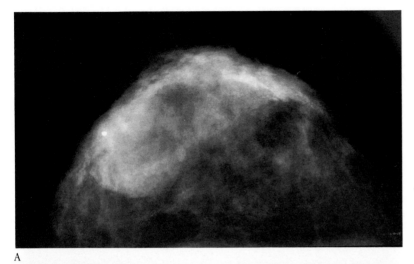

A

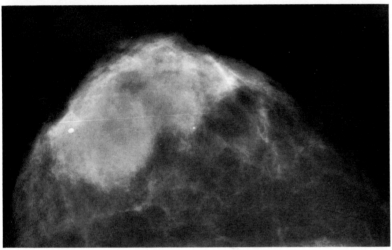

B

FIGURE 11-13 **A.** Large smoothly outlined cyst, proven with ultrasound. **B.** The same cyst 1 year later under tension, exhibiting ragged borders.

lobulated mass of about the same density as surrounding glandular tissue. They sometimes can have a "raspberry"-like configuration[1] (Fig. 11-14). Papillomas can present clinically with a spontaneous unilateral discharge and are usually only evident mammographically with ductography. They are benign lesions; however, when active (i.e., when they present with a discharge), biopsy is recommended because they have malignant potential.

Radial Scar   Radial scars are unrelated to surgical scars. They present as a stellate mass with radiolucent centers (Fig. 11-15 and 11-16). A radial scar should always be biopsied because of its mammographic similarities to carcinoma. Despite their usual large size, they are rarely palpable. (See further comments under Benign Diseases, above).

Other Lesions Presenting as Mass Densities

Hematoma (Contusion)   A hematoma can occur following injury or surgery when bleeding occurs within the breast. A new hematoma can appear as a mass density (Fig. 11-17). It will be round, well circumscribed, and more dense than surrounding glandular structures. A resolving hematoma can appear

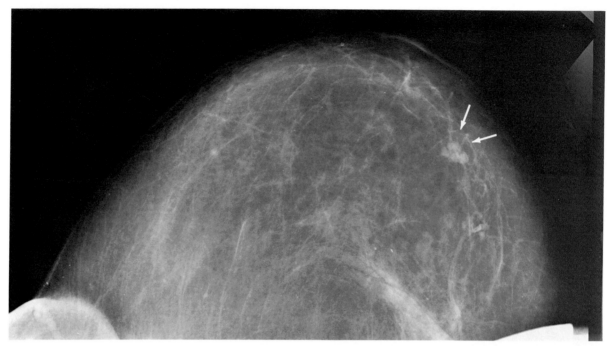

FIGURE 11-14   A papilloma that has grown large enough to be visible with mammography, exhibiting a typical "raspberry"-like configuration.

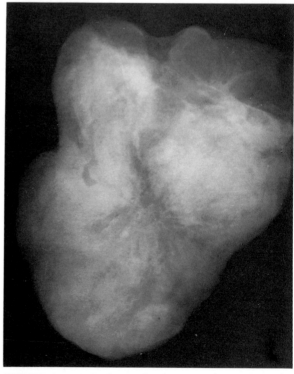

FIGURE 11-16   Radiograph of a surgical specimen of a radial scar exhibiting radiating lines from a radiolucent center.

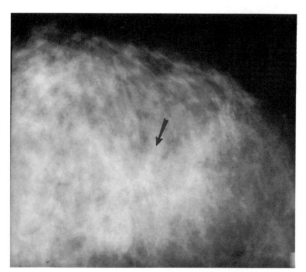

FIGURE 11-15   Radiating lines extending from a zone of radiolucency are typical of a radial scar (arrow).

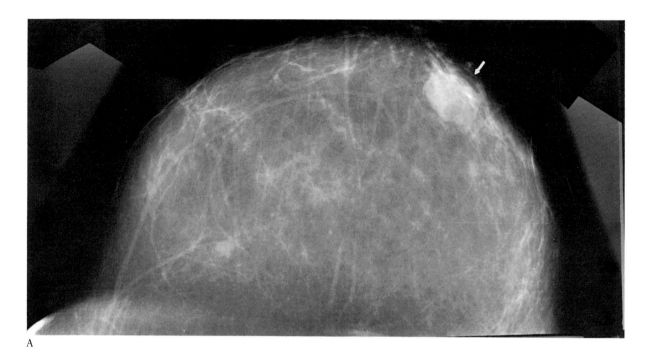

A

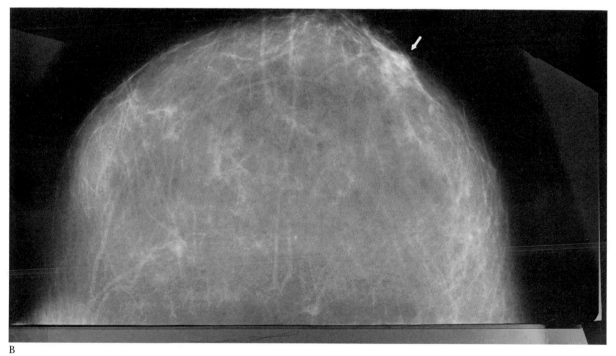

B

FIGURE 11-17   Smoothly outlined hematoma (arrow) (**A**) that is resolving 1 year later (**B**).

dense and stellate and can often calcify, imitating carcinoma.

Lymph Nodes   Intramammary lymph nodes are not uncommon. They present as a smoothly outlined, sometimes lobulated mass with a zone of lucency corresponding to the hilus (see Chapter 10). Their density is usually that of surrounding glandular tissue; however, they can appear more dense.

Gynecomastia   Benign proliferation of the breast tissue of the male breast can occur both bilaterally and unilaterally. It presents clinically as a palpable mass. Mammographically it can appear as a mass or as prominence of the ductal pattern. It is often much more pronounced in one breast.

Abscess   An abscess presents mammographically as a well-circumscribed mass with a density greater than surrounding glandular structures. An abscess is a localized infection.

Skin Changes

Lesions on the skin can appear mammographically as mass densities. They can even be calcified or calcifications can be imitated when a topical ointment is applied.

Skin Moles   Skin moles most often appear mammographically with a density similar to that of surrounding glandular tissue. Occasionally they can appear more dense. Often there is a lucency that surrounds the mole as a result of air being trapped between the film tray and the skin (Fig. 11-18). Labeling of skin moles on a diagram to accompany the completed mammogram will help to avoid confusion of mammographic findings.

Sebaceous Cysts   Sebaceous cysts occurring in the oil glands of the skin sometimes imitate carcinoma mammographically (Fig. 11-19). Infected cysts can appear dense and smooth in outline. Physical inspection to rule out a sebaceous cyst is important.

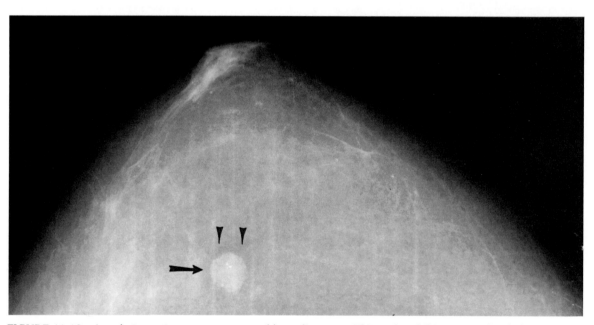

FIGURE 11-18   A mole (arrow) presents as a smoothly outline mass. This mole exhibits a typical radiolucency (arrowheads) caused by air trapped between the skin and the film tray or compression plate.

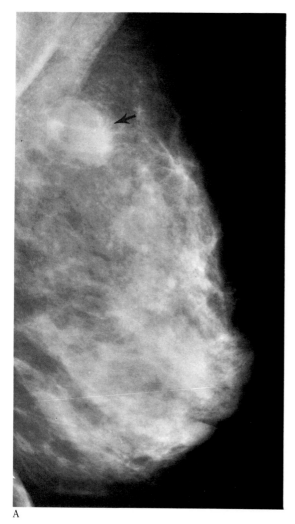

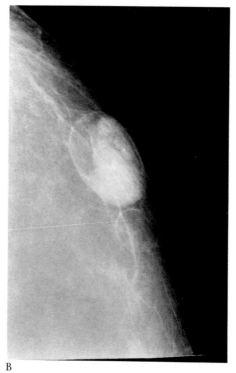

A   B

FIGURE 11-19   **A.** A sebaceous cyst was noted on the skin correlating to this mass (arrow) seen on the 45° oblique projection. **B.** A tangential view of the sebaceous cyst showed this to be the same mass seen on the 45° view.

Calcifications

Calcifications of the breast can occur with both benign and malignant processes. About 40%–50% of calcifications represent malignant disease (Fig. 11-20). Calcifications occur in the breast as a result of inspissated secretions (i.e., secretions within the ductal structures that have become thickened and dried) or as a result of necrotic processes.

The radiologist will consider certain mammographic characteristics of calcifications *in conjunction with* clinical and historical information to determine whether calcifications should be biopsied. These characteristics include (Table 11-2):

Shape
Density
Distribution
Definition

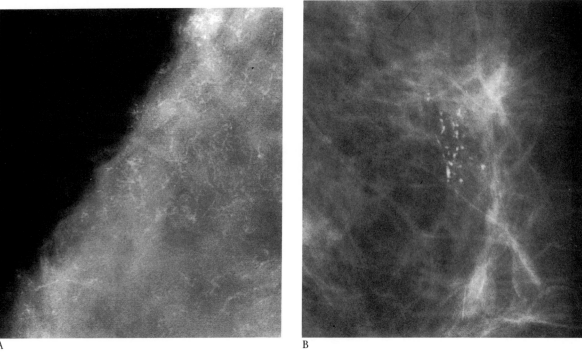

A   B

FIGURE 11-20   Two examples of maligant calcifications. Note differences in size, shape, and density.

TABLE 11-2   Mammographic Characteristics of Calcifications

	Benign	Malignant
Shape	Round, ring-like	Varying shapes
Density	Same density	Varying densities
Distribution	Scattered; benign Ca^{++} can also be clustered	Clustered
Definition	Well-defined borders	Poorly defined borders
Unilateral or bilateral	If the same type of calcifications occur in both breasts, they are more likely benign	Unilateral
Surrounding tissue	If the calcium is seen within a benign-appearing mass or if the tissue surrounding the calcium appears normal, this is a benign indicator	If there is architectural or parenchymal distortion associated with calcium, malignancy must be considered
Increasing in number from prior mammogram	Can be benign	Not an indicator alone but, when considered with other characteristics, can indicate malignancy
Size	Can be large or small	Most often small

Unilateral or bilateral
Surrounding tissue or associated mass
Increase in number
Size

Benign Calcifications

Certain types of calcifications in the breast are almost always benign.

Popcorn-Type Calcifications   Large, thick, dense, popcorn-shaped calcifications are a result of involuting fibroadenomas and occasionally other benign processes (Fig. 11-6).

Rim Calcifications   Rim calcifications occur along the border of a benign mass (Fig. 11-21).

Milk of Calcium   Milk of calcium calcifications occur in microcysts when the cyst contains radiopaque particles mixed with the fluid. On the craniocaudad projection they appear faint, ill-defined, and smudgy (Fig. 11-22). A true lateral projection (and sometimes the 45° oblique projection) will reveal the true characteristics of milk of calcium. These calcifications are clustered or scattered, and as the particles settle to the dependent portion of the microcysts the crescent shape of milk of calcium is evident.

Arterial Calcifications   Resulting from arterial atherosclerosis, arterial calcifications will be seen within the easily identifiable blood vessel (Fig. 11-23).

Skin Calcifications   Skin calcifications typically are round with radiolucent centers (Fig. 11-24).

Diffuse Accentuation of the Glandular Tissue

Diffuse accentuation of the glandular tissue presents as an overall prominence of the ductal structures (Fig. 11-25). The following conditions can present mammographically as diffuse accentuation:

Infection
Carcinoma

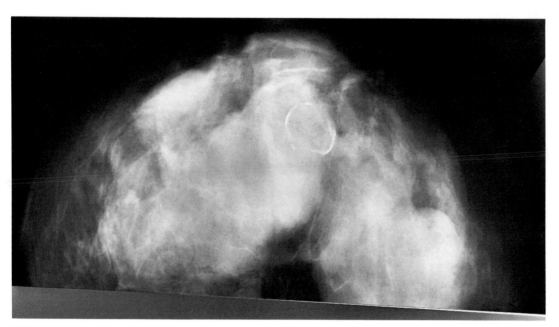

FIGURE 11-21   Rim calcification, occurring here in a cyst, is considered benign.

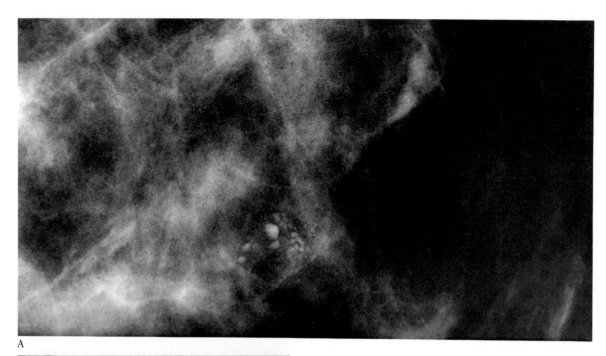

A

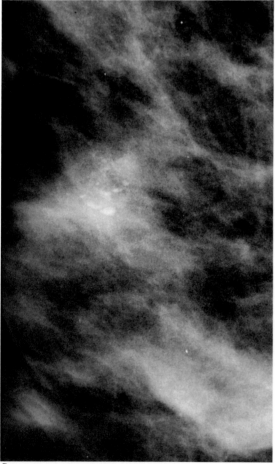

B

FIGURE 11-22   Smudgy appearing calcifications (**A**) that exhibit layering on the lateral or 45° oblique projections (**B**) are known as "milk of calcium."

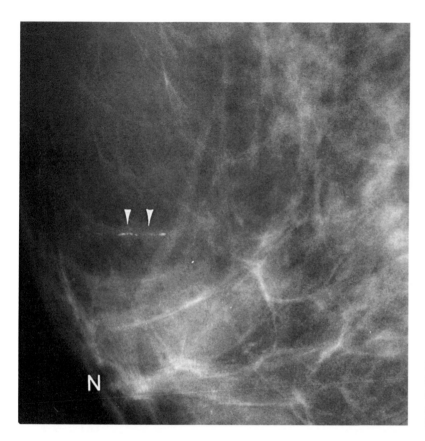

FIGURE 11-23 Arterial calcifications (arrowheads) evident within a blood vessel. Another indication that these are not ductal is that they are not heading toward the nipple (N).

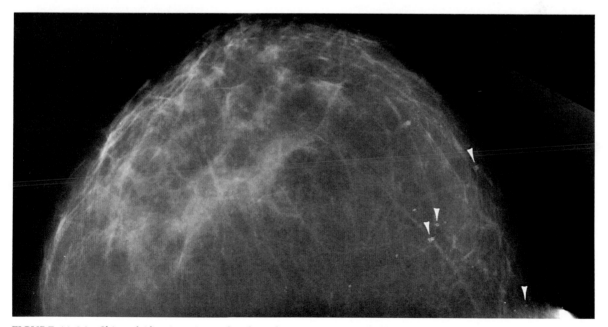

FIGURE 11-24 Skin calcifications (arrowheads), often appearing medially, are typically ring-like with radiolucent centers.

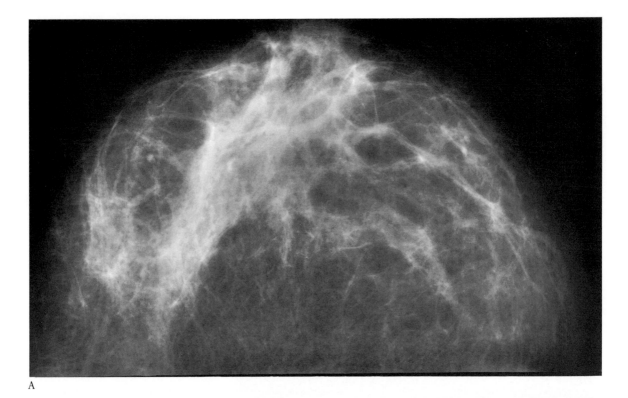

A

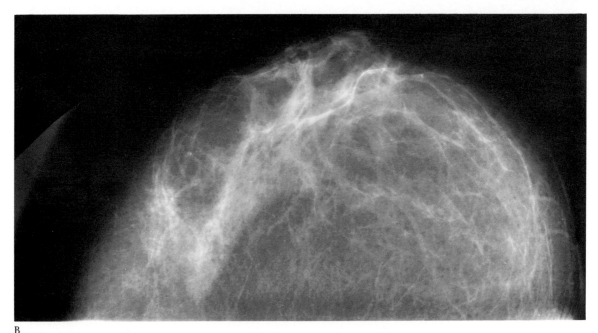

B

FIGURE 11-25   Diffuse accentuation of the glandular tissue can indicate a pathologic process. **A.** A craniocaudad view shows diffuse accentuation due to infection. **B.** The breast tissue has returned to normal after treatment with antibiotics.

Effects of medications
Effects of caffeine
Systemic disease
Trauma (contusion)
Radiation therapy

In some cases the breast is edematous and skin thickening is evident upon mammography.

Summary

Many pathologic processes can occur in the breast, some benign and some malignant. Discerning benign from malignant disease is very complicated, because these disease processes so often imitate one another. Realizing this, technologists can better appreciate the radiologists' need for quality mammographic images.

References

1. Tábar L, Dean PB: *Teaching Atlas of Mammography,* ed 2. New York, Thieme Inc, 1985.
2. Shaw-de Parades E: *Atlas of Film-Screen Mammography.* Baltimore, Urban & Schwarzenberg, 1989.
3. Kopans DB: *Breast Imaging.* Philadelphia, JB Lippincott Co, 1989.
4. Wolfe JN: *Xeroradiography of the Breast.* Springfield, IL, Charles C Thomas, 1972.
5. Page DL, Anderson TJ: *Diagnostic Histopathology of the Breast.* Edinburgh, Churchill Livingstone, 1987.
6. Azzopardi JG: *Problems in Breast Pathology.* London, WB Saunders, 1979.
7. Wellings SR, Jensen HM, Marcum RG: An atlas of subgross pathology of the human breast with special reference to possible precancerous lesions. *J Natl Cancer Inst* 1975;55:231.
8. Haagensen CC: *Diseases of the Breast.* Philadelphia, WB Saunders Company, 1986.
9. Lanyi M: *Diagnosis and Differential Diagnosis of Breast Calcifications.* New York, Springer-Verlag, 1986.
10. Hoeffken W, Lanyi M: *Mammography.* Philadelphia, WB Saunders Company, 1977.

Kathleen M. Willison

12

Mammographic Positioning

The objective of mammography is to adequately demonstrate the entire breast. In most cases this is accomplished with the two-view mammogram,[1] that is, the craniocaudad and the (45°) oblique positions. However, often a woman's body build and/or anomalies will require alterations of the standard views or additional films. By tailoring the exam to the woman's body, the breast tissue can be demonstrated in its entirety. Tailoring the exam may necessitate eliminating one of the standard views and replacing it with an alternate view or, in some instances, adding a third view (see Chapter 13). **It is the responsibility of the technologist performing the mammogram to ensure visualization of the entire breast.** This cannot be overstated. The technologist is the only person who has physically seen what portion of the breast was under the compression plate.

Guidelines for Positioning

The following guidelines for screen-film mammography should be applied to satisfactorily position and image the breast.

Skin Detail

Before technical improvements in mammography allowed sufficient visualization of the detail of the glandular tissue, the low contrast of these films enabled demonstration of both the skin and the glandular components (Fig. 12-1). Because the radiologist was not seeing the glandular tissue well, cancers were very difficult to diagnose radiographically and visualization of skin thickening and retraction was necessary even to "see" very large carcinomas.

With the many developments in screen-film mammography, especially the move to a very high-contrast study, the very minute changes in the glandular tissue that indicate early carcinoma are finally seen. This allows the radiologist to diagnose carcinomas as small as 5 mm, in most cases before skin thickening and retraction occurs. With this high-contrast imaging, demonstrating the skin line means underexposing the glandular tissue and missing information necessary to diagnoses. It should be necessary in most cases for the radiologist to use a "bright-light" with the mammogram in order to see skin detail.

If the *contrast* of the majority of films produced by a mammography facility allows for equal visualization of glandular tissue and skin detail, four tech-

163

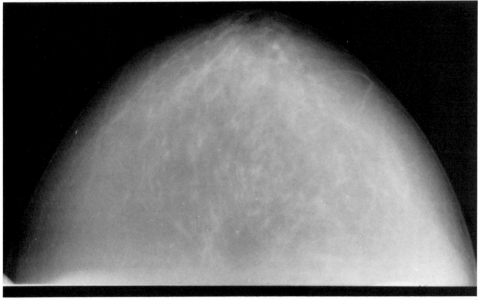

A

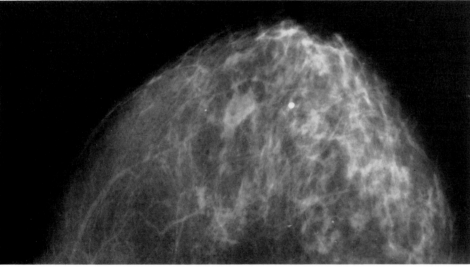

B

FIGURE 12-1   Two craniocaudad mammograms of the same woman in 1976 (**A**) and 1990 (**B**). The older study (**A**), which demonstrates skin line, does not image the glandular tissue adequately. The more recent mammogram (**B**), while not demonstrating the skin line, offers excellent detail of the glandular tissue, where cancers arise. It should be necessary in most cases to "bright-light" the image to see skin detail.

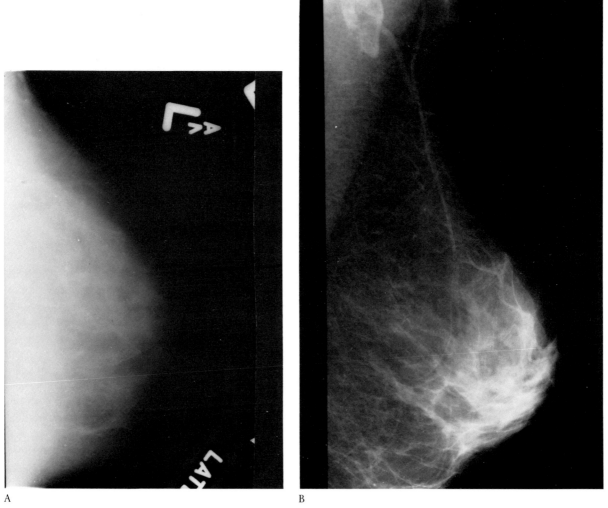

A   B

FIGURE 12-2   **A.** A lateral view of the breast with little or no compression and a technique that allows for visualization of the ribs. **B.** A 45° projection of the same patient with improved compression and technique. The latter method significantly increases the image quality of the breast tissue.

nical improvements should be considered: decrease in peak kilovoltage being used, addition of a mammographic grid, change of screen-film combination, or use of the proper filter for the kilovoltage range in which the facility works. (For a thorough discussion of technical improvements, see Chapter 5.)

Ribs

If one is to perform state-of-the-art screen-film mammography, the ribs must be excluded from the film (Fig. 12-2). In order to visualize the ribs, little or no compression must be coupled with a curved compression plate; this combination does not allow adequate demonstration of the breast tissue. Xeromammography had the latitude to demonstrate the entire breast, from ribs to nipple; screen-film, does not. Exposing the film with enough technique to demonstrate the ribs overexposes the breast tissue, resulting in poor-quality mammograms.

Skin Wrinkles

Eliminating skin wrinkles from under the compression plate is a practice held over from xeromammography, in which the edge enhancement effect of the skin wrinkle would obliterate surrounding breast tissue. This problem does not exist in screen-film mammography; skin wrinkles rarely interfere with the interpretation of the mammogram (see Fig. 12-9). Every effort should be made to smooth the skin of the breast out, but when smoothing a wrinkle means pulling breast tissue out from under the compression and out of view, the skin wrinkle should be left alone. When trying to eliminate a skin wrinkle, gently work it out toward the nipple, pulling forward away from the chest wall, rather than pulling the tissue out posteriorly (Fig. 12-3).

Nipple in Profile

The practice of bringing the nipple into profile resulted from the older method of screen-film mammograms, on which distinguishing the nipple from a mass was difficult. In addition, if the nipple was not in profile when performing a xeromammogram, edge enhancement effect (just as with skin wrinkles) again would obliterate surrounding information. *Centering attention on the nipple on the two-view mammogram*

may lead to missing a cancer elsewhere in the breast. In most women, the nipple falls into profile; if it does not, repositioning the breast to bring the nipple into profile is not recommended. This would sacrifice tissue either superiorly or inferiorly, and medially or laterally, depending on the position and the location of the nipple on the breast. The tissue that is being pulled out of the field may not be visualized in another view, and a cancer could be missed. If the patient has a suspected lesion in the subarealor region, if the radiologist cannot distinguish the nipple from a mass, or if needle localization of a lesion is indicated, a third view would be taken with the nipple in profile. (For further discussion, see Chapter 9.)

Posture

It is easier on both the patient and technologist if the patient is standing rather than sitting for the mammogram. For almost all mammographic views the best posture for a patient to assume is a poor posture. Positioning and compression will be easier if the patient can assume a "sloppy" stance. If the patient slumps from the waist, the breast naturally falls forward (Fig. 12-4). In addition, while the patient should be encouraged to grasp the hand rail with one hand or the other, it is especially important she does not have a "death grip" on it. This tightens the pectoral muscle and adds to the difficulty of positioning and compression.

Motorized Foot Control for Compression

Whenever possible, motorized foot control of the compression plate should be utilized during the *first* stages of compression. This allows for both hands to be free for better positioning of the breast.

The Craniocaudad Position

The craniocaudad position (Fig. 12-5*) is best used to visualize the subareolar, central, and medial portions of the breast.[1] The craniocaudad position is

*The schematic drawings accompanying the various positions are meant as immediate orientation of the breast to the C-arm and are not position models.

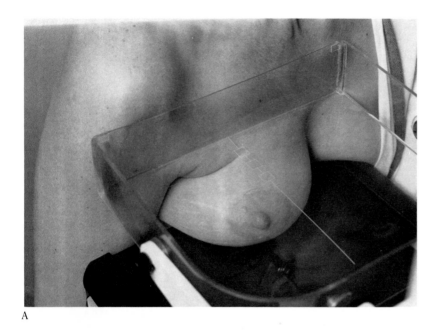

A

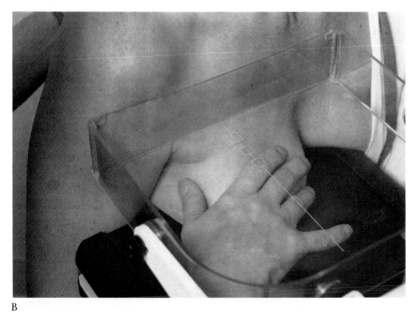

B

FIGURE 12-3   Smooth skin wrinkles (**A**) toward the nipple (**B**) so that breast tissue is not pulled out from under the compression plate.

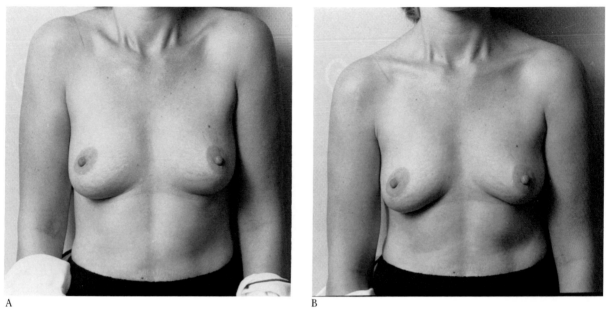

A   B

FIGURE 12-4   The breast will be easier to position if the patient can assume a poor posture. **A.** The patient's shoulders are raised and she is standing erect. **B.** The same patient "slumped" forward, demonstrating how the breasts naturally fall forward when the body is relaxed.

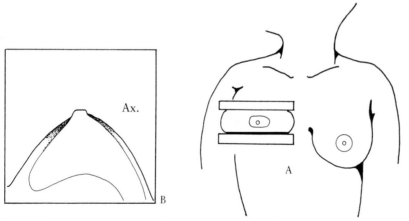

FIGURE 12-5   **A.** Schematic of the orientation of the breast to the C-arm for the craniocaudad projection. **B.** Schematic demonstrating the amount of the "glandular island" usually shown with this view.

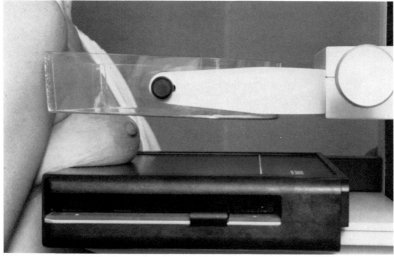

A

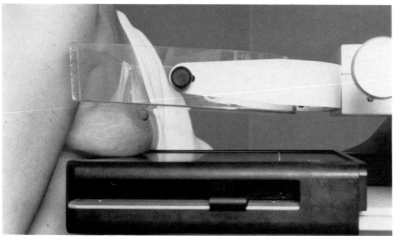

B

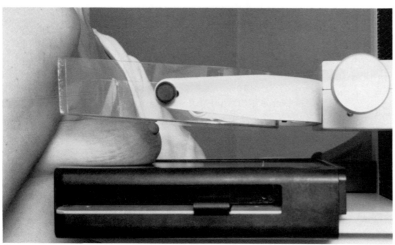

C

FIGURE 12-6 **A.** If the film tray is raised too high inferior and posterior tissue will be missed. **B.** If the breast is allowed to droop superior and posterior tissue will be missed. **C.** The film tray should be raised to meet the inframammary crease, forming a right angle with the chest wall.

achieved by placing the film inferior to the breast and directing the beam superiorly to inferiorly. There is no angulation of the C-arm. The patient's body should be facing forward with her feet toward the machine.

The film tray should be raised to form a right angle with the chest wall at the inframammary crease. If the film tray is raised too high, inferior and posterior tissue of the breast will not be visualized when properly compressed. In the same respect, if the film tray is not raised to meet the inframammary crease and the breast is allowed to droop, superior and posterior tissue will not be visualized (Fig. 12-6). This is generally determined from the lateral aspect of the breast, however some methods recommend using the medial aspect. With either method, a common sense approach must be applied; the lateral aspect should not be raised so high as to be pulling tissue out of view, nor should the film tray be so low as to allow a wide gap between breast and film on the medial side.

The breast must be lifted and pulled forward onto the film gently but firmly. The patient's ipsilateral arm should be kept close at her side and her shoulders must be relaxed. An elevated shoulder tightens the pectoral muscle and pulls up on the breast. This not only pulls breast tissue off the film but also makes compression and positioning difficult.

The patient's body should be rotated slightly so the medial and posterior tissue of the breast is visualized even if this means not visualizing all lateral tissue (which is best imaged with the oblique view). **This is the most important aspect of the craniocaudad position. If medial tissue is not imaged with the craniocaudad mammogram, it may well be eliminated from the study.** Even though every effort is made to demonstrate medial tissue on the oblique view, it is not always possible. In addition, medial detail can be lost on the oblique view because of superimposition of glandular tissue and because of its distance from the film (Fig. 12-7).

To adequately bring the medial tissue of the breast onto the film, check the patient's body position. This can influence the ease of positioning and create a more comfortable stance for the patient. The patient should be turned forward to face the machine, turning her head slightly to the side that is not being radiographed and curving her neck and head around and toward the unit, often around the tube head (Fig.

12-8). If possible, bring the opposite breast up onto the film tray (but out of the x-ray field). Have the patient lift her chin slightly. If the chin is tucked in, the chest wall is drawn away from the film. An effort should be made by the technologist to have the patient lean into the unit, reminding the patient to keep her shoulder rested and back. This brings the chest wall closer to the compression device and brings more medial and posterior tissue onto the film.

Have the patient hold onto the bar provided with the hand opposite that of the breast being positioned. This not only stabilizes the patient, but also helps bring medial tissue closer to the film tray. While pulling forward, lifting and holding the breast in place, and smoothing skin wrinkles toward the nipple, bring the compression plate down. The technologist can place one hand gently on the woman's back to prohibit the natural pull away from the compression. After the medial aspect of the breast is secured, pull the lateral aspect of the breast forward and onto the film. This was suggested by Dr. László Tábar (personal communication, December 1990) to compensate for lost lateral tissue when positioning for the medial aspect of the breast.

If the technologist and radiologist are uncomfortable with visualizing less of the lateral tissue on the craniocaudad view and the "Tábar" modification does not help, it may be useful at first for a third view (either 30° oblique or exaggerated craniocaudad) to be taken on those women with dense tissue.

If the technologist is having difficulty pulling the breast forward, two factors should be considered:

1. Remembering posture—the patient is probably standing too straight and erect. Have the patient take on a poor posture, drooping her shoulders. This relaxes the muscles and lets the breast fall forward onto the film tray. Rather than telling the patient to "relax," different words such as "slump," "droop," and "forget good posture" may be more helpful in attaining the results necessary.
2. Many patients push their hips forward. Have them step back and lean forward from the waist.

To determine radiographically if the craniocaudad positioning has been done correctly, look for (Fig. 12-9A,B,C):

1. A skin thickening toward the cleavage of the breast.

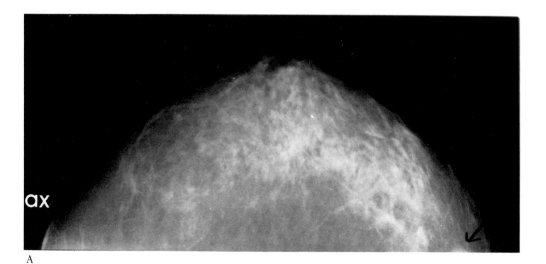

A

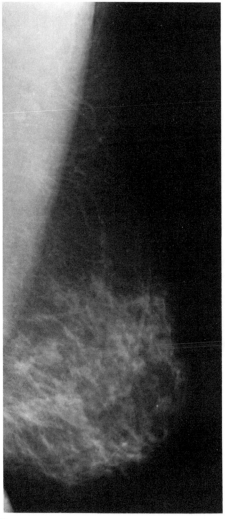

B

FIGURE 12-7 Visualizing medial breast tissue on the craniocaudad mammogram is critical, because this tissue may be omitted from or distorted on the 45° oblique projection. This medial lesion visualized on a craniocaudad mammogram (**A**) is not seen, whether because of distortion or omission, on the oblique projections (**B**).

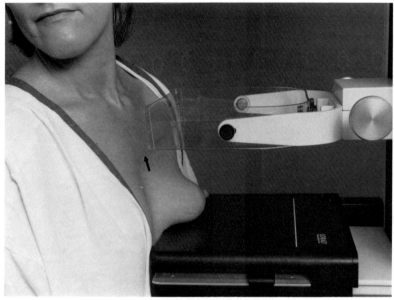

A

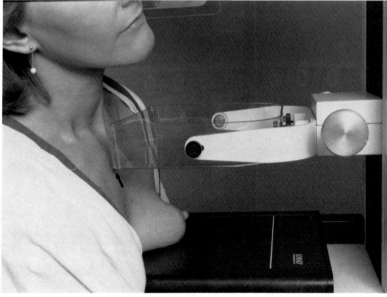

B

FIGURE 12-8   **A.** Positioning for the craniocaudad projection with the patient's head turned to the side. **B.** By turning her head forward and around the tube head or face plate, the chest wall is brought closer to the film, visualizing more medial and superior tissue.

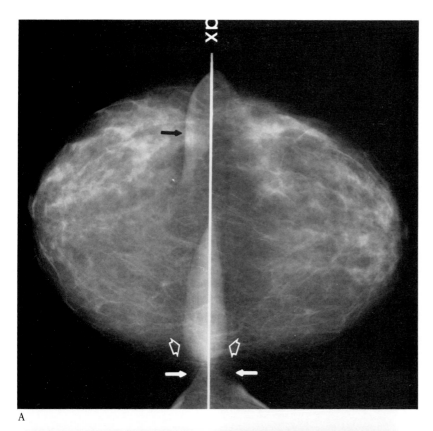

A

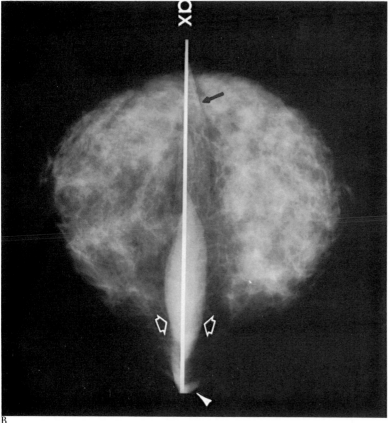

B

FIGURE 12-9 Three sets of well-positioned craniocaudad mammograms demonstrating various landmarks: skin thickening (white arrowheads), cleavage of the breast (white arrows), and pectoral muscle (open white arrows). In addition, skin wrinkles (folds) can be seen (black arrows). Some skinfolds can be eliminated by working them out toward the nipple. Others cannot; pulling back on these skin wrinkles would pull posterior and lateral tissue out from under the compression plate.
(*Figure continues.*)

173

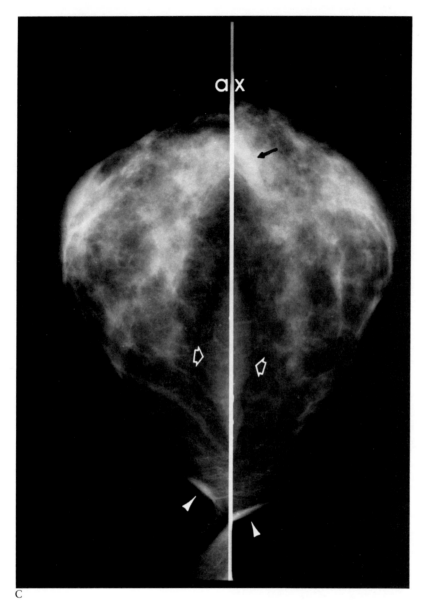

C

FIGURE 12-9   (*Continued*)

2. The cleavage of the breast.
3. The pectoral muscle, a radiopaque density of varying size that sometimes is mistaken for the patient's chin or a skinfold. It often has a triangular shape and, when seen bilaterally, its appearance is mirrored. More importantly, it can be perceived as a carcinoma when seen unilaterally (Fig. 12-10). When this occurs a third view needs to be included with the exam. A reverse oblique of 5–20° demonstrating more of the pectoral muscle will aid the radiologist in a differential diagnosis (Fig. 12-11).

One or all of these indicators may be absent in one or both mammograms as a result of anatomic differences from one woman to another and from the left to the right breast. The technologist should use discretion in deciding whether another view is necessary.

Summary of Craniocaudad Positioning

Figure 12-12A–J shows the step-by-step positioning process for the craniocaudad mammogram.

Variations of the Craniocaudad Position

Exaggerated Craniocaudad Position The exaggerated rotated craniocaudad position is best used to visualize posterolateral tissue of the breast (Fig. 12-13). However, this position will not "open up" the structures in the same way as the 30° oblique, nor is it always possible to image as far posterolaterally as needed.

To achieve the exaggerated craniocaudad position direct the beam superiorly to inferiorly as for a standard craniocaudad view. Turn the patient's body so that her feet are turned toward the side not being ra-

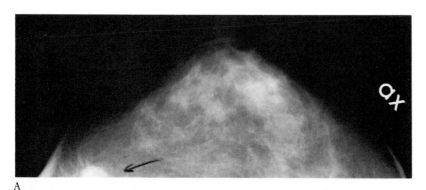
A

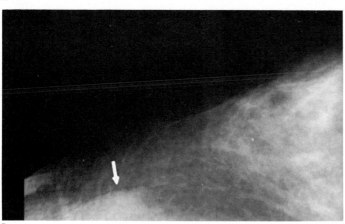
B

FIGURE 12-10 **A.** The pectoral muscle when seen unilaterally on the craniocaudad view can imitate a carcinoma. **B.** An extra reverse oblique view (in this case a 10° reverse) shows more of the pectoral muscle (arrow).

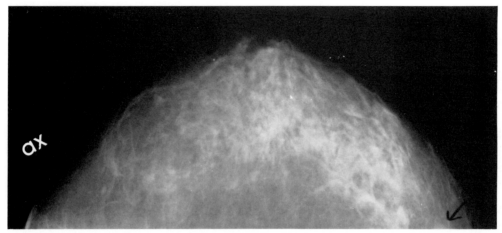

A

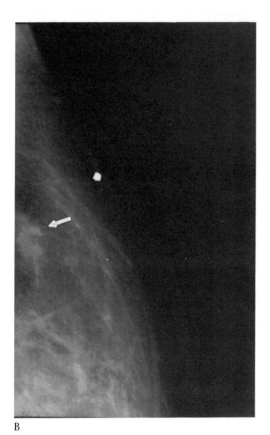

B

FIGURE 12-11   **A.** A density in the posterior medial aspect on this craniocaudad mammogram could be the pectoral muscle. **B.** A reverse 30° oblique mammogram shows this to be a true mass (arrow) and not the pectoral muscle. This was carcinoma on biopsy.

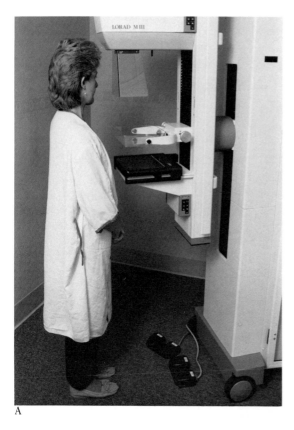

FIGURE 12-12A
1. Have patient stand with her feet toward unit.

A

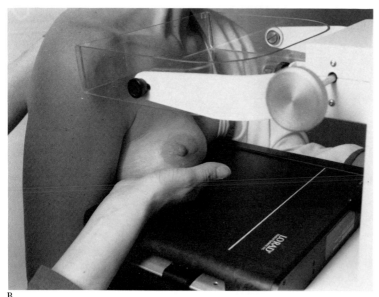

B

FIGURE 12-12B
2. Bring breast to rest on film tray.
3. Have patient relax her arm of the side being radiographed comfortably at her side (or over her abdomen).

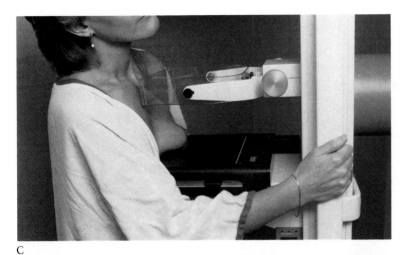

C

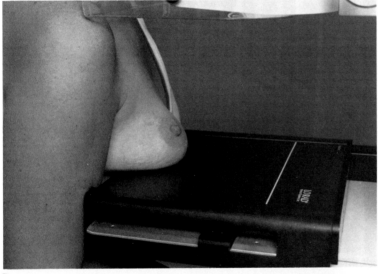

D

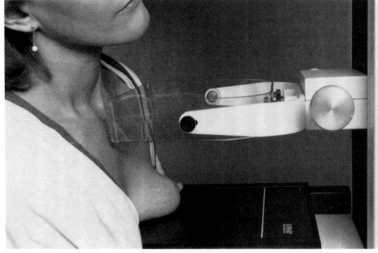

E

FIGURE 12-12C

4. For balance the patient should hold onto the machine with the hand opposite to the side being positioned.

5. Have patient rest her shoulders down, taking on a "droopy posture."

FIGURE 12-12D

6. Adjust film tray to meet inframammary crease perpendicular to chest wall.

FIGURE 12-12E

7. Have patient bring head inward around face plate or tube head, bringing the chest wall closer to the film tray so that medial tissue is visualized.

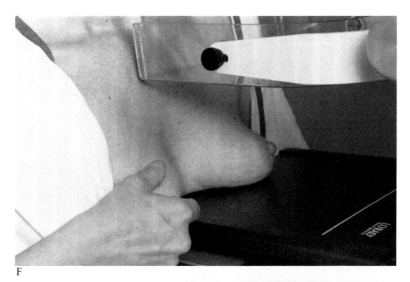

F

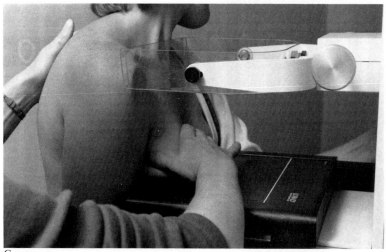

G

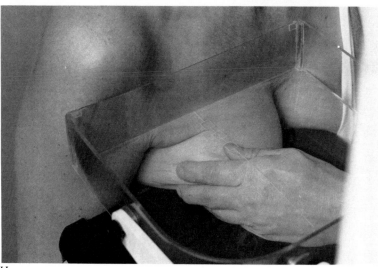

H

FIGURE 12-12F

8. Bring opposite breast onto film tray (to help visualize medial tissue) but not within x-ray field.

FIGURE 12-12G

9. Gentle placement of the technologist's hand on the patient's back will prohibit backward reaction to the compression.

FIGURE 12-12H

10. Pick up and gently pull breast forward. While applying compression, implement the Tábar modification and pull lateral tissue forward under the compression plate.

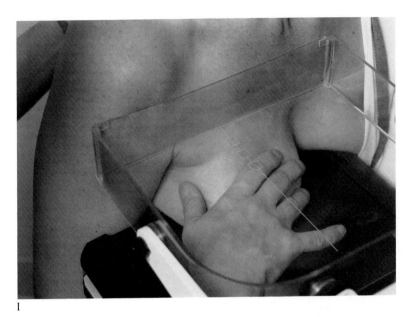

FIGURE 12-12I
11. Bring compression plate down, smoothing wrinkles toward the nipple (never pull skin wrinkles posteriorly).

I

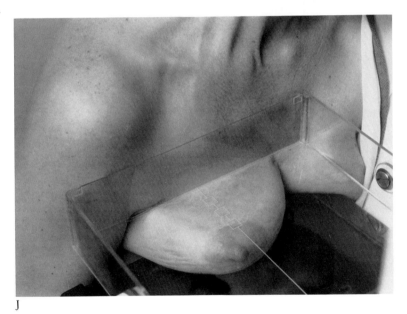

FIGURE 12-12J
12. Completed craniocaudad position.

J

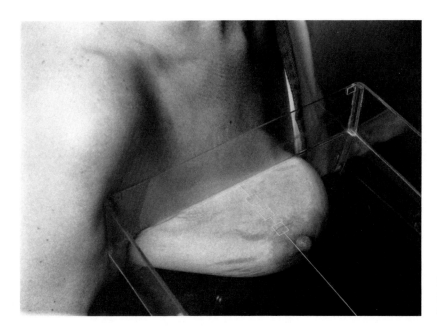

FIGURE 12-13 Completed positioning of the exaggerated craniocaudad projection.

diographed. The lateral aspect of the breast being imaged should be closest to the film tray. Gently pick up the breast and bring the outer half to rest on the film tray. Raise the C-arm up to meet the posterolateral tissue. Have the patient lean back slightly toward the side being radiographed, relaxing her shoulder down and back. Pull the breast forward and apply compression (Fig. 12-14).

Summary of Exaggerated Craniocaudad Positioning
1. Direct beam superior to inferior.
2. Turn patient away from side being radiographed.
3. Pick up and gently pull forward the outer portion of the breast, bringing it onto the film tray.
4. Raise C-arm so that the posterolateral breast comes to rest on the film.
5. Have patient lean back slightly toward side being radiographed.
6. Have patient relax her shoulder down and back.
7. Holding breast in place, apply compression.

"Pushed-Up" Craniocaudad Position This position is best used to visualize breast tissue high on the chest wall. The pushed-up craniocaudad position becomes an option when two opposing views are called for when localizing a nonpalpable lesion seen only on the 45° oblique or lateral projections.

To achieve the pushed-up craniocaudad position, direct the beam superiorly to inferiorly as for a standard craniocaudad view. The patient should be turned forward, facing the machine. Position the patient as for a standard craniocaudad view, having her slump forward and lean in toward the unit. Then raise the C-arm so that the film tray is *above* the inframammary crease, pushing breast tissue up and thereby visualizing tissue high on the chest wall. Gently pull outward and forward on the breast and apply compression.

Summary of "Pushed-up" Craniocaudad Positioning
1. Direct beam superiorly to inferiorly.
2. Face patient toward unit, feet forward.
3. Bring inferior aspect of breast onto the film tray.
4. Turn patient's head slightly toward side not being radiographed.
5. Bring patient's head and neck around tube head or face plate.
6. Lean patient inward and have her relax her shoulders.
7. Raise C-arm above inframammary crease, pushing breast tissue up and bringing superior tissue under the compression plate.
8. Pull breast outward and forward and apply compression while holding the breast in place.

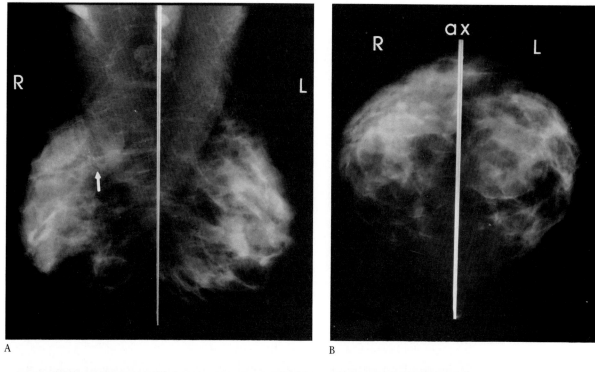

A

B

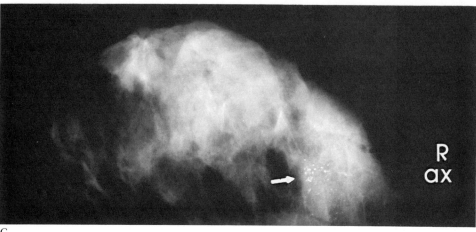

C

FIGURE 12-14   **A.** Right and left 45° oblique mammograms demonstrating calcium superiorly in the right breast. **B.** This calcium was not visualized on the craniocaudad view. **C.** An exaggerated craniocaudad view demonstrated the posterolateral aspect of the breast, including the calcium not visualized by the standard craniocaudad view (arrow).

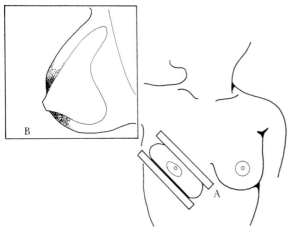

FIGURE 12-15 **A.** Schematic of the orientation of the breast to the film tray for the 45° oblique projection. **B.** Schematic demonstrating the amount of the "glandular island" usually shown with this view.

The (45°) Oblique Position

The (45°) oblique position (Fig. 12-15) is best used to demonstrate the posterior and upper outer quadrants of the breast. The (45°) oblique position is a mediolateral projection that was first introduced by Lund-gren.[2] It is the position of choice over the true lateral, whether a lateral-medial or medial-lateral lateral, because of its effectiveness in visualizing the posterior and upper outer quadrant breast tissue. This is intrinsic to the anatomy of the breast, which lies anterior to and follows the line of the obliquely coursing pectoral muscle. When the arm is raised to shoulder level the oblique line of the pectoral muscle approximates a 45° angle. By positioning parallel with this oblique line virtually all the glandular tissue can be demonstrated, because one is not fighting the natural course of the tissue.

It is important to match the angle to the patient's body build. Draw an imaginary line from shoulder to midsternum (Fig. 12-16) and match this angle with the film tray. In most women this will be about 45°; in others the angle will run more obliquely (as steep as 60° for very thin patients) and in others less obliquely (as flat as 30° for overweight patients). By "adjusting" the angle to the patient's build, the technologist can best demonstrate all the glandular tissue.

To achieve the 45° oblique position, turn the C-arm to the determined obliquity mediolaterally. Have the patient stand just in front of the film tray. Her feet and body should be turned toward the unit. Raise the patient's arm to shoulder level, forming a right angle with the body. Lifting the arm higher will

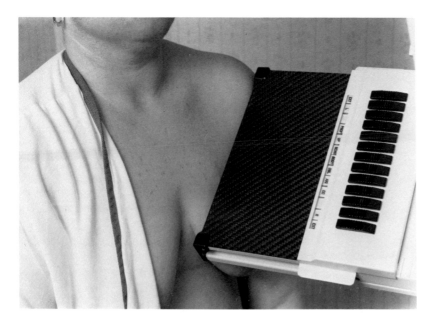

FIGURE 12-16 When positioning for the oblique projection, it is important to adjust the angle to the patient's body build. Draw an imaginary line from the shoulder to midsternum and match this line with the film tray.

pull tissue back and out of view and also tightens the skin, making positioning and compression more difficult. Place one hand behind the shoulder on the side to be positioned and the other posterolateral to the breast tissue. Lift and pull the breast gently but firmly upward and outward, and bring the lateral portion to rest on the film tray. It will help to have the patient relax her shoulders, taking on a poor posture. The corner of the film tray should rest just posterior to the axilla (Fig. 12-17). (Some methods recommend that the corner of the film tray be placed in the Axilla. If following this method, be sure the film tray is placed posteriorly in the axilla. Special attention must be directed to pulling lateral tissue around and forward to include this area on the oblique projection.)

With the lateral aspect of the breast on the film, the patient should be rotated so that the compression plate touches the sternum. Again, the technologist should be pulling the breast outward and upward at all times, ensuring visualization of posterior tissue

and the inframammary crease. In addition, pulling up and out on the breast ensures that the ductal structures will be properly represented. If the breast is left to droop, the ductal structures will fall upon themselves, and the detection of architectural distortion (a tell-tale sign of cancer) will be more difficult, if not impossible (Fig. 12-18). The compression plate should be lowered just enough to hold the posterior aspect of the breast in place, while the technologist moves the supporting hand anteriorly toward the nipple in order to prevent drooping and loss of tissue. Once this has been done, an extra effort can be made, by rotating the patient's hips inward, to include the inframammary crease. The patient may have to gently hold the other breast back and out of the way to avoid superimposition. Care should be taken that the patient does not pull too tautly on this breast, as tissue will be pulled away from the breast that is being positioned. The technologist should run a hand between the patient's back and the film tray to make certain that no posterior tissue is excluded. The skin should feel tight.

To determine radiographically if the oblique positioning has been done correctly, examine the mammogram for the following elements (Fig. 12-19):

1. The breast should not droop on the film.
2. The pectoral muscle should be demonstrated as far down as the line of the nipple. This may not be possible on all patients; however, it should be the rule rather than the exception. Judgment on the part of the technologist will determine if any posterior and lateral tissue has been omitted; if so, a third view needs to be taken (refer to Chapter 13).
3. The inframammary crease should be demonstrated.

The above are guidelines; if one or two of these elements are not demonstrated as stated, it is up to the technologist to determine whether a third view is necessary.

Often, the technologist can identify two lines on the patient's body resulting from the compression plate and film tray, one from behind the breast running obliquely, superiorly to inferiorly and laterally to medially, and the other at the medial aspect near the sternum. All breast tissue should be included within these lines. One can easily see if any tissue has

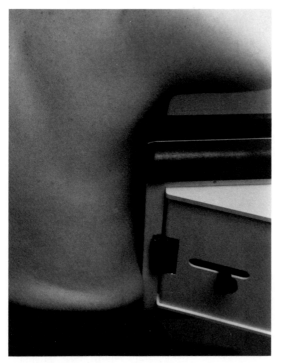

FIGURE 12-17   The corner of the film tray should rest not in the armpit, but just posterior to it.

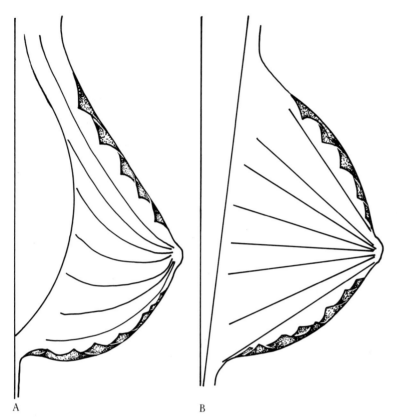

A   B

FIGURE 12-18   When positioning for the 45° oblique view, the breast should be pulled upward and outward (**B**) in order to properly demonstrate ductal structures. If left to droop (**A**), the ductal structures are not properly represented and detection of architectural distortion will be more difficult if not impossible.

been missed either medially or laterally. It will not be possible on all patients to include all the medial tissue on the (45°) oblique view. However, the lateral line should be behind the lateral and posterior tissue of the breast. If not, or if the pectoral muscle is not seen on the (45°) oblique, an extra view must be taken to demonstrate this area of the breast (see Chapter 13).

Summary of (45°) Oblique Positioning

Figures 12-20 and 12-21 illustrate the step-by-step process of correct patient positioning for the (45°) oblique view in a woman with small breasts (Fig. 12-20) and in a woman with large breasts (Fig. 12-21). The basic steps are listed here.

1. Determine the degree of obliquity needed and turn C-arm to this angle.

2. Have patient stand slightly in front of the film tray with feet turned inward toward the unit.

3. Have patient raise her arm to shoulder level.

4. Pick up breast, pulling upward and outward, and rest the lateral aspect of the breast and posterior axilla on the film tray, making sure that the corner of the film tray next to the patient's body is just posterior to the axilla.

5. Patient's upper body and shoulders should be relaxed.

6. Pick up breast and gently pull forward, checking posteriorly for "taut" skin between the patient's side and film tray.

7. With the breast held upward and outward, the compression plate should be brought down snugly.

8. Still holding the anterior portion of the breast in

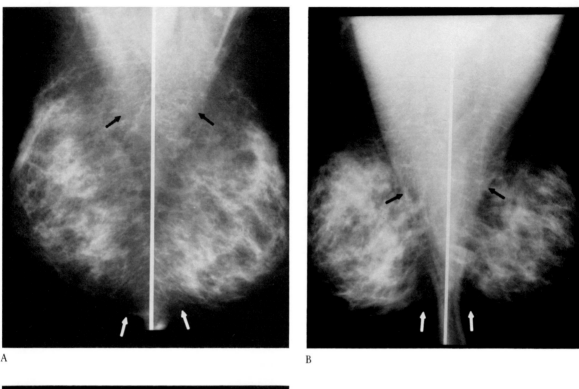

A

B

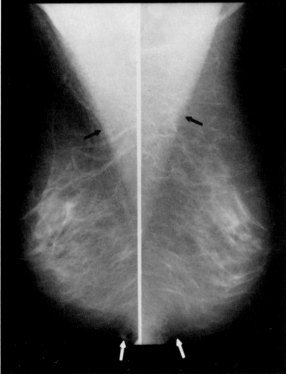

C

FIGURE 12-19   Three sets of well-positioned 45° oblique mammograms demonstrating varying degrees of pectoral muscle (black arrows) and the inframammary crease (white arrows). Note the breasts do not droop on the film, but rather are pulled upward and outward.

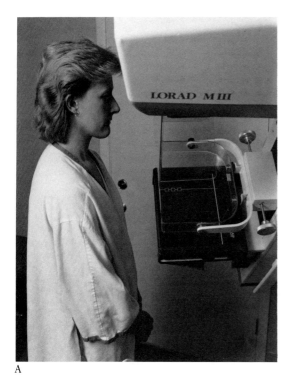

A

FIGURE 12-20 Step-by-step positioning of the 45° oblique projection for a small-breasted patient. A, Have patient stand slightly in front of film tray.

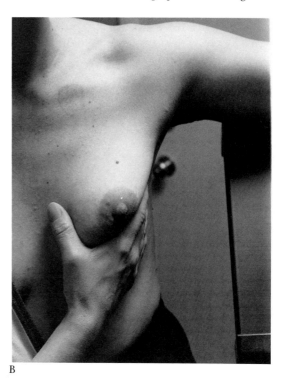

B

FIGURE 12-20B Place one hand posterolateral to breast tissue.

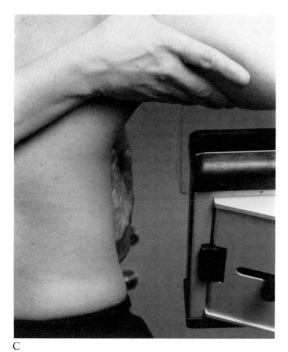

C

FIGURE 12-20C Place one hand behind the shoulder on the side to be positioned.

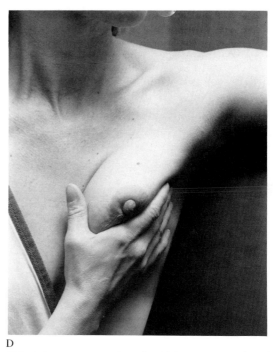

D

FIGURE 12-20D Lift and pull breast upward and outward and bring lateral portion to rest on film tray.

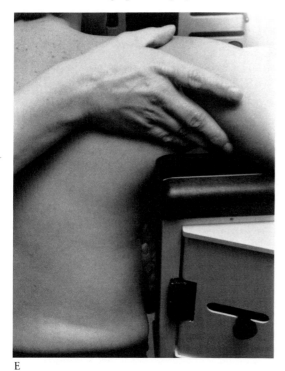

E

FIGURE 12-20E Ensure that corner of film tray rests just posterior to armpit, not in it.

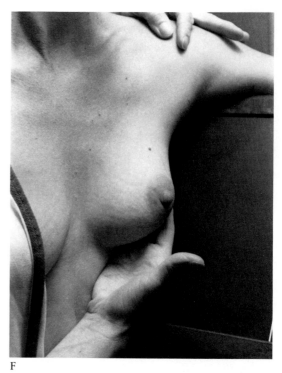

F

FIGURE 12-20F Rotate patient so compression plate touches sternum, continuing to pull breast upward and outward.

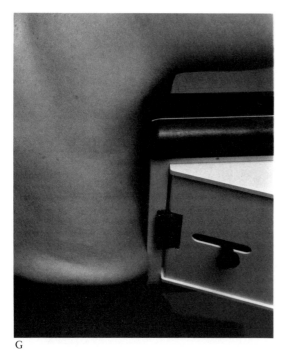

G

FIGURE 12-20G Check posteriorly to see that patient's skin is taut between her side and the film tray.

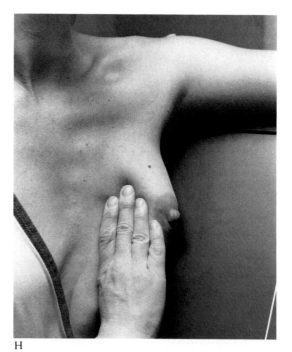

H

FIGURE 12-20H Move supporting hand anteriorly to prevent drooping and loss of tissue.

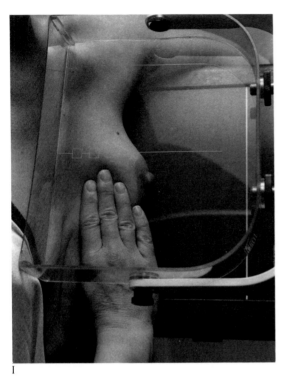

I

FIGURE 12-20I   Bring compression plate down and turn patient toward unit to visualize inframammary crease.

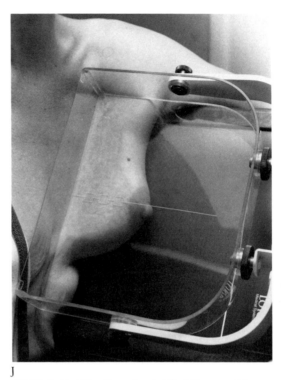

J

FIGURE 12-20J   Completed 45° oblique position.

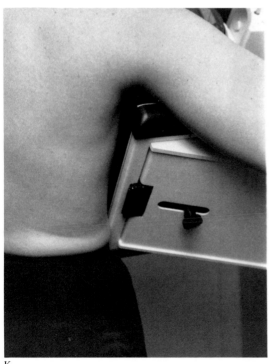

K

FIGURE 12-20K   Posterior view of completed positon.

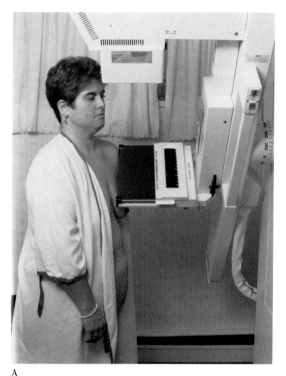

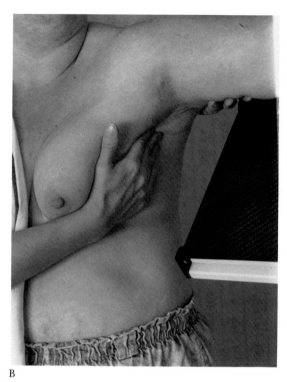

A

FIGURE 12-21 Step-by-step positioning of the 45° oblique projection for a large-breasted patient. A, Have patient stand slightly in front of film tray.

B

FIGURE 12-21B   Place one hand posterolateral to breast tissue.

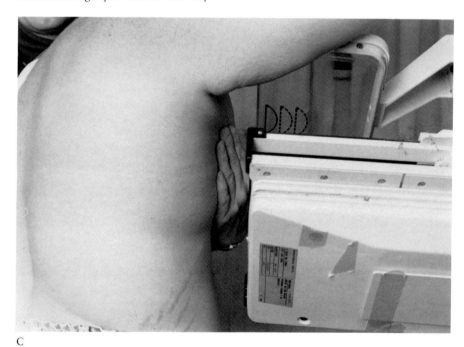

C

FIGURE 12-21C   Ensure that corner of film tray rests just posterior to armpit, not in it.

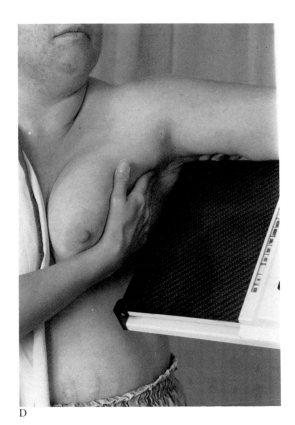

FIGURE 12-21D   Lift and pull breast upward and outward and bring lateral portion to rest on film tray, supporting the upper arm and shoulder.

D

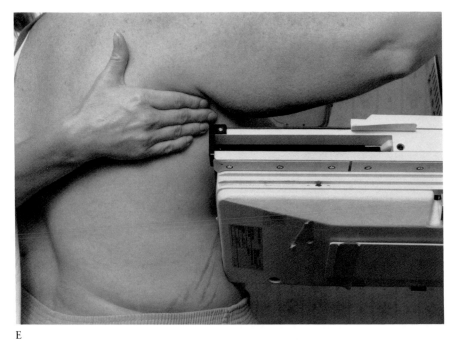

E

FIGURE 12-21E   Check posteriorly to see that patient's skin is taut between her side and the film tray.

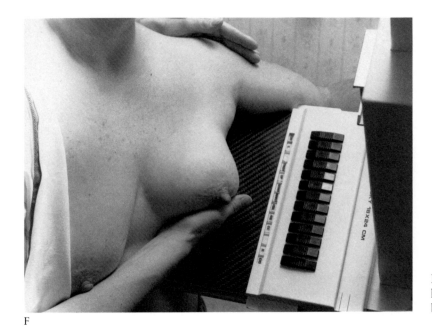

F

FIGURE 12-21F Move supporting hand under breast, continuing to pull breast upward and outward.

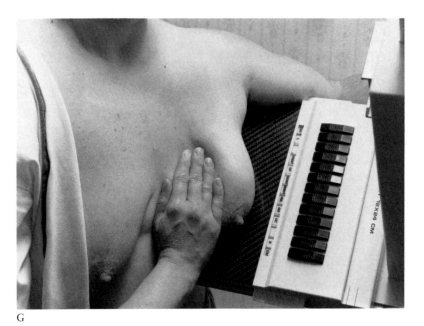

G

FIGURE 12-21G Move supporting hand anteriorly to prevent drooping and loss of tissue.

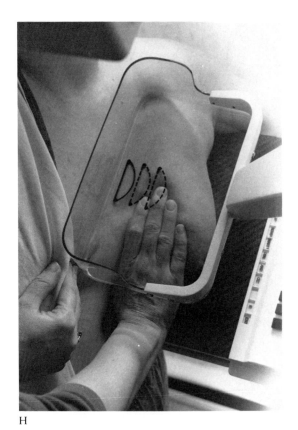

H

FIGURE 12-21H   Bring compression plate down and turn patient toward unit to visualize inframammary crease.

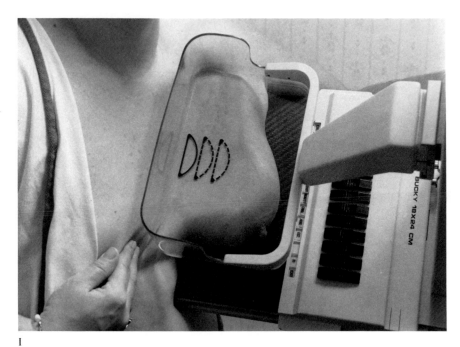

I

FIGURE 12-21I   Completed 45° oblique position.

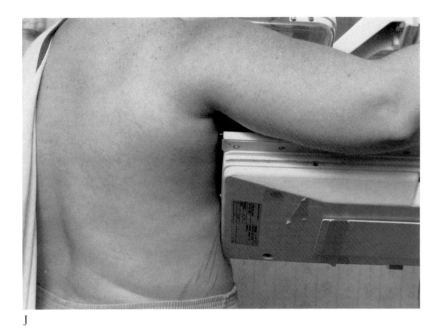

J

FIGURE 12-21J   Posterior view of completed position.

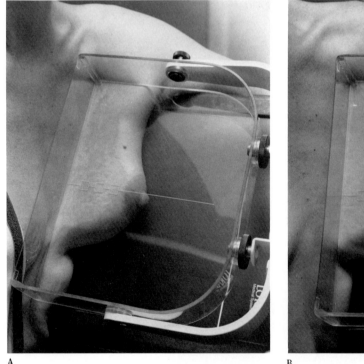

A

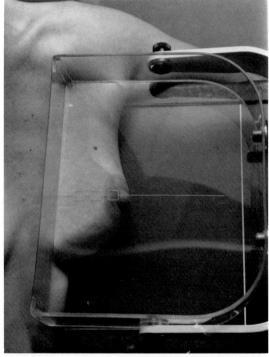

B

FIGURE 12-22   **A.** Small-breasted woman correctly positioned for 45° oblique projection. **B.** The same woman incorrectly turned, eliminating medial tissue and inframmary crease from visualization.

place turn patient toward unit to visualize infra-mammary crease (Figs. 12-22 and 12-23).

9. Slowly bring the compression plate down, and re-move supporting hand as the compression takes over the job.

Other Oblique Positions

The 30° Oblique Position   The 30° oblique posi-tion (Fig. 12-24), is a mediolateral projection, is best used to visualize the upper outer quadrant of the breast. However, it has many applications. Mam-mograms made using this position (Fig. 12-25) dem-onstrate the entire sheet of glandular tissue without superimposition of medial over lateral tissue, as oc-curs with the (45°) oblique position. It does not image posterolateral or posteromedial tissue as well as the craniocaudad or (45°) oblique positions and should not be used as a replacement for one of these in a two-view study. However, when performing a single-

view mammogram because of a patient's young age, for follow-up, and in similar situations, it is the po-sition of choice.

The 30° oblique position does "open" up the glan-dular tissue, separating overlapped structures. There-fore it is used for a third view when more information is needed about a possible lesion seen on a (45°) oblique projection (see Chapter 15). The 30° oblique position is used for a third view on both an unaf-fected and an irradiated breast in patients who have had breast cancer. These patients have an increased risk of either developing another carcinoma in the unaffected breast or of recurrence in an irradiated breast. A third view gives the radiologist and patient an advantage in early diagnosis (Fig. 12-26).

To position the patient for a 30° oblique projection the C-arm is turned to an approximately 30° angle mediolaterally. With the patient's feet pointed toward the unit (as for a craniocaudad projection) and her torso turned slightly outward with the lateral aspect

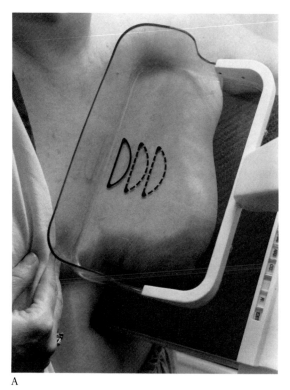
A

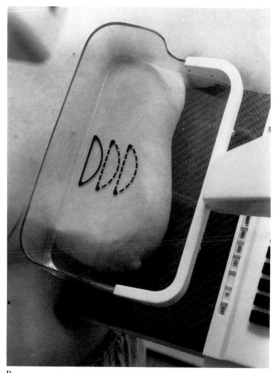
B

FIGURE 12-23   **A.** Large-breasted woman correctly positioned for 45° oblique projection. **B.** The same woman incorrectly turned, eliminating medial tissue and inframammary crease from visualization.

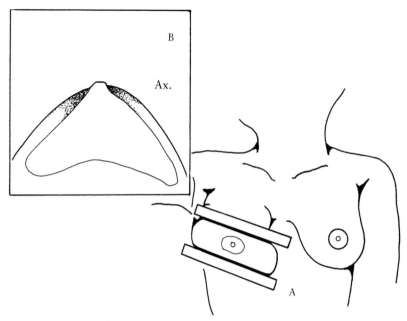

FIGURE 12-24   **A.** Schematic of the orientation of the breast to the film tray for the 30° oblique projection. **B.** Schematic demonstrating the amount of the "glandular island" usually shown with this view.

of the breast toward the unit, the breast is rested on the film tray. Turn the patient's head sideways in either direction, whichever best allows for patient comfort and the most visualization of posterior tissue on the film. Raise the C-arm so that posterolateral tissue comes to rest on the film tray. Have the patient relax her shoulder to better image the upper outer quadrant.

The objective of this view is to flatten the glandular tissue out as much as possible. *This sometimes necessitates a reduction in obliquity (20°–25°) or a "rolling" of the breast tissue in one direction or another.* The patient should press in toward the unit, but be careful that she does not lean sideways and back toward the film tray and the side being imaged, because the resulting image will imitate the (45°) projection of the glandular tissue. Gently pull the breast outward and forward. While holding the breast in place, apply compression (Fig. 12-27).

Summary of 30° Oblique Position
1. Turn C-arm to approximately 30° mediolaterally.
2. Have patient stand with feet facing unit, turning her upper torso slightly away toward side not

being imaged. Bring the breast to rest on the film tray.
3. Turn the patient's head to whichever side best allows for the breast to be positioned adequately and maintain patient comfort.
4. Raise the film tray to meet posterolateral breast.
5. Have the patient relax her shoulders.
6. Roll the breast flat or adjust obliquity.
7. Pull the breast outward and forward, holding in place, and apply compression.

Lateromedial ("Reverse") Oblique Position   The lateromedial projection (Fig. 12-28), sometimes referred to as a "reverse" oblique, best demonstrates the upper inner and lower outer quadrants of the breast. It has two applications, in the tangential position and as a third view in women with encapsulated implants. When performing a tangential study (see later discussion), the angle of obliquity will depend upon the location of the lesion. A reverse angle of 45° is used for a third view in women with encapsulated implants (when using the Eklund modified compression technique is not possible). Imaging the breast with implants in three views assures that some

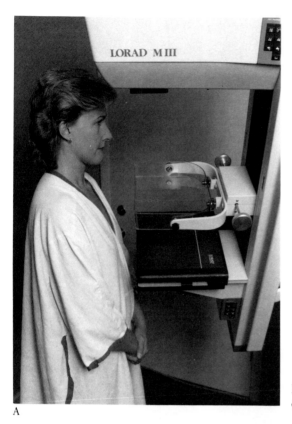

A

FIGURE 12-25   **A.** Orientation of the C-arm rotation for a 30° oblique of the left breast. **B.** The completed 30° oblique position.

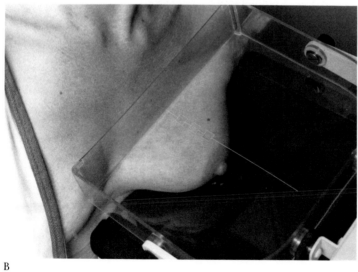

B

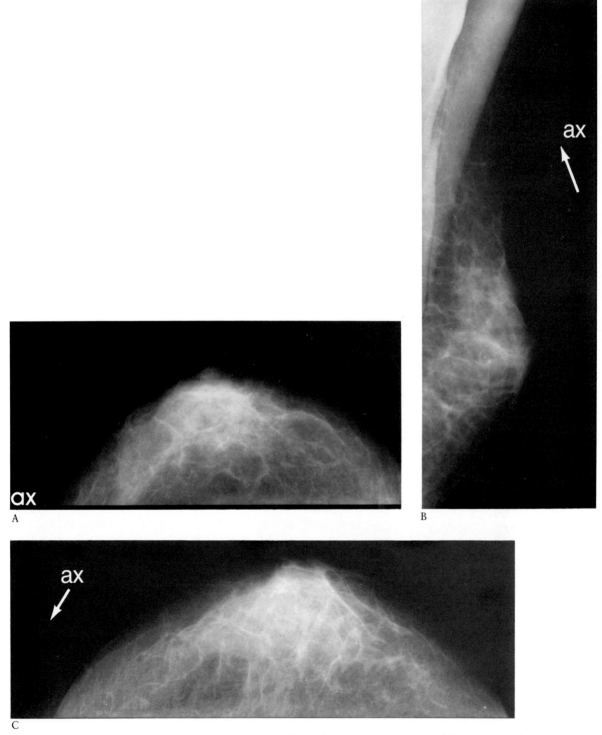

FIGURE 12-26   Craniocaudad (**A**), 45° oblique (**B**), and 30° oblique (**C**) projections of the remaining breast in a woman who has had a mastectomy. The 30° oblique projection will demonstrate (in most cases) the entire glandular island and give the radiologist a different projection of the glandular tissue.

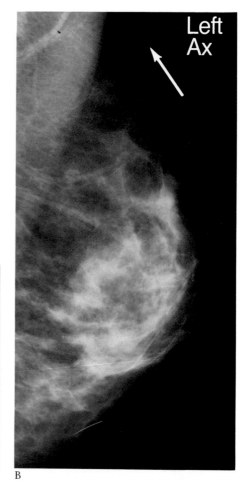

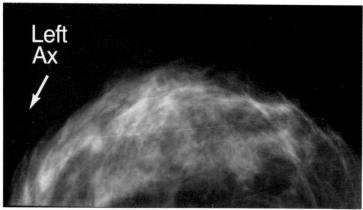

A

B

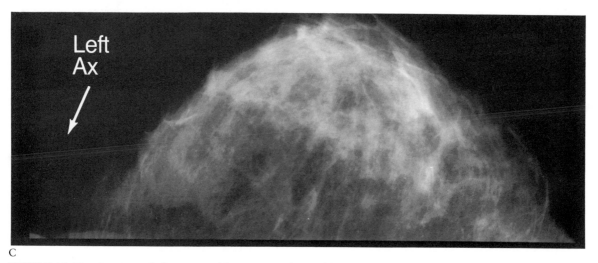

C

FIGURE 12-27   Craniocaudad (**A**), 45° oblique (**B**), and 30° oblique (**C**) projections of the left breast. The 30° oblique projection, visualizing the entire glandular island (in most cases), demonstrates the glandular tissue free of the superimposition of the 45° oblique projection.

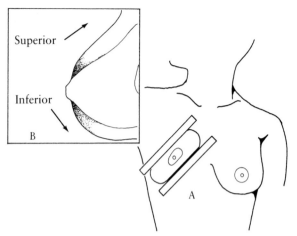

FIGURE 12-28 **A.** Schematic of the orientation of the breast to the C-arm for the "reverse" oblique projection. **B.** Schematic demonstrating the amount of the "glandular island" usually shown with this view.

part of the upper inner and lower outer quadrants is visualized (Fig. 12-29). These areas are not seen free of superimposition of the implant in either the craniocaudad or the (45°) oblique view (Fig. 12-30).

To complete a reverse (45°) oblique, as for implants, the technologist must angle the C-arm approximately 45° lateromedially (opposite to that for

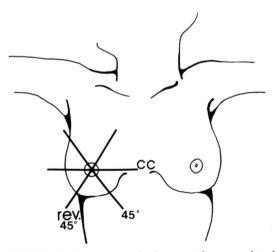

FIGURE 12-29 Imaging the breast with encapsulated implants in three views—the craniocaudad (CC), 45° oblique (45°), and lateromedial 45° oblique (rev. 45°)—assures that some part of all four quadrants are visualized.

a regular (45°) oblique projection). The patient should stand with her feet pointing toward the unit and the edge of the film tray should be placed at the sternum. The patient should hold on to the handrail with the opposite hand. The height of the C-arm should allow the mid-breast to rest over the photo cell or center of the film. Lift the breast and pull outward and upward, bringing the medial portion of the breast to rest on the film. Compress, holding the breast in place (Fig. 12-31).

Again, posture is a key factor for an excellent mammogram; having the patient lean forward from the waist sometimes helps with this view. Check to make sure that the shoulder has not superimposed the field; placing the patient's hand on her hip sometimes helps keep the shoulder back.

Summary of Lateromedial ("Reverse") Oblique Position
1. Turn the C-arm to approximately 45° so that the medial aspect of the breast will rest on the film tray.
2. Have patient face the unit, her arm at her side.
3. Place film tray at sternum, and have patient hold onto handrail with opposite hand.
4. Have the patient slump forward or hunch over, tilting her in the direction of the film tray.
5. Bring the medial aspect of the breast to rest on the film.
6. Adjust the height of the film tray so that breast is centered over the photo cell.
7. Lift the breast and pull outward and upward.
8. Compress, holding the breast in place.

Lateromedial Oblique Position, Arm Up and Over
The lateromedial (reverse) oblique position with the arm up and over is used for a right-angle view to the 45° oblique (see Chapter 15). It is achieved as is the reverse oblique position, but the arm of the side that is being radiographed is brought up and over so that the upper arm rests on the end of the film tray. This brings the upper outer quadrant into view (Fig. 12-32).

Summary of Lateromedial (Reverse) Oblique Position, Arm Up and Over
1. Turn the C-arm to approximately 45°.
2. Have patient face the unit.

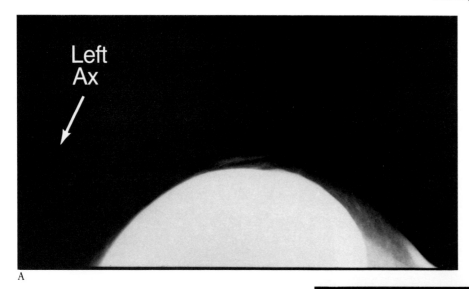

A

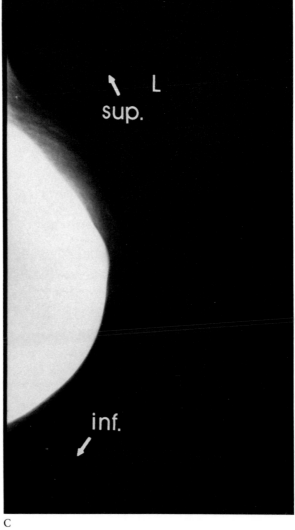

FIGURE 12-30 Craniocaudad (**A**), 45° oblique (**B**), and reverse 45° oblique (**C**) views of a woman with encapsulated implants.

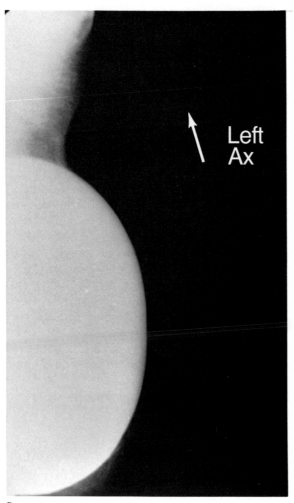

B

C

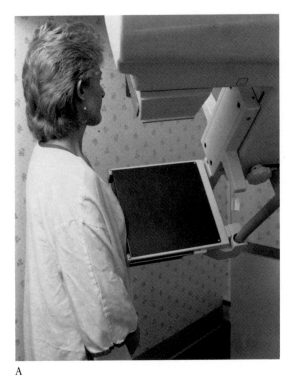
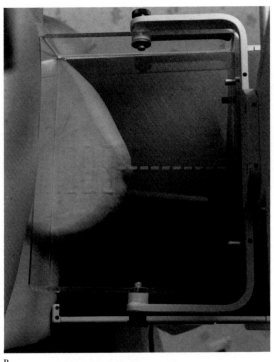

A   B

FIGURE 12-31   Orientation of the C-arm rotation for a lateromedial oblique (reverse 45°) projection of the right breast (**A**) and a completed lateromedial oblique (**B**) for a woman with encapsulated silicone implants.

3. Place film tray at sternum.
4. Have patient raise her arm up and over the film tray, resting the upper portion of the humerus on it.
5. Have the patient slump or lean forward from waist.
6. Bring the medial aspect of the breast to rest on the film.
7. Adjust height of the film tray so that the breast is centered over photo cell.
8. Lift breast, pulling outward and upward.
9. Bring compression plate down along posterior and lateral ribs, including as much lateral tissue as possible.
10. Compress, holding breast in place.

True Lateral Position

The true lateral position (Fig. 12-33) in the two-view mammogram has been largely replaced by the

(45°) oblique position. However, "tailoring" the exam to a patient's specific body build may in fact require replacement of the oblique with the true lateral. In this case, the lateromedial lateral position is more efficient than the mediolateral lateral position in demonstrating breast tissue. In fact, the image from a lateromedial lateral position will often imitate the results of the oblique position. However, this is a more cumbersome position for the patient and, more importantly, the upper outer quadrant of the breast (where 50% of carcinomas arise) is a greater distance from the film, leading to distortion of this area.

The true lateral position is also necessary for localization of a nonpalpable lesion, and may be used as a third view to further examine a suspected lesion (see Chapter 15).

The variations of the true lateral position are outlined below.

Mediolateral Lateral Position

To achieve the mediolateral lateral position (Fig. 12-34), turn the C-arm 90° so that the lateral aspect of

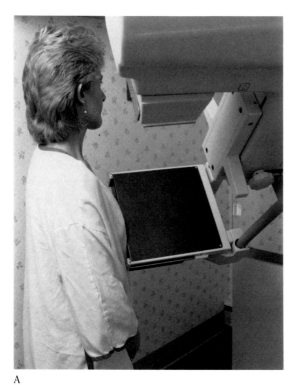 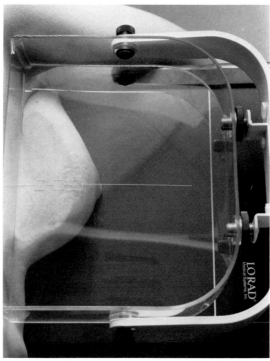

A   B

FIGURE 12-32   **A.** Orientation of the C-arm rotation for a lateromedial oblique (reverse 45°) projection with the arm up and over. **B.** Completed lateromedial oblique positioning with the arm up and over.

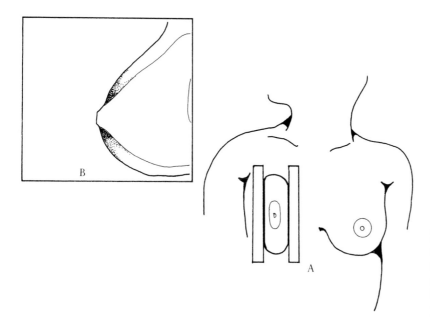

FIGURE 12-33   **A.** Schematic of the orientation of the breast to the C-arm for the true lateral projection. **B.** Schematic of the amount of the "glandular island" usually shown with this projection.

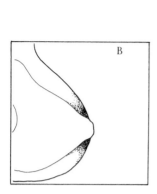

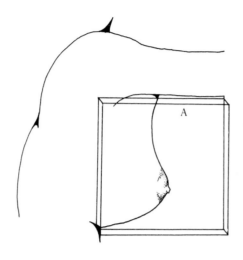

FIGURE 12-34 **A.** Schematic of the orientation of the breast to the C-arm for the mediolateral lateral projection. **B.** Schematic of the amount of the "glandular island" usually shown with this projection.

the breast will rest against the film tray. The patient should face the unit with her feet forward. Have the patient raise her arm to shoulder level (a larger size film tray may require the arm to be raised higher) and lean forward from the waist to facilitate easier compression. Place the edge of the film tray as far posterior to breast tissue as possible. Adjust the height of the C-arm so that the mid-breast is centered to the appropriate photo cell. Lift the breast and pull upward and outward. Lower the compression as the breast is held in place (Fig. 12-35).

Summary of Mediolateral Lateral Position
1. Turn C-arm to 90°.
2. Patient should face unit with feet forward.
3. Have patient raise her arm to shoulder level (possibly higher to accommodate film tray). Have patient lean forward from the waist.
4. Bring posterolateral tissue to rest on film tray.
5. Adjust height of C-arm.
6. Pull breast upward and outward.
7. Apply compression.

Mediolateral Lateral Variation A variation of the mediolateral lateral position is appropriate for localization of anterior lateral lesions. If the lesion is anterior enough, the arm does not have to be raised and may be left comfortably at the patient's side; other positioning steps are the same as described above. Always bring the nipple into profile when the view is being done for localization purposes (Fig. 12-36).

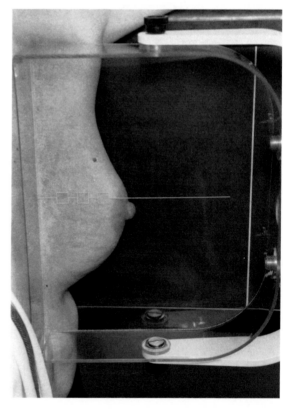

FIGURE 12-35 Completed mediolateral lateral position.

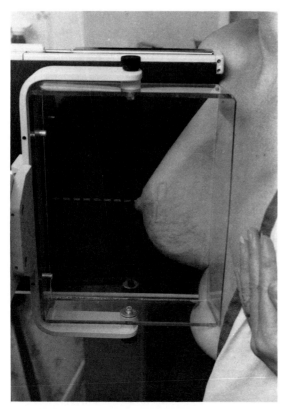

FIGURE 12-36 Completed variation of the mediolateral lateral position with the arm down. The nipple should always be brought into profile when used for localization of a lesion.

Lateromedial Lateral Position

To achieve the lateromedial lateral position (Fig. 12-37), rotate the C-arm 90° so that the medial aspect of the breast rests against the film tray. The patient should stand with her feet facing the unit and the edge of the film tray should be placed at the sternum. Have the patient lift her arm up and over the film tray, letting the upper arm rest on the tray edge. Adjust the height of the C-arm so that the breast is centered over the photo cell. Pick up the breast and pull up and outward, slightly rotating the patient inward toward the film tray so that more lateral tissue will come under the compression plate. Pulling upward and outward and holding the breast in place, bring the compression plate down just posterior to the axilla, to include all lateral breast tissue and the inframammary crease. Bring the compression plate down while holding breast in place (Figs. 12-38 and 12-39).

Summary of Lateromedial Lateral Position
1. Rotate the C-arm 90° so that the medial aspect of the breast will rest on the film tray.
2. Patient should stand with her feet toward unit.
3. Have patient lean in from the waist.
4. Place edge of film tray at midsternum.
5. Raise the arm of the side being radiographed up and over the film tray.
6. Bring the upper arm to rest on top of the film tray, bending the patient's elbow and resting her hand on the opposite shoulder.
7. Adjust the height of the film tray.
8. Pick up the breast, pulling upward and outward.

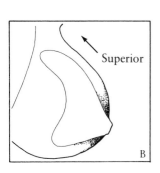

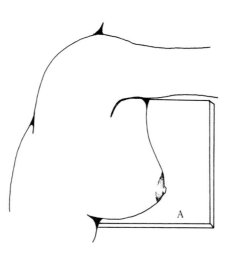

FIGURE 12-37 **A.** Schematic of the orientation of the breast to the C-arm for the lateromedial lateral projection. **B.** Schematic of the amount of the "glandular island" usually shown with this projection.

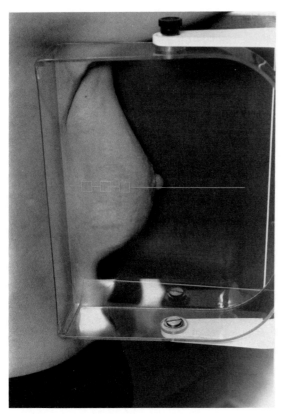

FIGURE 12-38   Completed lateromedial lateral position with the arm up and over.

9. Bring the compression plate down just posterior to the axilla, to include all lateral tissue and inframammary crease.

Lateromedial Lateral Variation   A variation of the lateromedial lateral position is appropriate for localization of anterior medial lesions. If the suspected lesion is anterior enough, the patient's arm can be left at her side; other positioning steps are the same as described above. Always bring the nipple into profile when completing this view for localization purposes (Fig. 12-40).

Cleopatra Position

The cleopatra position (Fig. 12-41) is best used to visualize the upper outer quadrant (tail) of the breast. It

has virtually been replaced by the 30° oblique position, for this use which more efficiently demonstrates this area with less superimposition. However, the cleopatra position is very useful in demonstrating very posterior, central lesions.

To achieve the cleopatra position, the C-arm is not rotated. It is best to have the patient seated. Have the patient raise her arm up and rest her hand behind her head. Bring the inferior-lateral aspect of the breast to rest on the film tray. Pick up the breast and pull outward, lowering the compression plate (Fig. 12-42).

Modified Compression Technique (Eklund Method)

Eklund et al.[3] recently reported a new method for imaging the breasts of women who have had implants.[4] They reported that by pulling the breast tissue away from the implant while displacing the implant posteriorly to exclude it from view (Fig. 12-43), better visualization of the breast tissue was possible. Increased compression and lack of superimposition over the implant could now be achieved, showing an improvement of tissue imaging in 99% of the cases. The modified compression technique can be accomplished regardless of whether the implant is posterior or anterior to the pectoral muscle, as long as the implant remains soft and free of encapsulation.

The Eklund method is an addition to the routine two-view mammogram and not a substitution, because it is not meant to image the most posterior portions of the breast. According to Eklund et al.[3] mammography for women with implants should include the following four views (Fig. 12-44):

1. Routine craniocaudad
2. Routine (45°) oblique
3. Craniocaudad with modified compression
4. (45°) oblique with modified compression

To accomplish the modified compression technique, the patient should be positioned as if to obtain the view intended (craniocaudad or oblique). Pick up the breast and feel for the anterior portion of the implant. Place the thumb and forefinger between the breast tissue and the implant. Bring this portion of the breast to rest on the film tray, still holding it be-

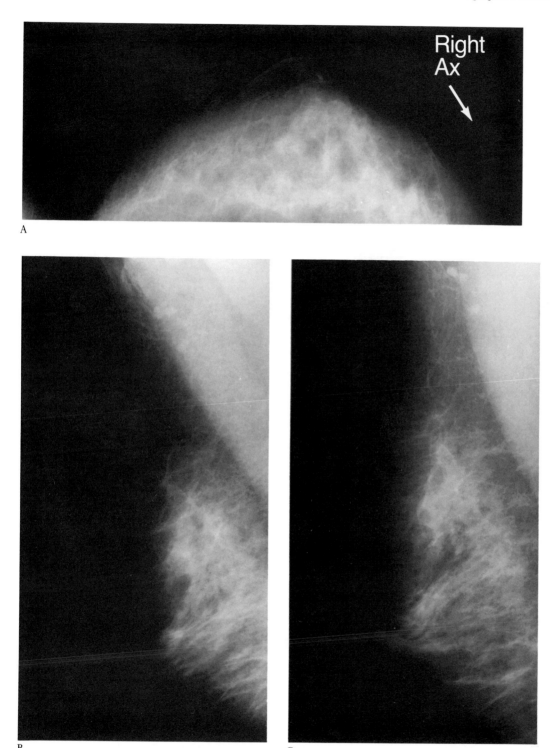

FIGURE 12-39   Craniocaudad (**A**) and 45° oblique (**B**) mammograms of a woman with pectus excavatum. The 45° oblique image shows glandular tissue running off the film. A lateromedial lateral projection (**C**) (with the arm up and over) visualizes more posterior tissue and completes the study. *Note:* The lateromedial lateral view is labeled with superior (sup.) and inferior (inf.) direction, because there is no axilla orientation.

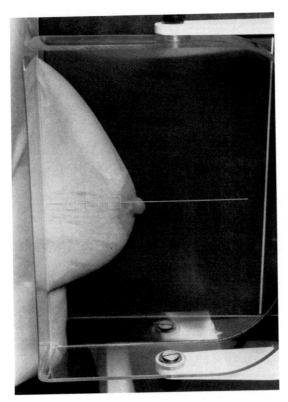

FIGURE 12-40   Completed variation of the lateromedial lateral position. *Note:* The nipple should always be presented in profile when used for localization purposes.

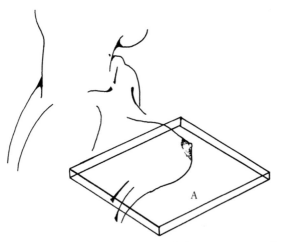

FIGURE 12-41   **A.** Schematic of the orientation of the breast to the C-arm for the cleopatra position.

tween the thumb and forefinger. Bring the compression plate down while pulling the breast tissue forward and outward, allowing the implant to be displaced posteriorly. (In some cases it helps to have the patient hollow out her chest wall.) Compress as usual. Phototiming may be used to image the breast.

Axilla Position

The axilla position, an anterior-posterior projection, is best used to visualize the axillary contents. The axilla view is included as a *unilateral* study ie: only one side is done on the affected side of women who have had breast cancer and on those women who are suspected to have inflammatory carcinoma. A *bilateral* study is obtained in those women presenting with lymphadenopathy (swollen lymph nodes), for comparative purposes. If the lymph nodes prove to be enlarged unilaterally, then an occult breast cancer is suspect. If the lymph nodes prove to be enlarged bilaterally, the cause is more likely systemic. A bilateral study is also routine when searching for a primary cancer in a patient who has had a positive biopsy for a cancer elsewhere in the body, with undifferentiated tumor cells.

To achieve the axilla position, rotate the C-arm 70–90°; it may be necessary to adjust this while positioning in order to best accommodate the patient's body. The patient should at first stand with her feet parallel to the unit. Have the patient extend her arm and lift it to shoulder level (remembering to slouch). Move her whole body toward the unit, bringing the posterior aspect of the shoulder to rest against the film tray. The arm can be kept straight or be bent at the elbow and should rest on the C-arm. Have the patient bend at the waist and lean in laterally toward the unit, so that the resulting image will include the glenoid fossa. If possible allow the rib cage to be included in the view. Demonstrating ribs is not adverse in this view, because it assures that all axillary tissue has been demonstrated; metastases in the lymph nodes can occur very low and close to the rib cage. The height of the film tray should allow visualization of the head of the humerus. Have the patient turn her feet and body inward toward the film tray so that more medial tissue is imaged. Compression should be

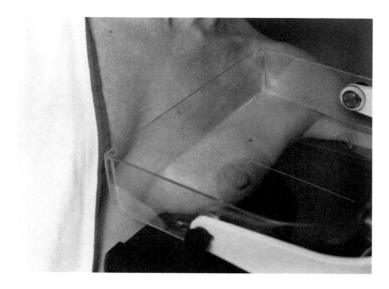

FIGURE 12-42   Completed cleopatra position. The C-arm has no angulation.

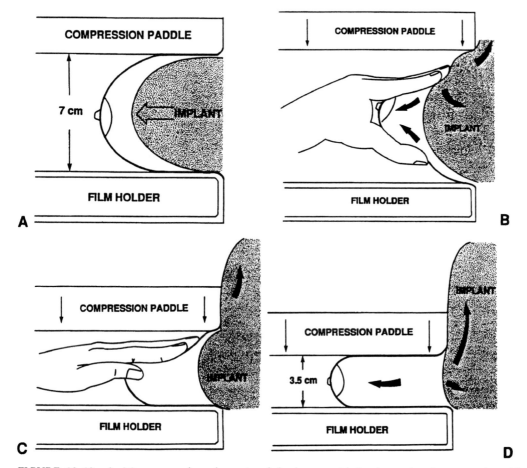

FIGURE 12-43   **A.** Mammography schematic of the breast with implants showing normal positioning and compression. **B–D.** Use of the *modified compression technique*, in which the implant is displaced posteriorly and superiorly, to image the breast free of superimposition and with better compression.

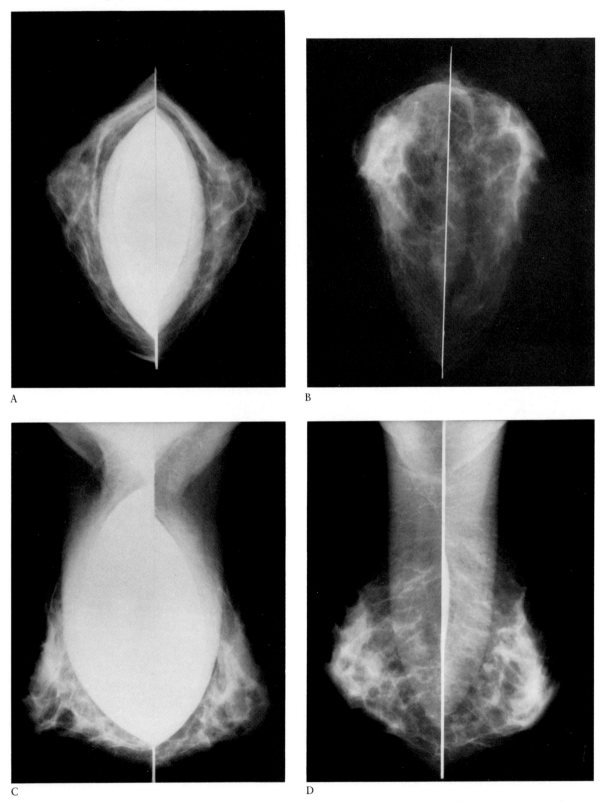

A

B

C

D

FIGURE 12-44   Craniocaudad (**A**) and 45° oblique (**C**) projections of a woman with silicone implants, and modified compression views in the same projections (**B** and **D**).

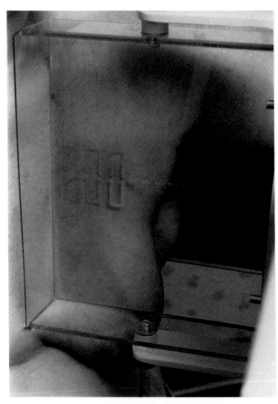

FIGURE 12-45   Completed axilla position.

applied just to hold the tissue in place (Figs. 12-45 and 12-46). Since this view is sometimes used for patients who have not had mastectomy, it is sometimes necessary to bring the breast under the compression plate.

The axilla view requires that a grid be used. The amount of tissue and bone visualized with this view requires that peak kilovoltage and milliamperage be increased. Average kilovoltage ranges from 33 to 35 kVp at 200–300 mAs depending on the specifications of the unit.

Summary of Axilla Position

1. Rotate the C-arm 70–90° to accommodate the patient's body.
2. Have patient stand at first with feet parallel to the unit.
3. Extend the patient's arm and lift to shoulder level.
4. Bring the posterior aspect of the shoulder to rest against the film tray.

5. Adjust the height of the film tray to allow visualization of the head of the humerus.
6. Have the patient bend at the waist and lean in laterally toward the unit.
7. Bring rib cage into view if possible.
8. Turn the patient's feet and body inward toward the unit so that more medial tissue is imaged.
9. Apply compression if possible, just enough to hold the tissue in place.

Tangential Position

The tangential position is best used to visualize suspected lesions, palpable or nonpalpable, free of surrounding glandular structures. However, it is especially useful for visualizing palpable lesions not seen on the two-view mammogram and for demonstrating areas of interest in a dense breast. By situating the lesion adjacent to subcutaneous adipose tissue, the resulting increase in subject contrast enhances its radiographic characteristics. The tangential view is the best image for a suspected lesion because it demonstrates an area free of superimposition and often brings it closer to the film, for optimum detail. In order to obtain a tangential view the lesion must be palpable or, if nonpalpable, must be visualized on any two views so that approximate location can be determined.

To achieve a tangential position, draw an imaginary line from the nipple to the lesion. Turn the C-arm so that the film tray parallels this line. Rules of thumb for determining the direction of the C-arm are:

Lesions seen in the upper inner or lower outer quadrant require a lateromedial (reverse) oblique angulation of some degree depending on the location of the lesion (Fig. 12-47A).

Lesions seen in the upper outer or lower inner quadrant require a mediolateral oblique angulation of some degree depending on the location of the lesion (Fig. 12-47B).

Lesions that approximate 12:00 or 6:00 are best visualized with a true lateral projection.

Lesions that approximate 3:00 (left) or 9:00 (right) are best visualized with an exaggerated craniocaudad projection.

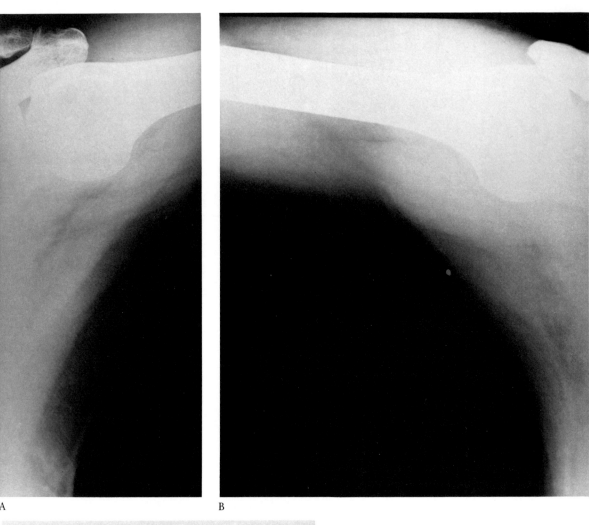

A

B

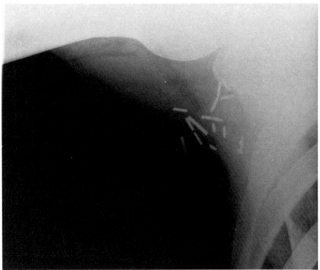

C

FIGURE 12-46   Variations of well-positioned axilla views.

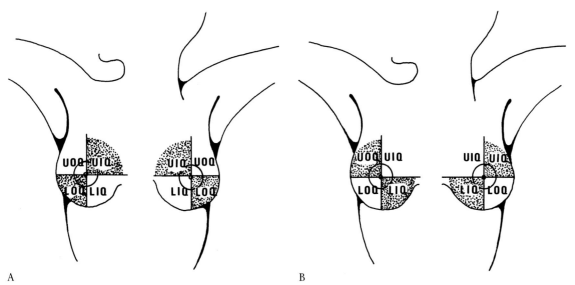

A

B

FIGURE 12-47   Guidelines for doing a tangential view. **A.** Areas seen in the upper inner quadrant (UIQ) or lower outer quadrant (LOQ) require a lateromedial oblique angulation of some degree. **B.** Areas seen in the upper outer quadrant (UDQ) or lower inner quadrant (LIQ) require a mediolateral oblique angulation of some degree.

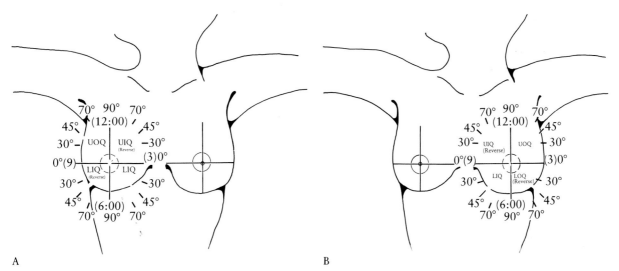

A

B

FIGURE 12-48   Correlation of the location of the lesion with the degree of angulation of the C-arm. Note that a certain angulation of the film tray will demonstrate both an upper quadrant and a lower quadrant lesion tangentially.

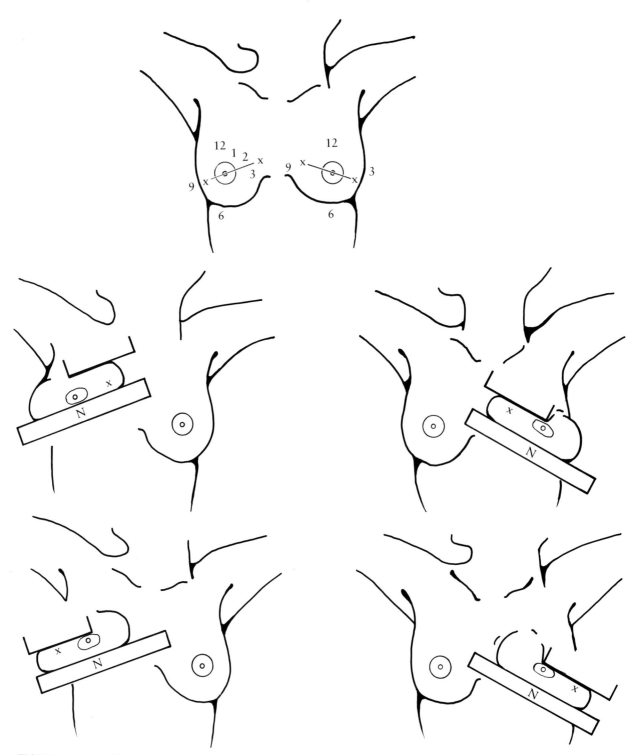

FIGURE 12-49A   If the "lesion" lies at 2:30 or 8:30 in the right breast or 9:30 or 3:30 in the left breast then a lateromedial (reverse) oblique projection of about 15° will demonstrate these areas tangentially. Again note that a certain angulation illustrates both an upper quadrant and lower quadrant lesion tangentially.

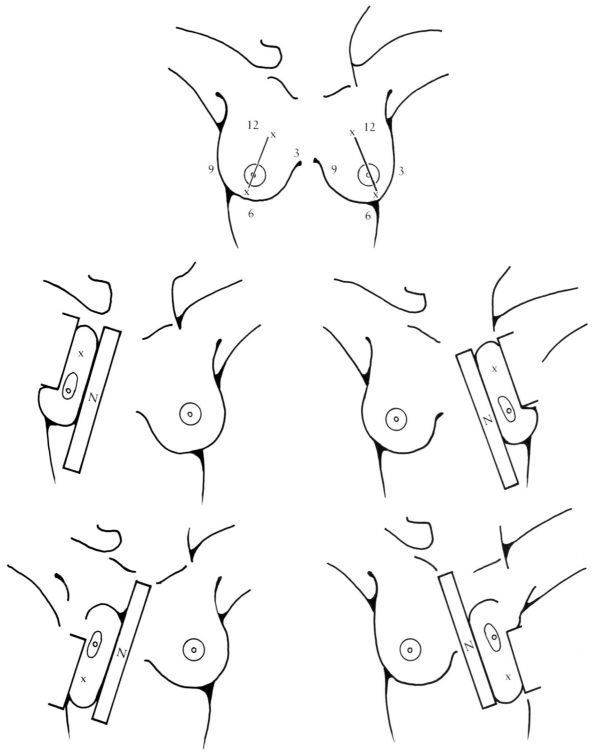

FIGURE 12-49B   If the "lesion" lies at 1:00 or 7:00 in the right breast or 11:00 or 5:00 in the left breast then a lateromedial (reverse) oblique projection of about 70° will demonstrate these areas tangentially.

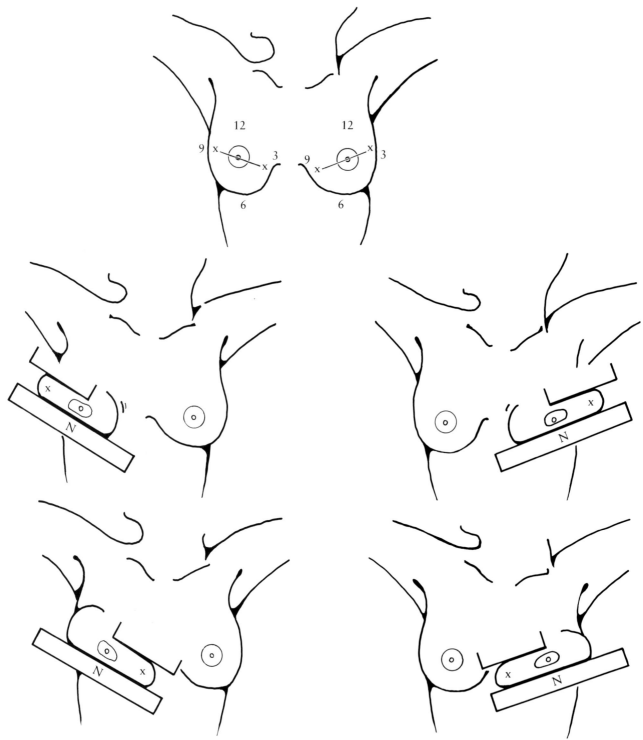

FIGURE 12-50A   If the "lesion" lies at 9:30 or 3:30 in the right breast or 8:30 or 2:30 in the left breast then a mediolateral oblique projection of about 15° will demonstrate these areas tangentially. Again note that a certain angulation illustrates both an upper quadrant and lower quadrant lesion tangentially.

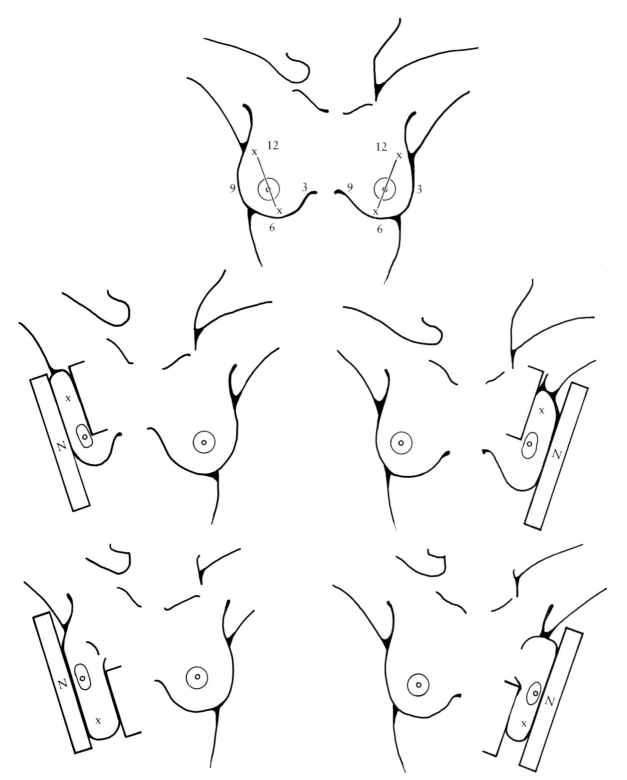

FIGURE 10-50B   If the "lesion" lies at 11:00 or 5:00 in the right breast or 1:00 or 7:00 in the left breast then a mediolateral oblique projection of about 70° will demonstrate these areas tangentially.

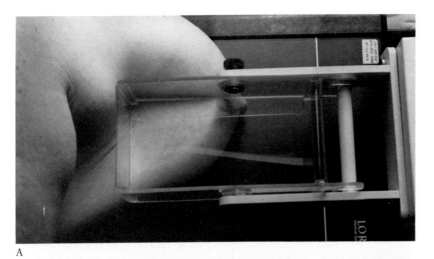

A

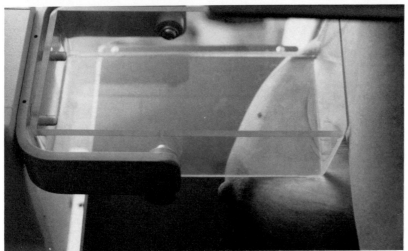

B

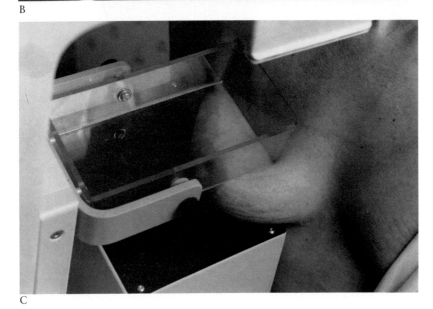

C

FIGURE 12-51 Three examples of positioning for the tangential view. **A.** A reverse 70° oblique for the 5:00 area of the right breast. **B.** A reverse 45° oblique for the 10:30 area of the left breast. **C.** A 20° oblique for the 9:30 area of the right breast.

Figure 12-48 illustrates correlation of the location of the lesion with the degree of angulation of the C-arm, and Figures 12-49, 12-50 and 12-51 give examples of the application of tangential positioning.

Mammographic Positioning for Investigating "Mass Effect" (Pseudo-Carcinoma)

The following three positions are all used to determine if a "mass" seen mammographically is a true lesion. In addition the slight oblique and rolled positions can be used to determine a lesion's approximate location by the direction it moves. For application of these positions, refer to Chapter 15.

Slight Oblique Position

The slight oblique position is best used to clear up the question of superimposition when a suspicious area is seen on a craniocaudad view (Fig. 12-52). An angle of 5–20° is employed in a reverse oblique or regular oblique position depending on the location of the area in question and the makeup of surrounding tissue. Sometimes both obliques need to be done to prove an area is truly overlapped tissue. (These same principles can be applied when there is a question of a pseudo mass on the (45°) oblique. The patient should be positioned as for the 45° oblique and then the C-arm rotated approximately 15° upward and 15° downward.)

"Spot Compression" Position

The spot compression position is used to clear up the question of superimposition on a craniocaudad or (45°) oblique projection. The same view that showed the suspected lesion is retaken using a spot compression device (if the lesion is seen on both views then both should be done). It should be noted that without a rotation of the breast, by either rolling the breast or rotating the C-arm, the risk of demonstrating the same overlap of tissue might occur even with the better compression. The increased compression usually allows the tissue to be spread more evenly. Superimposed structures will separate if in fact the "lesion" is not real. In addition, close collimation adds contrast to the image (Figs. 12-53 and 12-54).

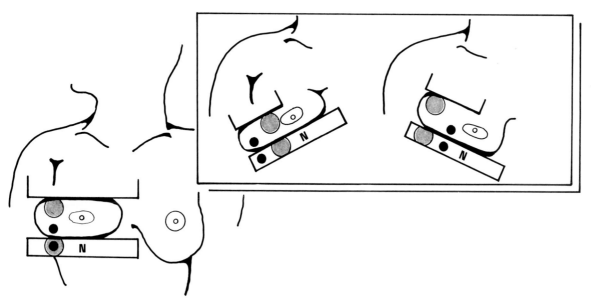

FIGURE 12-52   The question of overlapped tissue can be resolved with a slight oblique projection. Superimposed areas will "spread" apart whereas a true lesion will hold its shape.

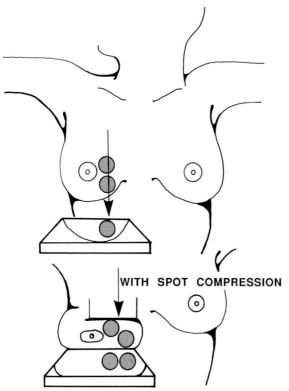

FIGURE 12-53   The question of overlapped tissue can be resolved with a coned-down "spot compression" view of the area. Localized compression over the area of interest spreads overlapped tissues apart.

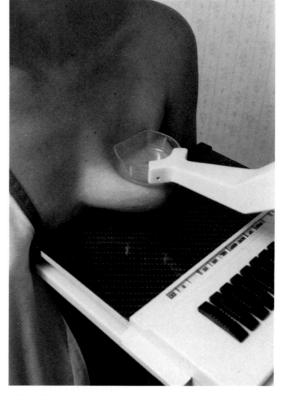

FIGURE 12-54   Completed spot compression position demonstrating localized compression over a specific area.

"Rolled" Position

The "rolled" position[58] is used to clear up the question of superimposition when a suspicious area is seen on a craniocaudad projection. Place the breast in the craniocaudad position. Rotate the top half of the breast in one direction while rolling the bottom half in the other. This allows for the separation of glandular structures (Figs. 12-55 and 12-56).

Coat Hanger Position

The coat hanger position is best used to image palpable masses that cannot be visualized or visualized well by conventional techniques:

1. Palpable lesions high on the chest wall.

2. Palpable lesions posterolateral next to the chest wall.

3. Palpable lesions that must be separated from a silicone implant (where the modified compression technique is not possible).

These are usually the lesions that "slip" out from under the compression plate.

Either corner of a standard household wire coat hanger is used to "capture" the mass. The coat hanger should be cut in half and the exposed cut edges covered with tape. By imposing it between the rib cage and the lesion or the implant and the lesion, the palpable mass can now be "caught" and held in place for imaging (Fig. 12-57).

Two people are required to achieve this position, one person (with lead apron and glove) to hold the "coat hanger" in place and the technologist to posi-

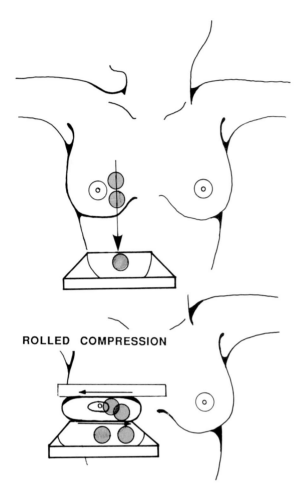

ROLLED COMPRESSION

FIGURE 12-55   The question of overlapped structures can be resolved with a "rolled" view. Rolling the top half of the breast in one direction and the bottom half in the other moves the structures away from one another.

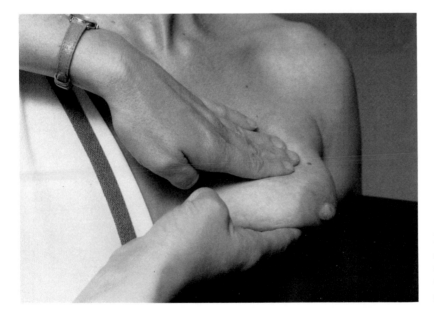

FIGURE 12-56   Rolling the superior and inferior aspects of the breast in opposite directions for the "rolled" view, to resolve areas of superimposition.

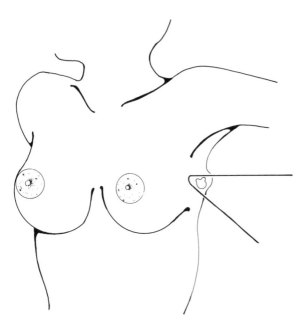

FIGURE 12-57 A schematic demonstrating the coat hanger position to image those lesions that slip out from under the compression plate.

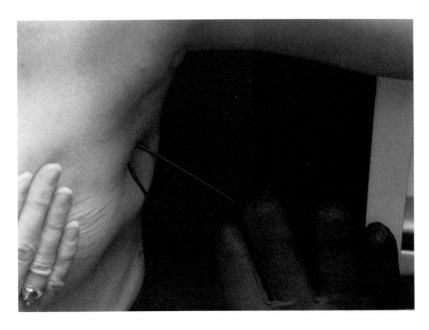

FIGURE 12-58 Completed positioning for the coat hanger view to "catch" the very slippery lesions.

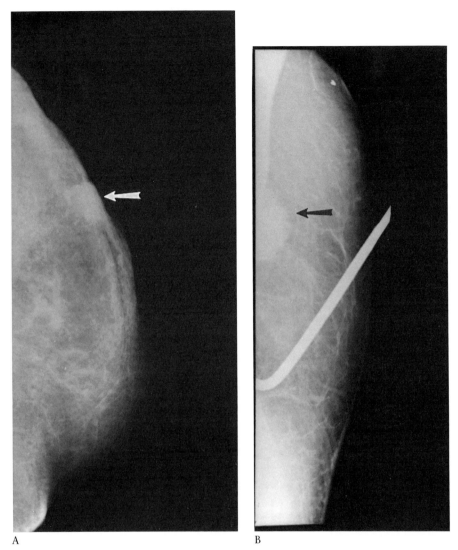

A   B

FIGURE 12-59   **A.** A palpable mass posterolaterally could not be imaged with a 45° oblique projection of the left breast after quadrectomy (the arrow points to the nipple). Other conventional extra views failed to image the lesion as well. **B.** A coat hanger view was successful in imaging this lesion (arrow) which was recurrent carcinoma on biopsy.

tion and make the exposure. It is important to consider state radiation health laws when holding the coat hanger. In some cases the patient can hold the coat hanger herself.

The angle of the C-arm is dependent on the location of the lesion to be imaged. The compression paddle should be removed; the coat hanger applies the compression. A very minimal pressure is necessary because the area caught by the coat hanger is very thin and small. Bring the patient to the film tray. Set the edge of the rib cage (or implant) next to the palpable mass against the edge of the film tray. Impose the "coat hanger" between the ribs or implant and the lesion, pressing against the film tray and bringing the lesion into view (Figs. 12-58 and 12-59). Coat hanger views are best made with magnification.

References

1. *Mammography—A User's Guide*, NCRP report No. 85. Bethesda, MD, National Council on Radiation Protection and Measurements, 1986.
2. Lundgren B: The oblique view at mammography. *Br J Radiol* 1977;50:626–628.
3. Eklund GW, Busby RC, Miller SH, et al: Improving imaging of the augmented breast. *AJR* 1988;151:469–473.
4. Logan WW, Janus J: Use of special mammographic views to maximize radiographic information. *Radiol Clin North Am* 1987;25(5):953–959.
5. Kopans DB: *Breast Imaging*. Philadelphia, JB Lippincott Co, 1989.
6. Gormley L, Bassett LW, Gold RH: Positioning in film-screen mammography. *Appl Radiol* 1988;00:35–37.
7. Swann CA, Kopans DB, McCarthy KA, et al: Localization of occult breast lesions: Practical solutions to problems of triangulation. *Radiology* 1987;3:577–579.
8. Sickles EA: Practical solutions to common mammographic problems: Tailoring the examination to the needs of the individual patient, in Feig SA (ed): *Breast Imaging*, Categorical Course Syllabus. Reston, VA, American Roentgen Ray Society, 1988, pp. 59–67.

13 Kathleen M. Willison

The Nonconforming Patient

This chapter is divided into two sections. A problem and solution guide for difficulties met in everyday work and, from the office of Wende Logan-Young, M.D., recommended views for a variety of patient situations.

It is important for the technologist to realize there are other options for the patient whose body build, anomalies, or medical treatment prohibits obtaining the routine four-view mammogram. To try to make every patient conform to the standard four views only leads to frustration on the technologist's part, increased discomfort for the patient, and usually an inadequate mammogram. Varying the angle or changing the position of the patient usually addresses the problem in most cases; in others an extra view *must* be taken.

The technologist is encouraged to try new techniques and most importantly to share new successful information with other technologists.

Difficulties in Positioning the Nonconforming Patient

Small-Breasted Patient

Problem   Failure to image posterior breast tissue on 45° oblique position.

Possible Solutions
1. Increase the angle of the C-arm to as much as 70°.
2. Have patient slump, drawing shoulders together. This lets the breast fall forward away from the chest wall.
3. Take another view. The 30° oblique or exaggerated C-C would image this tissue.

225

Large-Breasted Patient

Problem   Too much shoulder and axilla area included, resulting in too much compression superiorly and posteriorly on the oblique position and minimal compression anteriorly. The resulting mammogram will show a large band of pectoral muscle (and sometimes latissimus dorsi), but the anterior breast will droop dramatically.

Possible Solutions

1. Check the superior corner of the film tray—if it is too far posterior to the axilla, reposition to bring the corner just posterior to the axilla (see Chapter 12).
2. Film tray may be too high; lower the film tray and reposition.
3. Shoulder and upper arm not relaxed back; pick up the upper arm and roll the shoulder back.
4. Remember, the (45°) oblique view is for the posterior and upper outer quadrant of the breast. The uneven compression may be due to the patient's body build. An extra view needs to be taken to image the anterior breast. There is much superimposition of the anterior breast tissue on the (45°) oblique view. A 30° oblique would serve the dual purpose of imaging this tissue with better compression and opening up the structures normally overlapped on the (45°) oblique.

Problem   Inability to pull the breast up and outward to achieve proper ductal pattern visualization on the oblique view (see 1.).

Possible Solution   Reduce angle of the C-arm to as low as 30° and have the patient lean in and back so that the film tray is now supporting the breast. The net results will be the same because of the combination of C-arm and patient angle.

Problem   Inability to get full coverage of the breast even with the larger cassette size on craniocaudad view.

Possible Solution   Image as shown in Figure 13-1.

Problem   Inability to get full coverage of breast even with the larger cassette size on (45°) oblique view.

Possible Solution   Perform (45°) oblique view as usual in order to image posterolateral tissue. Then take an extra view imaging missed anterior tissue.

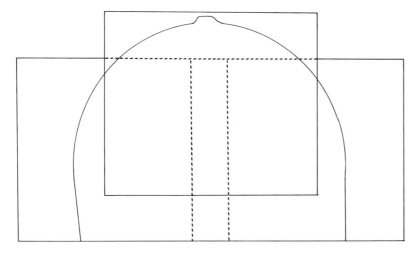

FIGURE 13-1   When imaging a breast too large for one cassette, three views should be taken as shown, allowing overlap to cover the entire breast.

Obese Patient (see also Large-Breasted Patient)

Problem   Abdomen protruding, making visualizing the posterior and inferior portion of the breast difficult if not impossible on the (45°) oblique view.

Possible Solutions
1. Bring patient to stand more anterior to the film tray.
2. Reduce angle of C-arm to as low as 30° and have the patient "lay" back. This brings the body more in line and lessens protrusion.
3. Press abdomen back and out of way without eliminating inframammary crease.
4. Have patient step away from unit, then lean forward from waist. (This also helps on craniocaudad view with these patients).

Barrel- (Pigeon) Chested Patient (Sunken Chest)

Problem   Impossible to image full breast on two views.

Possible Solution   Take three views:
1. A craniocaudad view for medial tissue (the nipple will fall very laterally on the film).
2. A 30° oblique view or exaggerated craniocaudad to image lateral tissue not included on first craniocaudad view.
3. An oblique view to image posterior tissue.

Patient with Pectus Excavatum

Problem   Failure to image medial tissue on craniocaudad or (45°) oblique projections.

Possible Solution   A third view—either a reverse 45° oblique or a lateromedial lateral needs to be added to the two-view mammogram. The technologist should judge which view will best image the nonvisualized medial tissue.

Patient with Kyphoscoliosis

Problem   Failure to image lateral tissue on oblique view.

Possible Solution   Replace oblique view with lateromedial lateral (with arm up and over) view.

Problem   Failure to image medial tissue on craniocaudad view.

Possible Solution   Add third view—lateromedial lateral—to image this tissue.

Patient With "Wrap-Around-the-Corner" Breasts (Breast Extends More Laterally into Axilla)

Problem   Failure to image posterior tissue on the oblique position.

Possible Solution   An extra 30° oblique view needs to be taken to image this missed tissue.

Male Mammogram

Problem   Breast slips out from under compression plate on craniocaudad view.

Possible Solutions
1. Reduce amount of compression.
2. Have patient hold onto handrail and pull himself closer to the unit.

Recommended Views for the Nonconforming Patient

Patient Who Has Had Breast Cancer

The patient who has had a previous breast cancer has a 50% greater chance of developing a breast cancer in the unaffected breast (usually a new primary and not a metastasis from the first cancer) than the average American woman, simply because she has had breast cancer. Whether the patient opts for a mastectomy or lumpectomy with or without irradiation and/or chemotherapy, it is no longer possible to make a comparison, either physically or mammographically, between two "mirror-image" breasts. With this in mind, a three-view study of the unaffected breast is recommended to give the radiologist a better op-

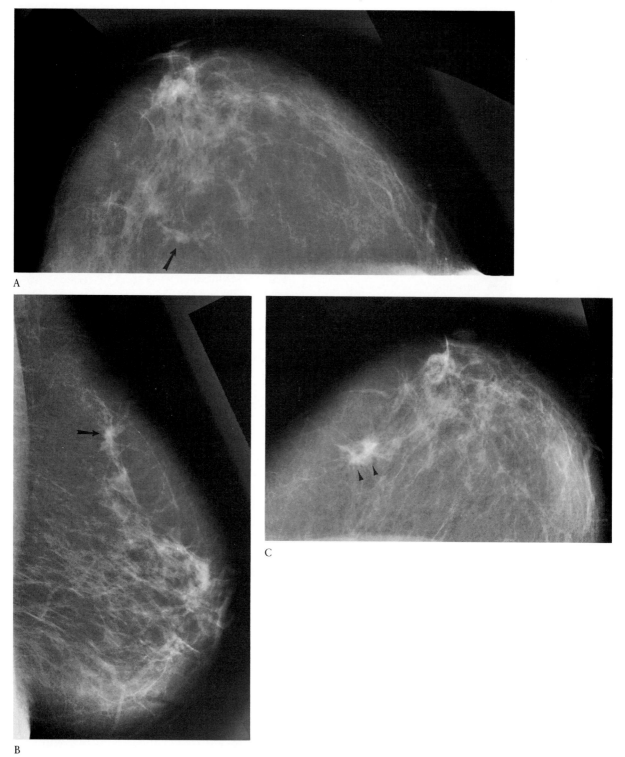

FIGURE 13-2   After breast cancer a three-view study of the unaffected breast is recommended. This three-view mammogram was completed on an asymptomatic woman who previously had a right mastectomy for breast cancer. The 30° oblique view (**C**) demonstrates a lesion (arrowheads) suspicious of being a carcinoma. This lesion could have been missed with the two-view mammogram (black arrows, **A** and **B**)

portunity to diagnose a new breast cancer (Fig. 13-2).

At the time of mastectomy or lumpectomy a lymph node sampling is performed. Because this sampling does not remove all the lymph nodes, imaging the axilla is necessary to enable the radiologist to pick up recurrence before the affected lymph node(s) become palpable (Fig. 13-3). In the same regard, if there is any remaining tissue at the mastectomy site, it needs to be imaged; use one or two angles to visualize as much of this tissue as possible.

Recommended Views following Mastectomy

Unaffected Breast	*Affected Side*
Craniocaudad	Axilla
45° oblique	Remaining tissue
30° oblique	

Recommended Views following Lumpectomy with Irradiation

Unaffected Breast	*Irradiated Breast*
Craniocaudad	Craniocaudad
45° oblique	45° oblique
30° oblique	30° oblique
	Axilla view

Mammography of the affected side is recommended postsurgically (after healing) and preradiation to determine:

1. If all affected tissue was removed.
2. Surgical changes—it is important to know what changes are due to surgery prior to radiation therapy.

Subsequent recommendations for mammography are:

Mammography of the irradiated breast every 6 *months* for at least 2 years.
Mammography of unaffected breast every year.
After 2 years, if all is well, mammography of both breasts every year.

Recommended Views following Postmastectomy Reconstruction

Reconstructed Breast	*Unaffected Breast*
Craniocaudad	Craniocaudad
(45°) oblique	(45°) oblique
Reverse (45°) oblique	30° oblique
Axilla view	

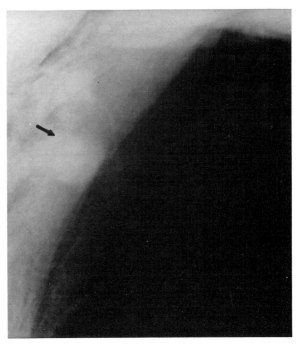

FIGURE 13-3 An axilla view is included routinely on the affected side of a woman who has had a breast cancer. Metastates to lymph nodes can then be seen before they are palpable, as in the above case (black arrow).

Patient With Implants (for Augmentation)

Encapsulated Implants

Craniocaudad
(45°) oblique
Reverse 45° oblique

Soft Implants   For implants anterior or posterior to pectoral muscle.

Craniocaudad
Craniocaudad using modified compression technique
    (see Chapter 12)
(45°) oblique
(45°) oblique using modified compression

If the technologist believes that the upper inner and lower outer quadrant tissue has not been imaged, a reverse (45°) oblique or true lateral view should be added to cover this area.

Patient with Possible Primary Carcinoma

The purpose of the mammogram for the patient who presents with an undifferentiated carcinoma found elsewhere in the body is to determine if she has a clinically occult breast cancer that has metastasized. In some cases the breast cancer will remain occult on the four-view study; bilateral axillas *help* to determine lymph node involvement. If there is nodal involvement unilaterally, a breast cancer would be considered. If involvement is bilateral then the possibility that the patient's metastasis is from the breast decreases markedly and the possibility of systemic disease increases.

Routine mammography for these patients involves obtaining the following views *bilaterally:*

Craniocaudad
(45°) oblique

Axilla
30° oblique if the patient has dense glandular tissue

Patient with Suspected Inflammatory Carcinoma

It is often difficult for the radiologist to distinguish infection from inflammatory carcinoma. Bilateral axilla views must be taken for comparative purposes. If there is lymph node involvement unilaterally on the affected side, the woman is more likely to have an inflammatory carcinoma.

Routine mammography for these patients involves obtaining the following views *bilaterally:*

Craniocaudad
(45°) oblique
Axilla

14

Kathleen M. Willison

Orientation of Mammographic Images

The mammogram is a two dimensional image of a three dimensional organ. The two-dimensional mammogram involves a great deal of overlap of medial over lateral tissue, superior over inferior tissue, and so forth. In addition, the projection of the glandular tissue (in relation to the nipple) changes from view to view. In order to locate a lesion for a special view (or palpation), determine the view that will best image that area, and solve mammographic uncertainties, orienting oneself to each image and relating it to the body position becomes critical. This can be accomplished by:

1. Using consistent viewing methods.
2. Knowing descriptive terminology.
3. Knowing what areas of the breast are superimposed on each mammographic view.
4. Knowing how lesions "move" from one view to another.
5. Knowing how to locate a lesion by using the above information.

Following these guidelines will allow the technologist to perform special views and correlative physical exam with accuracy.

Consistent Viewing

When viewing the mammogram, always hang the films consistently. Whether it be emulsion-side-up or emulsion-side-down, whether the images are hung side-by-side or back-to-back, it is important that the technologist determine what format works best both personally and for the radiologist, and then stay with it. By routinely conforming to the same method one will become more familiar with breast tissue distribution and with what is medial or lateral, right or left, etc. If this established format is used consistently, the technologist will be more apt to recognize patterns of pathology.

Descriptive Terminology

Each breast is divided into four quadrants: the upper outer quadrant (UOQ), upper inner quadrant (UIQ), lower outer quadrant (LOQ), and lower inner quadrant (LIQ). To explain exact location within the

231

breasts, they are viewed as two clocks (Fig. 14-1). Note that 2:00 o'clock in the right breast represents the UIQ, whereas the same time in the left breast represents the UOQ. This opposite labeling is the same for all other clock "times" in the breasts. A lesion's location should always be described in terms of quadrant and clock time for the radiologist (Fig. 14-2). The lesion's distance from the nipple should also be noted. If the lump lies beneath the nipple area, the lump is said to be *subareolar*.

Mammographic Superimposition

Each mammographic view is a summation of tissue. However, it is possible to demonstrate areas of the breast free of superimposition of other glandular islands. Awareness of tissue orientation with regard to superimposition and the nipple, the only point of reference in the breast, is critical not only to locating an area of interest but to also demonstrating it. Figures 14-3 through 14-7 demonstrate some of the more common views and their corresponding superimpositions. They also indicate areas seen free of superimposition in these views.

How Lesions "Move" From View to View

A lesion's relationship to the nipple will change from one projection to another. Acquainting oneself with how the lesion "moves" in this manner will aid in locating it, demonstrating it free of superimposition (if necessary), or finding it on a third view. By following a single lesion from projection to projection, an appreciation can be gained of how a lesion moves in relation to the nipple (Fig. 14-8). There are two rules of movement that hold true:

1. When comparing the (45°) oblique projection to the true lateral projection, a *medial* lesion will *move up* on the lateral from its position on the (45°) oblique (Fig. 14-9).
2. When comparing the (45°) oblique projection to the true lateral projection, a *lateral* lesion will

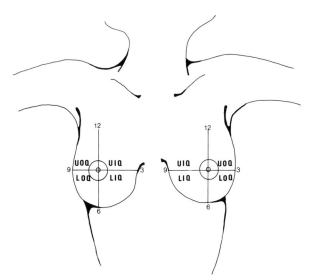

FIGURE 14-1   Each breast is viewed as a clock and is divided into four quadrants, the upper outer quadrant (UOQ), the upper inner quadrant (UIQ), the lower outer quadrant (LOQ), and the lower inner quadrant (LIQ).

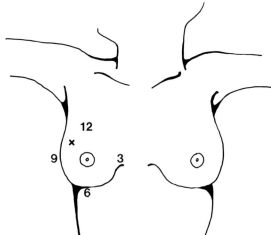

FIGURE 14-2   A lesion should always be described in a consistent manner. For example, the lesion denoted by the "x" is located in the right breast UOQ at approximately 10:30.

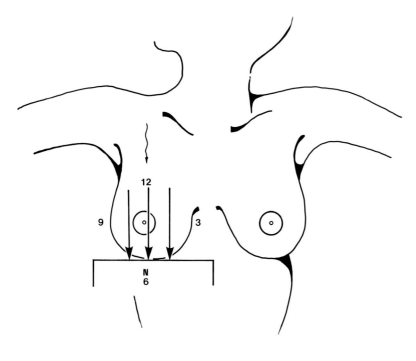

FIGURE 14-3 The craniocaudad projection superimposes superior over inferior tissue. This view shows a true orientation of the tissue to the nipple (i.e., measurement of a lesion's distance lateral or medial to the nipple is a true measurement).

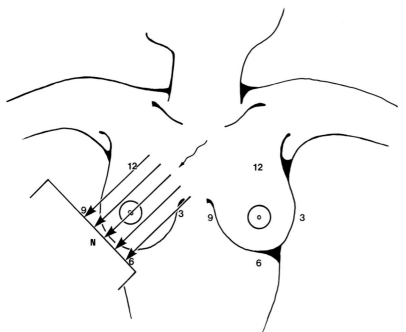

FIGURE 14-4 The 45° oblique projection superimposes medial over lateral tissue. Note that:
1. The 12:00–1:00 area in the right breast (and 11:00–12:00 in the left) is superimposed over the UOQ tissue.
2. A portion of the UIQ as it approaches 2:30–3:00 in the right breast (9:00–9:30 in the left) is actually projected below the nipple.
3. The LIQ of the breast is demonstrated free of superimposition.
4. The *lower* outer quadrant from 7:30 to 8:00 in the right and 4:30 to 5:00 in the left breast is projected *at the level of* the nipple.

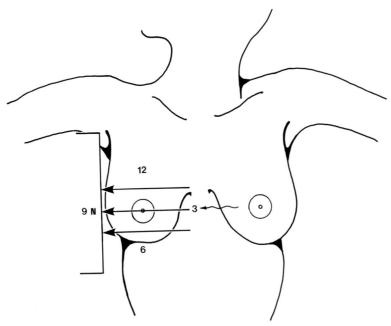

FIGURE 14-5   The true lateral projection superimposes medial over lateral tissue. This view shows a true orientation of the tissue to the nipple (i.e., measurement of a lesion's distance superior or inferior to the nipple is a true measurement). Note that:
1. A 12:00 lesion will be demonstrated free of superimposition.
2. A 6:00 lesion will be demonstrated free of superimposition.

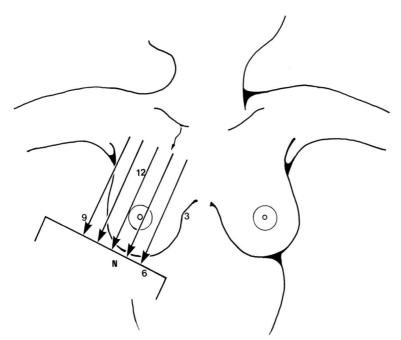

FIGURE 14-6   The 30° oblique projection superimposes superior over inferior tissue. Note that:
1. The UOQ is seen free of superimposition.
2. 12:00 lesions will be demonstrated lateral to the nipple.

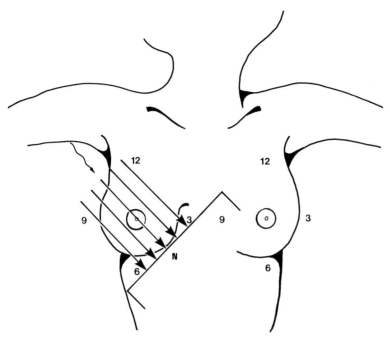

FIGURE 14-7   The reverse (lateral medial) 45° oblique projection superimposes lateral over medial tissue. Note that:

1. The UOQ 10:30 area in the right breast (UOQ 2:30 area in the left) will be projected at nipple level.
2. The *lower* inner quadrant 3:30–4:30 area in the right breast (7:30–8:30 in the left) is projected *above* or at the level of the nipple.
3. The UIQ and LOQ are projected free of superimposition.

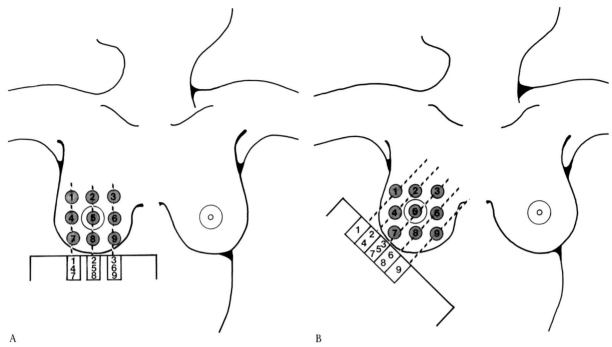

A   B

FIGURE 14-8   The lesions illustrated schematically here are arrayed in a grid corresponding to superior–mid-breast–inferior and lateral-central-medial locations. Their corresponding numbers are shown below on the film cassette outline. By following any numbered lesion from projection to projection, an appreciation of how a lesion "moves" (in relation to the nipple) can be gained. For example, lesion #3 is:

1. Projected medial to the nipple on the *craniocaudad* view (**A**).
2. Projected at the level of the nipple on the *45° oblique* view (**B**).
3. Projected superior to the nipple on the *true lateral* view (**C**). (*Note:* The lesion moved up from the 45° oblique to the lateral; this holds true for all medial lesions.)
4. Projected medial to the nipple (but in closer proximity to the nipple than on the craniocaudad view) on the *30° oblique* view (**D**).
5. Projected superior to the nipple free of superimposition on the *reverse 45° oblique* view (**E**).

In addition to illustrating "movement," these figures also demonstrate in which view a lesion is seen free of superimposition of other quadrants.

(*Figure continues.*)

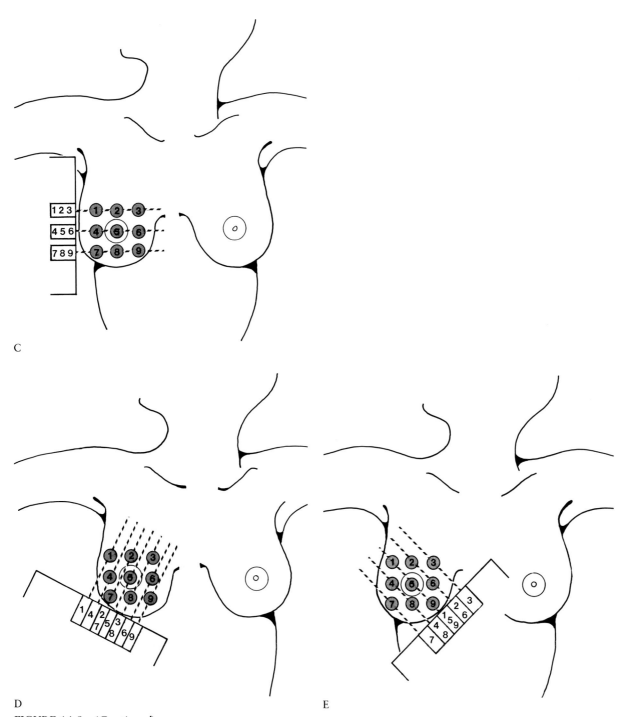

C

D

E

FIGURE 14-8   (*Continued*)

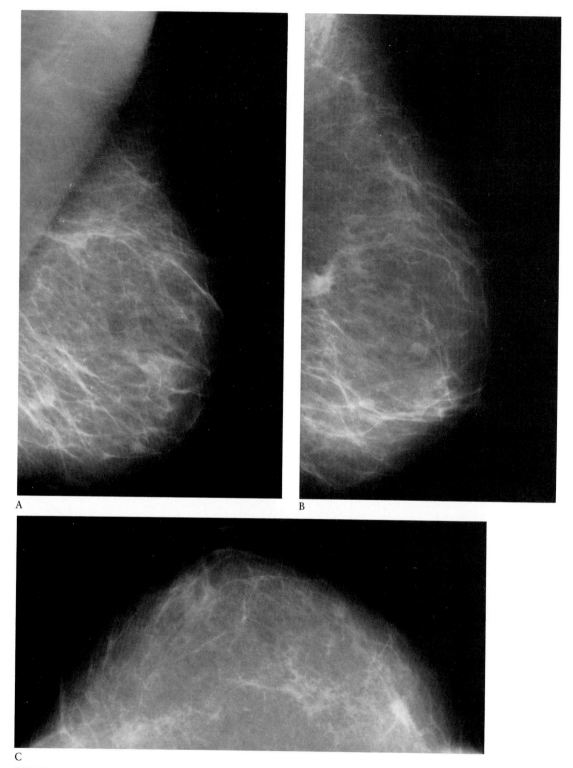

A

B

C

FIGURE 14-9   When comparing the 45° oblique projection (**A**) to the true lateral (**B**), a medial lesion will move up from its position on the 45° oblique. The craniocaudad view (**C**) is shown to verify that the lesion lies medially.

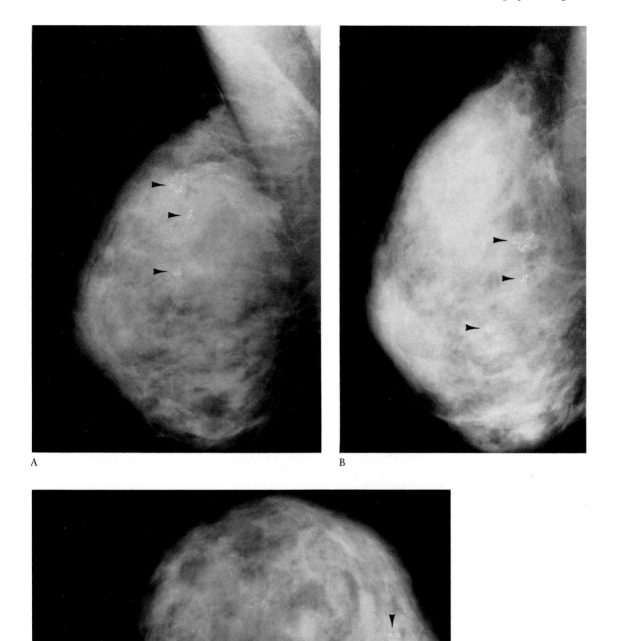

A   B

C

FIGURE 14-10   When comparing the 45° oblique projection (**A**) to the true lateral (**B**), a lateral lesion (arrows) will move down from its position on the 45° oblique. The craniocaudad view (**C**) is shown to verify that the lesion lies laterally.

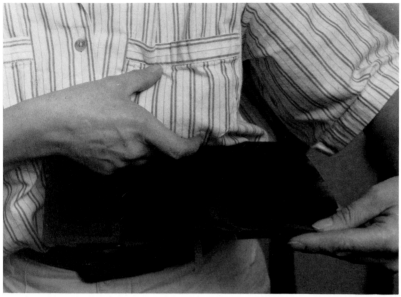

A

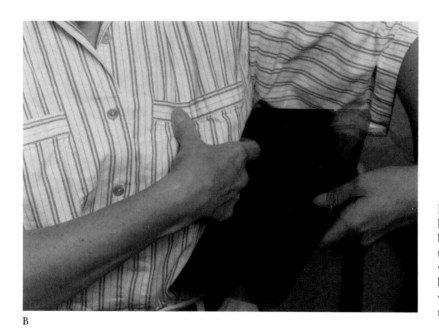

B

FIGURE 14-11 To approximate a lesion's location using one's own breast as a model, hold the image up to the body at the angle at which it was taken and follow the "lesion" back to the breast (**A**). Do the same with the second projection and correlate the findings (**B**).

move down on the lateral from its position on the (45°) oblique (Fig. 14-10).

A central lesion will have very little movement from (45°) oblique to true lateral.

Approximating Location (for Palpation and/or Extra View)

Approximating a lesion's location (or at the very least its quadrant) in the breast will guide the technologist in correlative palpation and in obtaining extra views, should they be necessary.

Two views are needed to determine approximate location. One method, and by far the simplest, is to use one's own breast as a model (regardless of size relationship). Hold one image up to the body in the angle it was taken (remember it is the nonemulsion, or shiny, side of single-emulsion films that is against the patient's body when performing the study) and follow the "lesion" back to the breast. Do the same

with the second projection and correlate the findings. In this way the lesion's approximate location can be determined (Fig. 14-11).

Approximating Location For a Lesion

When a "lesion" is first noted on one view, its approximate distance from the nipple is determined and the same plane (allowing for rotation of the nipple) is searched in the second view (Fig. 14-12). If this search does not reveal the lesion, a third view must be taken to find the lesion or to determine if the lesion is real (See Chapter 15).

Once the lesion has been found on two views, the following guidelines will help in specifying the location of an area of interest:

1. From the *craniocaudad* projection one can determine whether a lesion is *medial* or *lateral* to the nipple and its distance posterior from the nipple (Fig. 14-13A,B).
2. From the (45°) oblique projection one can determine whether a lesion is *superior* or *inferior* to the

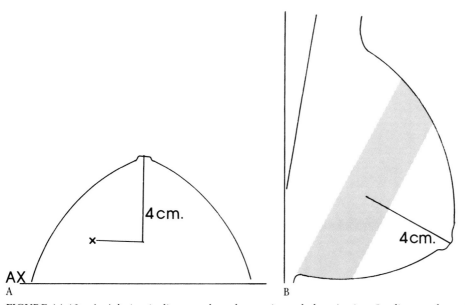

FIGURE 14-12   **A.** A lesion is discovered on the craniocaudad projection. Its distance from the nipple is determined to be 4 cm. **B.** To find the lesion on the second view (in this case a 45° oblique projection), a distance of 4 cm is measured back from the nipple; a wide area (to allow for nipple rotation) is then searched to find the lesion.

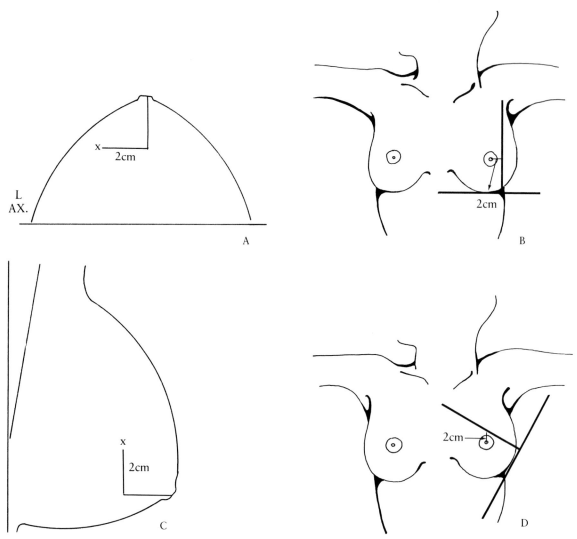

FIGURE 14-13   The craniocaudad projection will determine whether the lesion is medial or lateral and how far posterior from the nipple it lies. **A.** In this craniocaudad view the lesion is seen 2 cm back from the nipple and 2 cm lateral to the nipple. **B.** Measure 2 cm laterally from the nipple. The lesion lies somewhere along the line that represents the x-ray beam. (*Note:* superior or inferior location cannot be determined with the craniocaudad view.)

C. The 45° oblique projection will determine whether the lesion is superior or inferior to the nipple and how far posterior. In this view, the lesion is seen 2 cm back from and 2 cm above the nipple. **D.** Measure up 2 cm from the nipple. The lesion lies somewhere along the line that represents the x-ray beam. (*Note:* Medial or lateral cannot be determined with the 45° oblique view.)

E. The intersection of the two lines determined in B and D will approximate the location of the lesion within the breast.

(*Figure continues.*)

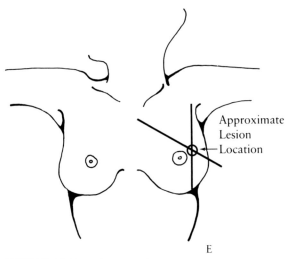

Approximate
Lesion
—Location

E

FIGURE 14-13   (*Continued*)

nipple and its distance posterior from the nipple (Fig. 14-13C,D). (True nipple orientation can only be determined with a true lateral view. Refer to Figure 14-4 for the distortion that takes place with the (45°) oblique view.)

3. A lesion will not change distance from the nipple. However, if the nipple is not in profile, this must be accounted for.

Conclusion

The skills described in this chapter are not acquired easily. However, given time, practice, and guidance from the supervising radiologist, the technologist can become adept at employing them.

15

Kathleen M. Willison

Practical Applications in Problem Solving

Detecting the suspected lesion is only half the job, proving the need for biopsy is quite another.

László Tábar

While it is the radiologist's ultimate responsibility to decide when to recommend a biopsy it is the technologist's responsibility to provide the radiologist with views necessary to make this diagnosis. The technologist working without a radiologist on site also has the added responsibilities of presenting a clear clinical picture as to correlate with the mammographic findings. A record of physical findings and history combined with an extra view if necessary can make the difference; for example, if a special coned down view of a palpable mass shows smoothly outlined tissue, the radiologist can follow it by repeating the extra view at intervals of 4–6 months. This added information can also mean saving the patient from preoperative needle localization of a "nonpalpable" lesion seen on a screening mammogram when correlation of the physical exam with a marked extra view is used to determine the location of the in fact palpable lesion. Wende W. Young, M.D., said that "We as mammographers are in a unique position to cor-

relate what we see with what we feel." It is important to take advantage of this.

A number of examples are presented in this chapter to show how various mammographic positions are applied in problem solving. Because all breasts are different and each case is unique, *no one view will address all needs and all problems.* There is more than one approach to problem solving, or more than one mammographic view that will in essence net the same results. Keeping this in mind, the best the technologist can do is:

1. Establish with the radiologist a protocol to follow when engaged in problem solving. The technologist must have a clear idea of his or her responsibilities regarding extra views and palpation.
2. Become familiar with patterns of pathology both physically and mammographically.
3. Become comfortable with the mammographic views and positions discussed in the previous chapters.
4. Recognize the orientation of breast tissue in relation to the nipple from one view to another (see Chapter 14).

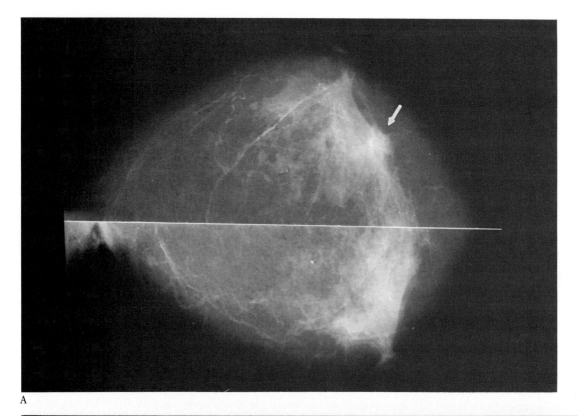

A

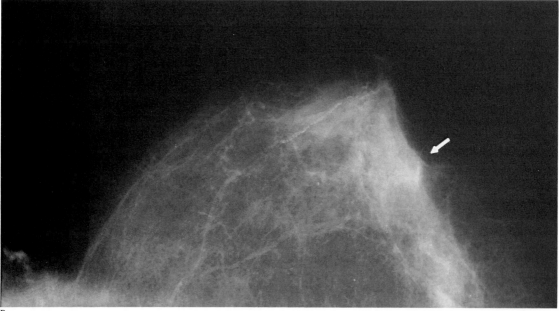

B

FIGURE 15-1   Having prior mammograms available for comparison is critical for distinguishing new lesions. A craniocaudad mammogram (**A**) demonstrates a change in the outline of the glandular tissue (arrow) in comparison to the previous mammogram 1 year ealirer (**B**). After further mammographic study, biopsy was recommended; biopsy proved carcinoma of the breast.

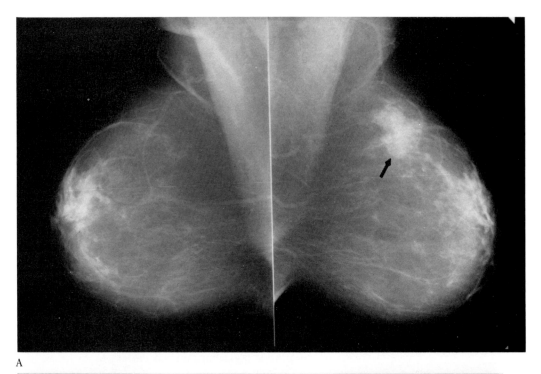

A

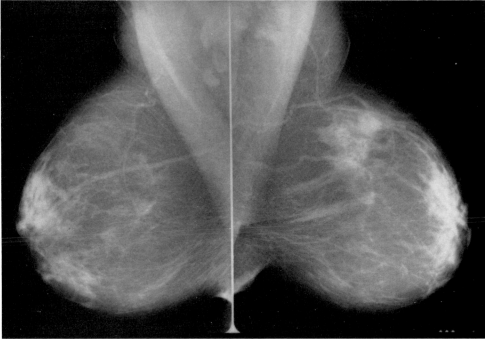

B

FIGURE 15-2   Having prior mammograms available for comparison will often eliminate the need for further study. An area of asymmetry (arrow) in the present mammogram (**A**) is shown to be unchanged in comparison to this patient's prior mammogram (**B**) one and one-half years earlier.

Establishing a Protocol

A suspected lesion will need a work-up to determine whether an interval follow-up or biopsy is necessary. Often an extra view is a part of this process. Taking into consideration the following steps in a protocol will help in the "what to do next" dilemma.

1. Obtain patient history
2. Review prior mammograms
3. Perform correlative physical exam
4. Determine whether the "lesion" is real (in the case of mass effect)
5. Perform ultrasound (if available)
6. Obtain extra views

Not all of these steps will be applicable in every case, nor will they necessarily be used in the order listed. Again, tailoring the exam to each patient's case becomes important to the outcome. The steps taken depend on the protocol set up by the radiologist and the technologist.

History

A clear clinical history should include at least the following information:

1. Reason or symptoms that prompted the mammogram.
2. Prior family history of breast cancer, including age of occurrence.
3. Prior biopsy (biopsy sites should be marked on a diagram and dated).
4. Nipple inversions that are recent.
5. Nipple discharge—spontaneous or expressed, bilateral or unilateral, color and how long the discharge has been present.
6. Moles and birthmarks (should be diagrammed).
7. All medications, including hormonal intake.
8. Date of last menstrual period.
9. Caffeine ingestion.
10. Prior infection.
11. Prior mammograms (where and when).
12. Recent or old trauma.

In addition to gathering the above information, it is critical to talk with the patient. Make sure she has not excluded a symptom that may indicate a problem; she may have hesitated from fear or because her own physician was not concerned about the area. The patient is usually the one who is most familiar with her body. It is essential to ask her if *she* has any concerns about her breasts. It is part of the technologist's responsibilities to create an atmosphere that allows the patient to speak about her fears. Otherwise, important clues to the correct diagnosis may be overlooked.

Prior Mammograms

It is recommended that prior mammograms be available for comparison with the present study, preferably at the time the patient is being seen. This is critical for distinguishing new lesions (Fig. 15-1) and for reassurance regarding normal variations in breast tissue. Comparison of old and present mammograms can determine the need for an extra view (Fig. 15-2). A look at the patient's prior films for breast size and composition will also aid in determining optimum technique for the patient's tissue.

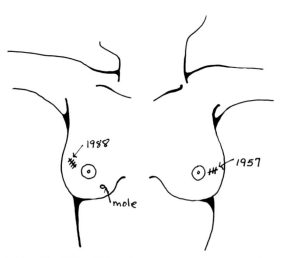

FIGURE 15-3 Skin changes (e.g., previous biopsies, moles, and scars) should be noted and diagrammed prior to mammography.

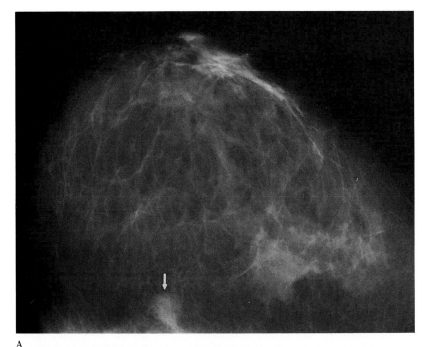

A

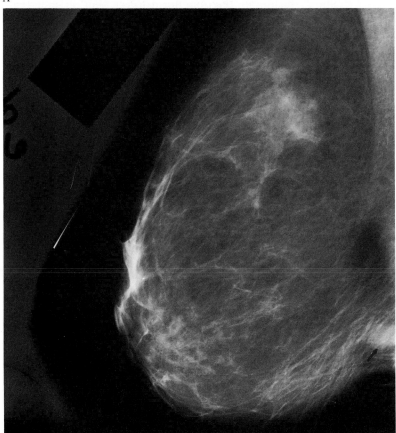

B

FIGURE 15-4 Physical inspection of the lower half of this woman's breast revealed an infected sebaceous cyst correlating to the density seen mammographically on two views (arrows).

Physical Exam

The physical exam is twofold and involves inspection as well as palpation.

Inspection

Before performing the mammogram, the technologist should diagram any skin changes or abnormalities (Fig. 15-3). Many skin abnormalities can look suspicious mammographically. After the mammogram, inspection involves correlating an area seen on mammography with what is seen on the skin (Figs. 15-4 and 15-5). Findings should be diagrammed.

Palpation

Before an extra view is obtained, even for the smallest of lesions, a correlative physical exam should be performed. If a lesion detected on a screening mammogram is palpable in retrospect, deciding on an extra view, if it is necessary, becomes easier (Fig. 15-6). Also correlation of what is seen with what is felt often eliminates the need for a needle localization prior to biopsy.

When the lesion is seen on two views, determine the quadrant and approximate time (see Chapter 14) and palpate this area. If it is seen on one view only, that one-half of the breast should be palpated. If the lesion is found to be palpable, this eliminates the need for another mammogram to "find" it; however, another view might be needed to prove its need for biopsy. In most cases a tangential view will yield the most information about a palpable suspect lesion.

Wende Logan-Young, M.D., reported that, regarding "nonpalpable" cancers found by mammogram, most were determined to be palpable in retrospect; many are palpable only with the patient upright, especially those in the upper one half of the breast. Logan-Young emphasizes the need to palpate in both the *upright* and *supine* positions. Keep in mind that very early malignant lesions can feel benign (i.e., soft, easily movable, not fixed to the skin or underlying tissue).

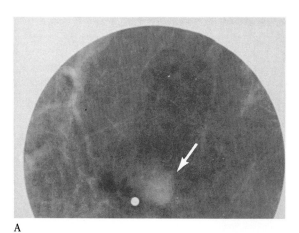

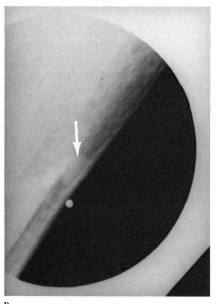

A   B

FIGURE 15-5   **A.** Biopsy was recommended of this mass density (arrow) based on the mammogram only. The patient sought a second opinion prior to biopsy. The technologist performing a magnified view of this lesion noted a sebaceous cyst on the skin at the area of interest. A tangential view (**B**) proved this lesion to be only a sebaceous cyst.

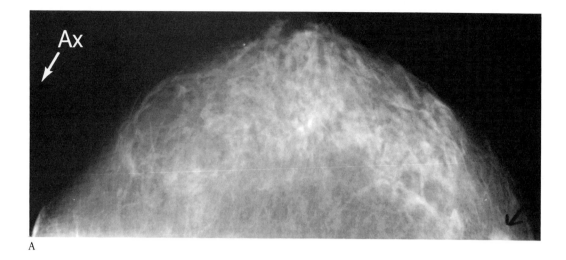

A

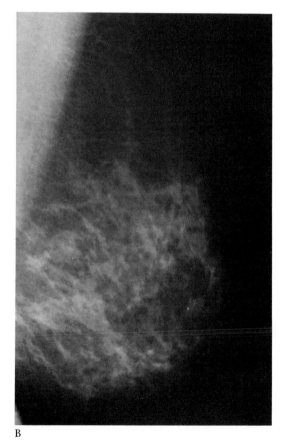

B

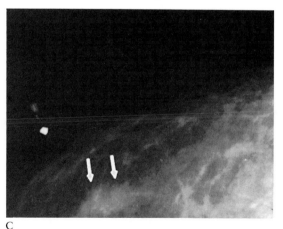

C

FIGURE 15-6   A correlative physical exam can help determine which extra view will best demonstrate a lesion. **A.** This left craniocaudad mammogram exhibits a density posteriorly and medially. **B.** The 45° oblique proved inconclusive. Palpation of the medial half of this woman's breast revealed a lump in the upper inner quadrant at about 10:30. **C.** A lead BB (arrowhead) was placed just posterior to the palpable mass, not directly over it (to avoid superimposing the marker over the lesion). A reverse 45° oblique magnified tangential view revealed the palpable mass (arrows) to be the ill-defined density seen originally on the craniocaudad mammogram.

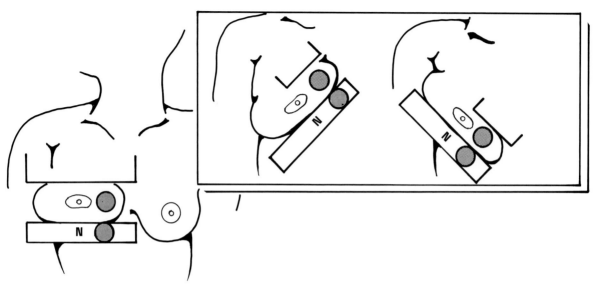

FIGURE 15-7   Cancer will keep its shape; it may be obscured by other glandular structures from view to view, or distorted because of its distance from the film, but it will not flatten under compression to the same extent as glandular tissue.

Mass Effect (Pseudo-Carcinoma) Versus Real Lesion

Overlap of ductal structures, the effects of Cooper's ligaments on tissue, and blood vessels coursing through the breast all contribute to the mammographic finding known as "pseudo-carcinoma" (mass effect). To decide whether a mass is a true lesion, keep the following criteria in mind:

A cancer mass will keep its shape; it may be obscured by other glandular structures from view to view, or distorted because of its distance from the film, but it will not flatten under compression to the extent that glandular tissue does. (Figs. 15-7, 15-8, and 15-9).

In some cases correlation of the craniocaudad and the (45°) oblique projections is enough to prove whether a "lesion" is real or is merely tissue overlap (Figs. 15-10 and 15-11). However, it is critical to note that *central* to *medial* lesions seen on the *craniocaudad* projection and *superior* lesions seen on the 45° *oblique* projection can often be obscured or distorted on the opposing view. This can be a result of the distance from the lesion to the film (geometric blurring) or tissue overlap. Difference in compression from one view to the next will be a factor as well. In such cases an extra view must be taken (Fig. 15-12). The following criteria will help in determining which view to obtain to prove a lesion is mass effect.

Lesion in a Fatty Breast

Large Lesion   A large lesion in a fatty breast cannot hide. A right-angle view will determine whether the "lesion" is mass effect or a true lesion (Fig. 15-13).

Small Lesion   Because it is so easy to "lose" a small lesion with too much rotation of the C-arm, a slight oblique angulation of 10–15° in one or both directions* from the position in which the lesion is best seen is used to determine whether the lesion is real (Figs. 15-14 and 15-15). The same results can be obtained in most cases with a rolled view.

*A slight oblique view is taken in one direction; if the area still looks worrisome, then a slight oblique view in the opposite direction is obtained.

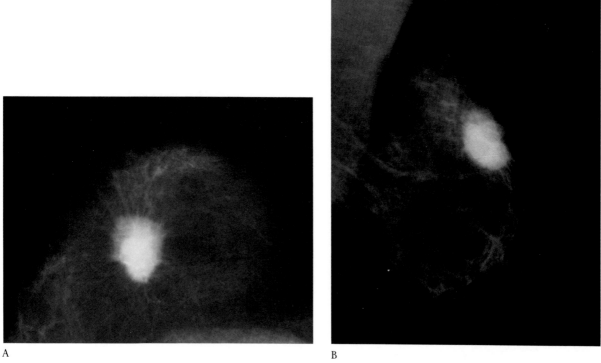

A   B

FIGURE 15-8   This left two-view mammogram provides a dramatic example of a cancer not spreading out under compression. Despite the use of vigorous compression in two directions, it holds its shape.

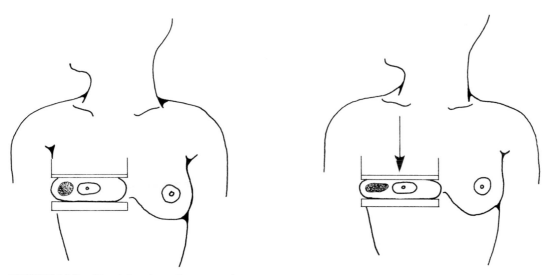

FIGURE 15-9   Glandular tissue flattens with vigorous compression.

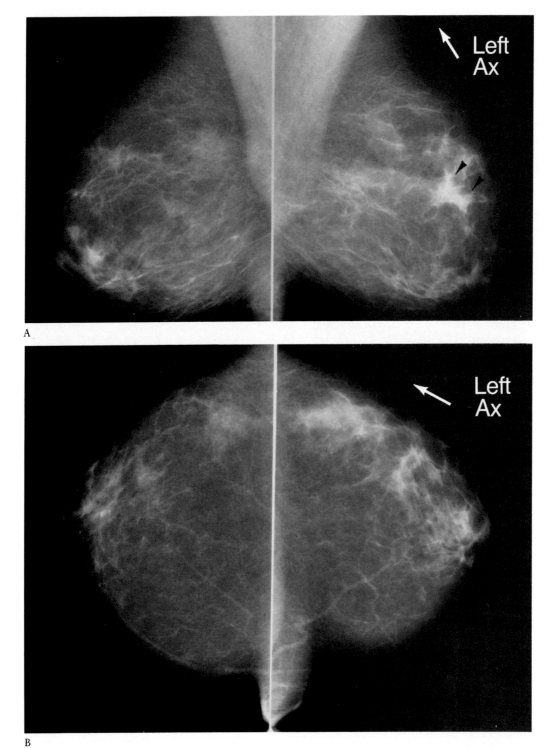

A

B

FIGURE 15-10   This four-view mammogram shows a large area of asymmetry (arrowheads) on the left 45° oblique view. (A). Correlation with the left craniocaudad view (B) shows that there is a greater amount of glandular tissue in the left breast as compared to the right and the lesion seen on the 45° oblique is not real, but a mass effect due to overlapped tissue.

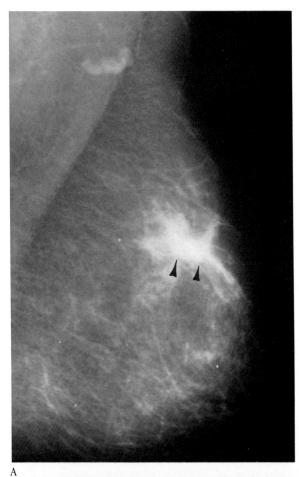

A

FIGURE 15-11 **A.** This left 45° oblique view shows a large area (arrowheads) that was asymmetric in comparison with the other breast. **B.** The craniocaudad view shows this to be mass effect due to overlapped tissue.

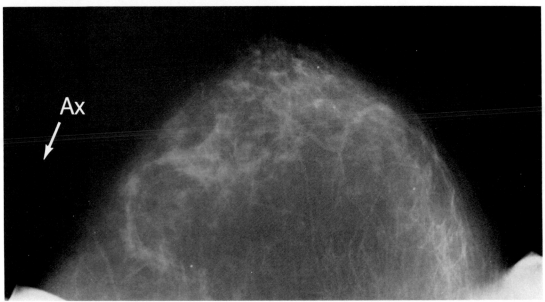

B

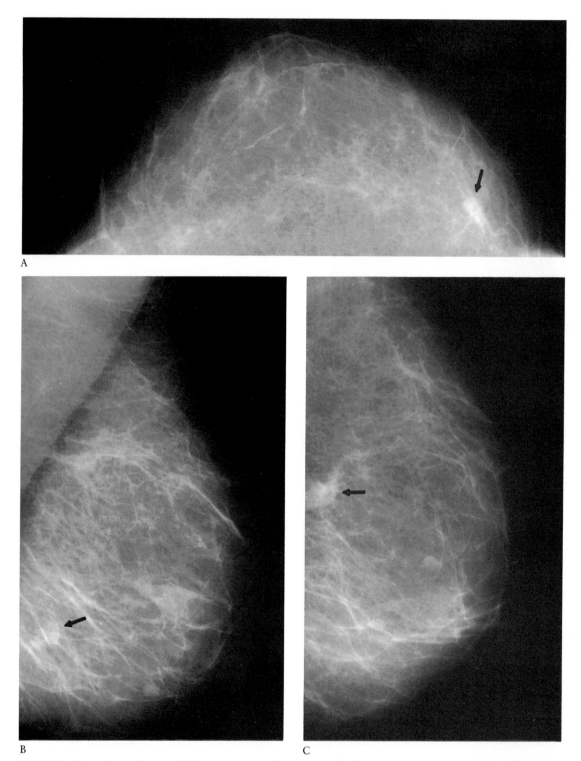

FIGURE 15-12   Central to medial lesions seen on the craniocaudad projection can be obscured on the oblique projection. A left craniocaudad mammogram (**A**) reveals a lesion (arrow) medially that is virtually obscured on the left 45° oblique view (arrow) (**B**). **C**. A third *lateromedial lateral* view (to bring the lesion in closer proximity to the film for optimum detail) clearly demonstrates this lesion (arrow).

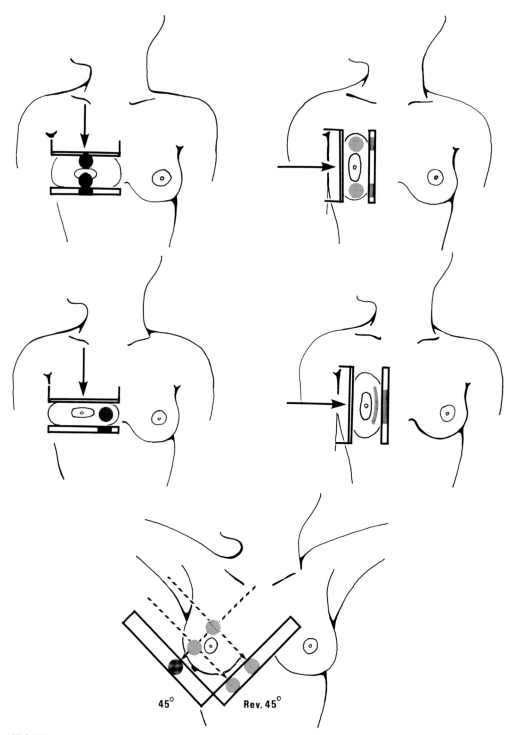

FIGURE 15-13   When determining whether a large "lesion" in a fatty breast is real, a right-angle view will help flatten (**B**) or separate (**A** and **C**) overlapped structures.

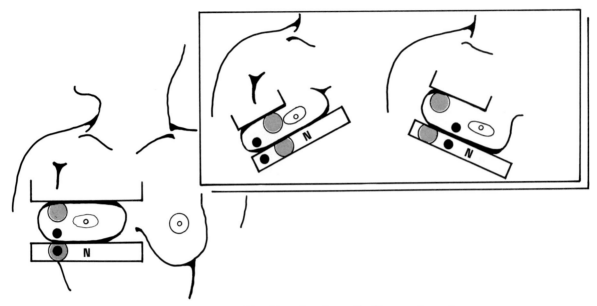

FIGURE 15-14   Slight oblique views at 10–15° in either direction will offset overlapped structures.

Lesion in a Dense Breast

Large or Small Mass   In dense tissue a small or a large lesion becomes obscured very easily. A slight oblique angulation of 10–15° in one or both directions* from the position in which the lesion is best seen will help in determining whether the lesion is real (Figs. 15-16 and 15-17). The same results can be obtained, in most cases, with a rolled view.

Ultrasound

If ultrasound is available it may very well eliminate the need for an extra view if it can definitely identify a lesion.

Extra Views

There are six primary purposes of an extra view:

1. To Demonstrate a Portion of the Breast Not Imaged on the Two-View Mammogram

(see Chapter 13)

2. To Determine If a "Mass" is Real

(as discussed above)

3. To Assist the Radiologist in Preoperative Needle Localization

Whenever a nonpalpable lesion is detected, a true lateral view with the nipple in profile is automatically obtained. A true lateral view in conjunction with the craniocaudad view will give true orientation of the lesion to the nipple.

4. To determine the Location of a Nonpalpable Lesion Visualized Only on One View

The radiologist cannot recommend biopsy of a nonpalpable lesion seen only on one view. If correlative palpation is negative and the "lesion" is real, additional views need to be obtained to find and locate the lesion. There are no set rules for "finding" a lesion on a third or sometimes subsequent views. Acquainting oneself with each mammographic projection and the area of the breast demonstrated with each view (see Chapter 14) will help in choosing the projection that will "find" a lesion seen only on one view (Figs. 15-18 and 15-19).

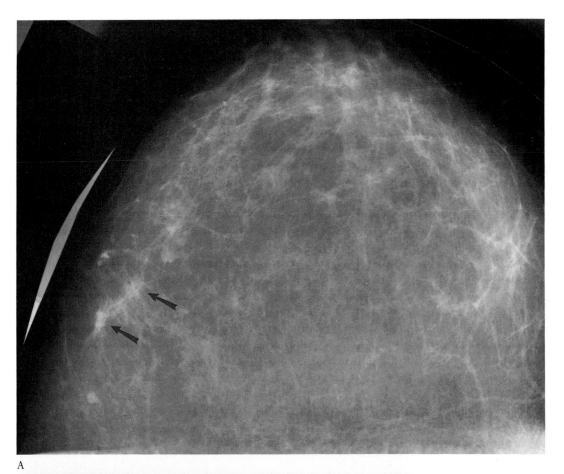

A

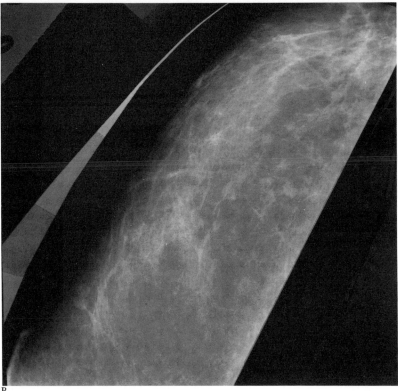

B

FIGURE 15-15   A slight oblique view at 10–15° can separate overlapped structures. **A.** Two stellate mass densities (arrows) are seen on this craniocaudad mammograms. **B.** A slight oblique view of 10–15° proves these areas to be pseudo-cancers.

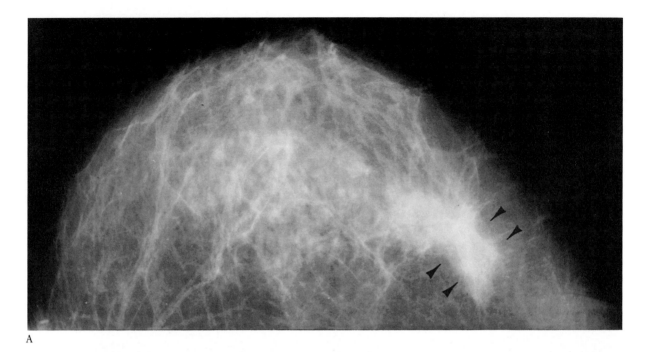

A

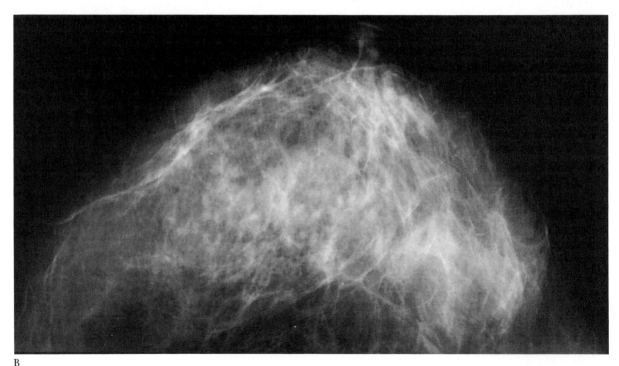

B

FIGURE 15-16   **A.** A craniocaudad mammogram exhibiting a large stellate "mass" medially (arrowheads) in a dense breast. **B.** An oblique view at 15° shows this "mass" to be overlapped structures.

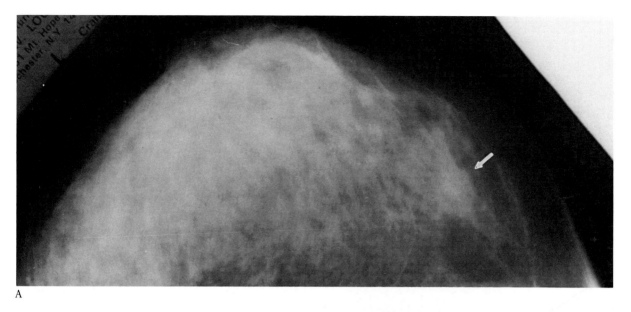

A

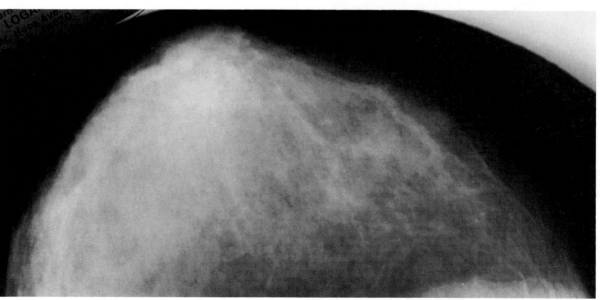

B

FIGURE 15-17 **A.** This craniocaudad view exhibited a mass density medially (arrow). **B.** A reverse oblique view at 15° shows this to be a pseudo-carcinoma.

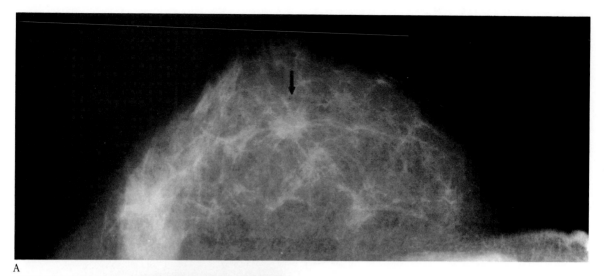

A

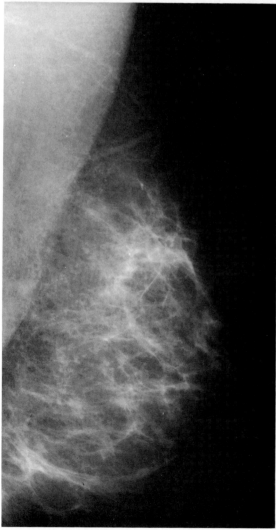

B

FIGURE 15-18 **A.** The left craniocaudad mammogram demonstrates a stellate lesion. **B.** The 45° oblique view is inconclusive for abnormality.

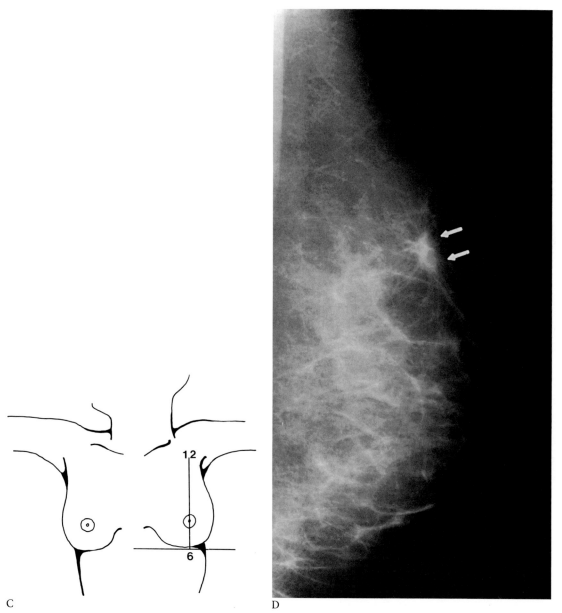

C   D

FIGURE 15-18   (*Continued*) **C.** A schematic illustrates the information obtained from the craniocaudad view. The lesion lies directly behind the nipple. It must lie somewhere along the vertical line, but whether it lies superior or inferior to the nipple cannot be determined. **D.** A true lateral view (which best shows the 12:00–6:00 areas) demonstrates the lesion (arrows).

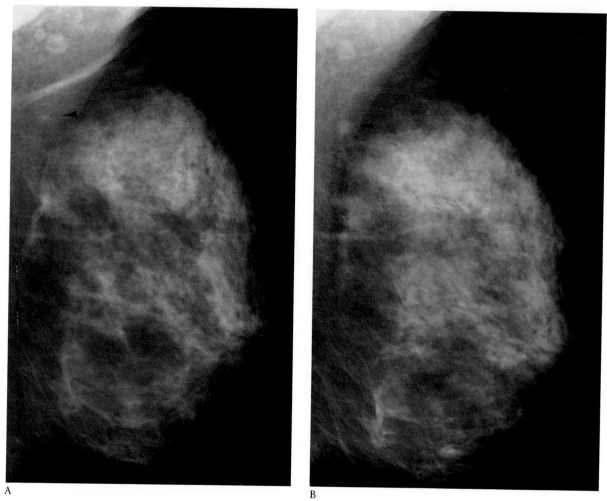

A   B

FIGURE 15-19   **B.** This 45° oblique mammogram demonstrates a stellate lesion that has increased in size since the mammogram 2 years earlier (arrowheads) (**A**). The craniocaudad view (not shown) did not reveal the lesion. From the 45° oblique, it can only be determined that the lesion lies superior to the nipple.

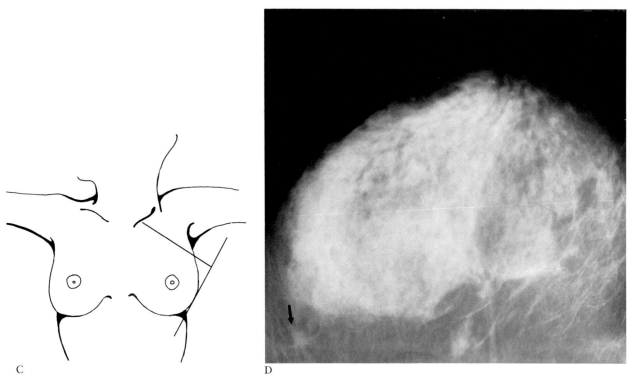

C   D

FIGURE 15-19   *(Continued)* **C.** A schematic demonstrates the information obtained from the 45° oblique view. The lesion lies superior to the nipple somewhere along the slanted line. The first thought is that this lesion lies in the upper outer quadrant of the breast because that is where the majority of carcinomas occur. **D.** A 30° oblique view, which best demonstrates this area free of superimposition, demonstrates the lesion (arrow). Had the lesion not been seen on this view, a lateromedial lateral would best image the 11:00–1:00 area high on the chest wall. This lesion was positive for carcinoma.

5. To Determine Radiographically Whether a Nonpalpable Suspicious Area Fits the Criteria for Biopsy

In order to determine whether a suspicious-looking area on a mammogram fits the criteria for biopsy, the radiologist must look at the borders of a mass or evaluate the characteristics of calcifications. This assessment must be handled differently for masses and calcifications.

Calcifications   The radiologist looks for certain criteria when considering biopsy of calcifications. The technologist should become acquainted with the following methods to aid the radiologist in obtaining the information necessary to decide whether to perform a biopsy or follow the patient radiographically.

Coned-down magnification—A coned-down magnified view will better delineate the characteristics of the calcifications and the surrounding tissue.

A tangential view—A tangential view is obtained to see if the calcifications are in the skin (Fig. 15-20).

Magnification of the contralateral breast—This is accomplished to see if there are calcifications of the same type in both breasts. If there are bilateral similar calcifications, they are most likely benign.

A true lateral view—This view is obtained to determine if the calcifications show fluid levels. This type of benign calcification is termed "milk of calcium." If the calcifications lie laterally, a mediolateral lateral projection would best demonstrate it; if the calcifications lie medially, a lateromedial lateral is obtained.

Masses   As with calcifications, there are certain criteria that a radiologist looks for when considering biopsy of a mass (Fig. 15-21). The technologist should become acquainted with the following methods to aid the radiologist in obtaining the information necessary to decide whether to perform a biopsy or follow the patient radiographically:

Slight obliques, rolled views, spot compression—These are obtained to determine whether the lesion is real or represents overlapped tissue.

Right-angle view—This is obtained to determine whether the lesion is real or represents overlapped tissue.

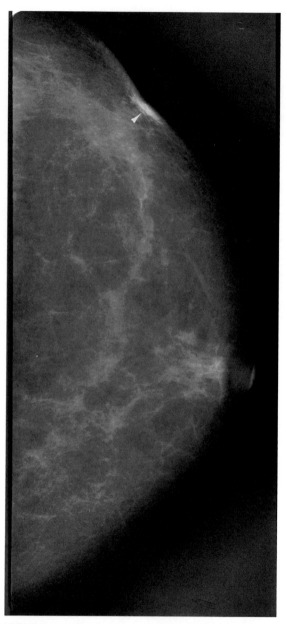

FIGURE 15-20   A tangential view demonstrates this calcium (arrowhead) seen on the craniocaudad and 45° oblique projections to be in the skin.

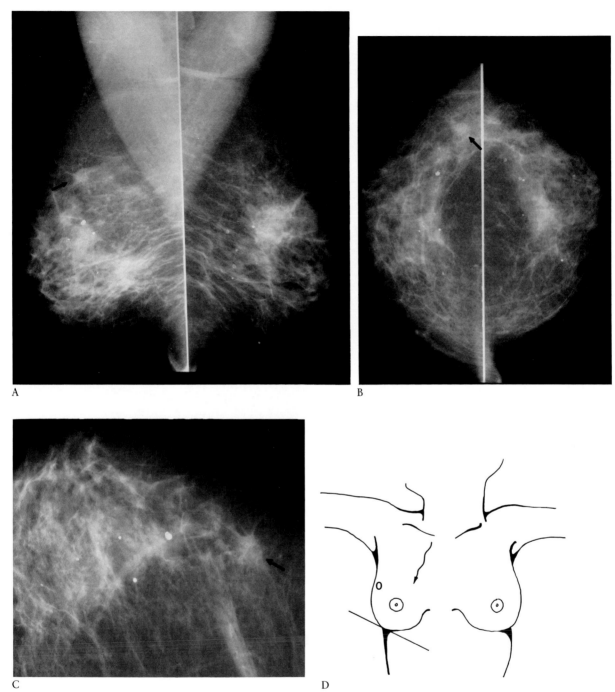

A

B

C

D

FIGURE 15-21   Even when a mass (arrows) is imaged on two views (**A** and **B**), another projection might be required for the radiologist to be comfortable recommending biopsy. In this case a lesion is seen in the upper outer quadrant at about 10:30. **C.** A 30° oblique view (which images this area free of superimposition) was taken yielding more information about this lesion. **D.** A schematic of the location of the lesion (0) and the angle of the film tray for the 30° oblique. This was cancer upon biopsy.

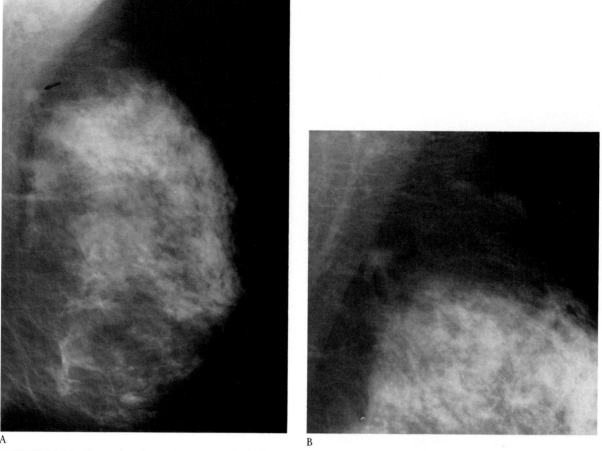

A   B

FIGURE 15-22   Repeating the projection in which the lesion was best seen while incorporating magnification
will yield necessary information about the characteristics of a mass. **A.** This 45° oblique projection shows a
stellate mass (arrow). **B.** A repeat 45° oblique was performed employing magnification. The magnified mass
shows characteristics suspicious for carcinoma. This was cancer upon biopsy.

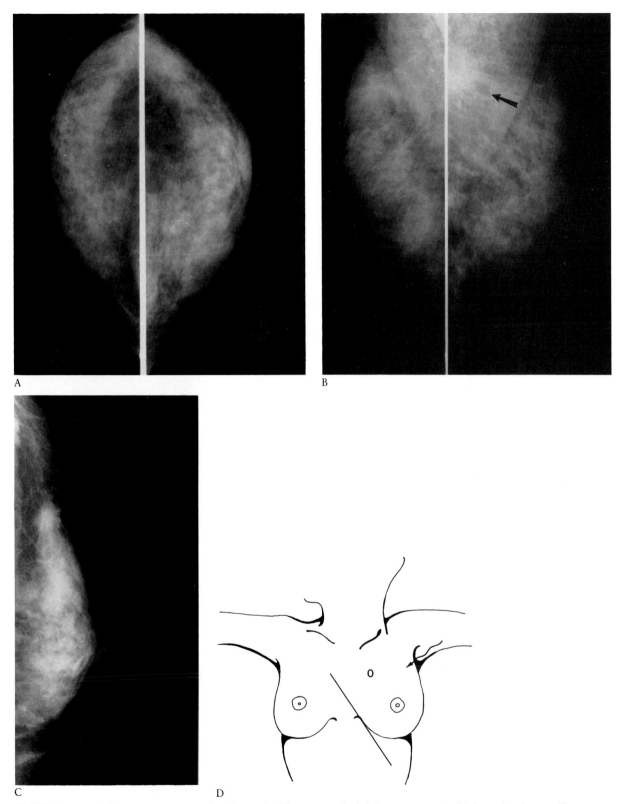

FIGURE 15-23   This patient presented with a palpable mass in the left breast at 10:30, high on the chest wall. The four-view mammogram (**A** and **B**) demonstrated a portion of this mass (arrow). **C.** A tangential view of the palpable area demonstrates the mass in its entirety (arrow). **D.** A schematic of the location of the lesion (0) and the angle of the film tray for the tangential view.

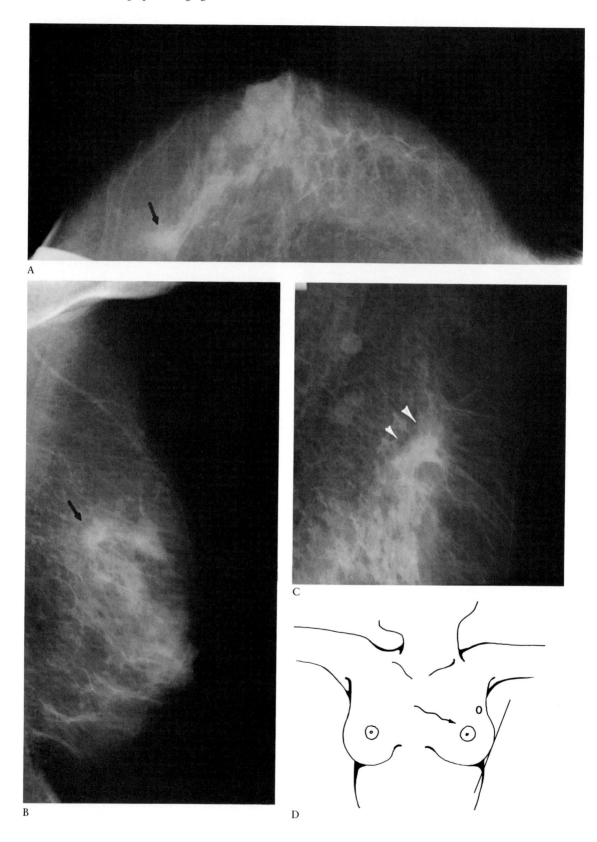

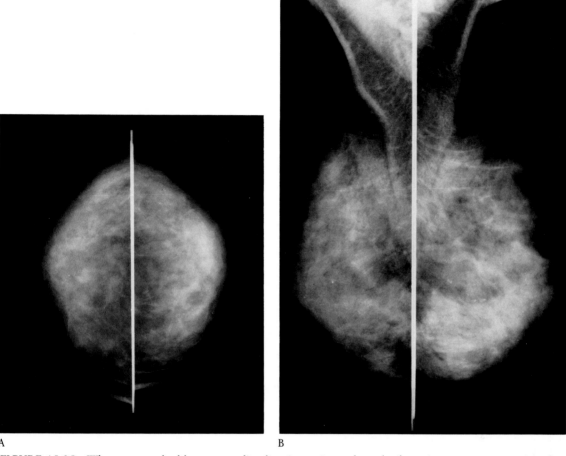

A   B

FIGURE 15-25   When a nonpalpable mass or dimpling is not imaged on the four-view mammogram (**A** and **B**) it *must* be imaged with an extra view. This patient presented with dimpling of the skin in the left breast in the 5:30 area.

FIGURE 15-24   A mass density (arrow) is visualized on both the craniocaudad (**A**) and 45° oblique (**B**) projections of this left breast. To better delineate the borders of this nonpalpable mass, the approximate location was determined (about 1:30 in the upper outer quadrant) and a 60° tangential view (**C**) was obtained, demonstrating this lesion (arrowheads) to be suspicious for carcinoma. This was cancer upon biopsy. **D.** A schematic showing the location of the lesion (0) and the angle of the film tray for the tangential view.

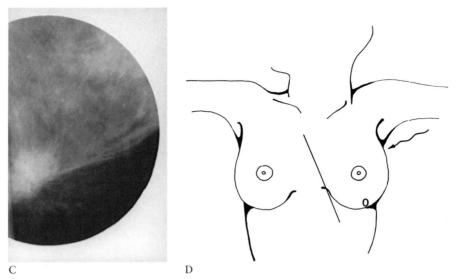

C   D

FIGURE 15-25 *(Continued)* **C.** A tangential view (a reverse 70° oblique) demonstrates an underlying mass suspicious for carcinoma. A schematic demonstrating the location of the lesion (**D**) and the angle of the film tray for the tangential view. This was cancer upon biopsy.

Coned-down magnified view—This view is obtained to better delineate the borders of a mass. It is usually made in the projection on which the lesion was best demonstrated in the two-view study (Fig. 15-22).

Tangential view—This view is obtained to better delineate the borders of a mass. The lesion must be palpable or evident on two views in order to obtain a tangential view. Magnification will always enhance this view; but when magnification is unavailable or unobtainable because of breast thickness or density, a tangential view will still offer the most information about a mass (Figs. 15-23 and 15-24).

6. To Determine Radiographically Whether a Palpable Lump or Dimpling Not Evident on the Two-View Mammogram Fits the Criteria for Biopsy

If a woman presents with a palpable mass that is not visualized on the mammogram, *an extra view must be obtained.* This is the most critical aspect of the technologists job. Taking an extra view can eliminate needless biopsies as well as find carcinomas. The best view to obtain is a coned-down magnified tangential view, because it shows the area free of superimposition (Fig. 15-25). A coat hanger view will help image "slippery" lesions that will not stay under the compression plate.

IV
Special Procedures

16

Kathleen M.
Willison and
Valerie Fink
Andolina

Special Procedures*

Ultrasonography

Ultrasound's value in breast imaging lies in its ability to distinguish a cyst from a solid lesion. Although it can identify a solid mass, it cannot determine whether the lesion is benign or malignant. For this reason, every solid mass must be viewed as a possible cancer until proven otherwise. In addition, sonography can reveal an intracystic lesion and localize a "nonpalpable" mammographically detected abnormality.

Indications for ultrasonography are:

1. A palpable mass and a mammogram that reveals dense glandular tissue or a smoothly outlined mass.
2. A nonpalpable radiographically detected mass.

Ultrasound is not used for screening because it is not sufficiently sensitive. Only when examining dense breast tissue does ultrasound's accuracy even begin

*Portions of this chapter are directly excerpted from the upcoming book *Breast Cancer: A Practical Guide to Diagnosis* by Wende Westinghouse Logan-Young and Nancy Yanes Hoffman.

to approach that of mammography in detecting a hidden cancer.[1–6] Mammography-positive/ultrasound-negative cancers are generally small, nonpalpable, and without regional lymph node spread; ultrasound-positive/mammography-negative cancers usually are larger, palpable, and more apt to have metastasized.[2–5,7,8] Mammography and physical examination are a much more effective diagnostic combination than ultrasound and physical examination in evaluating symptomatic and asymptomatic patients.

Cyst Aspiration

When and Why to Aspirate a Cyst

A cyst may be aspirated for one or more of six reasons:

1. When a patient is uncomfortable because a cyst is under pressure, it can be aspirated to give her relief. If a patient comes in for a mammogram and she has a large painful cyst, sonograph the cyst, drain it, and do the mammogram afterward. That

275

way the study is better: the tissue surrounding the cyst is more clearly visible, and the patient can tolerate vigorous compression better because she no longer is in pain.

2. When a cyst occupies so much space that it interferes with an accurate physical examination.
3. When the referring physician or the patient thinks that there may be a cancer. Aspirating a cyst quickly and simply alleviates the patient's discomfort and allays the referring physician's and the patient's fears.
4. When the sonogram reveals a localized area of internal echogenicity suggestive of an intracystic mass.
5. When the sonogram discloses a lesion with definite internal echogenicity throughout. These echoes could be either a sign of internal cellular proteinaceous debris or an indication that the lesion is a soft tissue mass.
6. When a mass is less than 5 mm in diameter, but the sonographic resolution does not permit differentiation between a small cyst and a soft tissue density.

Cyst Aspiration Procedure

During cyst aspiration (usually performed by the radiologist) the patient is most often supine, but occasionally she is asked to roll on her side because a lateral cyst is easier to palpate and fixate when the patient is in this position. Before aspirating the cyst, wipe the skin with alcohol. To immobilize the lesion, hold it firmly between the index and third finger of one hand while the other hand quickly introduces a 23-gauge butterfly needle into the center of the cyst to deter it from sliding away. At the same time, an assistant provides negative pressure with a 20-ml syringe. As the fluid is extracted, gently press the cyst to empty it. As the cyst collapses, the needle passes into the opposite cyst wall. Pull the needle back several millimeters into the cyst again, while the assistant maintains negative pressure. By doing this, a few more milliliters of fluid can usually be obtained. When no further fluid remains, withdraw the needle from the patient's breast.

To prevent bleeding, firmly press the aspirated area for several minutes. Although a 23-gauge needle rarely causes bleeding, thwarting it is important: bleeding could form a palpable hematoma and con-

fuse the issue for the clinician. Once the bleeding has definitely stopped, cover the area with a bandage.

Pneumocystography

Ultrasonography usually provides enough information to judge whether the breast is harboring an intracystic lesion. Occasionally, however, ultrasonography lacks the resolution to detect a subtle abnormality within a cyst. When ultrasound's resolution does not suffice, the cyst is aspirated, the aspirate is sent to the cytology laboratory for analysis, and then pneumocystography is performed. Its resolution is superior to that of ultrasound.

The indications for pneumocystography are as follows:

1. If ultrasound shows an intracystic lesion.
2. If the patient has a palpable cyst that ultrasound reveals to be solitary and larger than 1.5 cm.
3. If fluid rapidly reaccumulates in a cyst (within 2 months).
4. If the cyst aspirate contains bloody fluid and the patient has no history of trauma or previous aspiration.

Pneumocystography Procedure

Pneumocystography is a simple procedure, performed in much the same manner as cyst aspiration with one exception: before removing the needle from the cyst, replace the aspirated fluid with the same volume of air. After this, perform a craniocaudad and a *lateral* view mammogram. Most of the time introducing air produces no discomfort. If the patient feels uncomfortable, aspirate some of the air to relieve her, because it requires a week for all the air to be absorbed.

Fine-Needle Aspiration Cytology

Fine-needle aspiration cytology (FNAC) is a procedure in which a small amount of cells are aspirated from a lesion with a small-gauge needle. These cells are then sent for cytologic evaluation.

The indications for FNAC are as follows:

1. When carcinoma is strongly suspected. If the cytologic examination verifies the presence of malignant cells, the surgeon can discuss options for treatment with the patient before her surgery. The surgeon then can bypass lumpectomy and proceed directly to wedge resection or mastectomy.
2. When the patient's screening mammogram reveals a benign-appearing mass or area of asymmetric tissue.
3. When the sonographic appearance of a problematic area is not definitely characteristic of either a cyst or a solid mass.
4. When the patient's clinical examination discloses smooth elastic thickening of the glandular tissue that is more likely to be produced by increased hormonal levels, but might be caused by a diffuse intraductal carcinoma or a deep-seated cancer buried in glandular tissue.
5. When certain benign conditions alter the patient's physical examination. Such conditions include:
Infection
Burn
Contusion
Postsurgical change
Augmentation mammoplasty
Spontaneous fat necrosis
Incipient fibrocystic disease
Mondor's disease (thrombosis of a vein in the breast)
Weight gain or loss
Gynecomastia
Sebaceous cyst
Lipoma
Hamartoma
Fibrous disease
Fibroadenoma
Papilloma
Autoimmune disease
Caffeine consumption
Radiation therapy
Medications

It should be stressed that the decision to perform a biopsy or not is made based on the mammogram, ultrasound (if applicable), and physical exam, before FNAC is completed. FNAC is used to back the decision.

FNAC Procedure

For FNAC, the patient can be seated or supine, whichever position is best for the radiologist to palpate the lesion and fix it in place; usually she is in the supine position. No local anesthesia is used for FNAC. Desensitizing the area would necessitate introducing another needle into the breast, which would be as bothersome as the needle itself. Holding the needle with the dominant hand, the radiologist takes the lesion between the index and third fingers of the other hand, fixes it firmly in place, and pulls the skin tightly over the lesion to secure it and prevent it from sliding when the needle is inserted. If the lesion is small and slippery, the radiologist can prop the fourth finger of the hand grasping the needle against the far side of the lesion to keep it from slipping away.

The radiologist wipes the skin with alcohol and quickly inserts a disposable, 2-cm long, 23-gauge butterfly needle through the skin and into the area of palpable abnormality. An assistant holds a 20-ml syringe attached to the tubing of the butterfly needle. As soon as the needle passes through the skin, the assistant pulls the plunger back almost to the end of the barrel and holds it there until the aspiration is completed. The 20-ml syringe is necessary to attain strong negative pressure to draw the cellular material into the lumen. With the mass held firmly in place, the radiologist moves the needle back and forth 10 to 20 times while angling it to sample cellular material from all areas of the mass. With this maneuver, enough cellular material can usually be procured to prepare two slides for cytologic analysis. If the lesion is large, the radiologist should try to obtain cells from its periphery, because the cells in the center of a cancer tend to be more necrotic and thus more difficult for the cytologist to interpret.

When the radiologist finishes moving the needle back and forth, the assistant releases the syringe's negative pressure slowly and smoothly over a period of 2 seconds. Withdrawing the syringe slowly is important because releasing pressure suddenly might force the cells back through the needle. Only after the release of negative pressure does the radiologist withdraw the needle from the breast. The assistant applies firm pressure to the needle site for several minutes. The firm pressure is exceedingly important to prevent hematoma, which could obscure the border of the original lump.

In the meantime, the radiologist quickly detaches the syringe from the butterfly tubing, fills the syringe with air, and expels the cells from the needle onto the clear end of a slide that is frosted at one end for labeling. The radiologist repeats this process twice to express the remainder of the material onto a second slide.

To smear the cellular material, the radiologist touches the cellular-material sides of the two slides to each other and pulls them apart with only minimal pressure. This done, the slides are turned back-to-back with the cellular material on the outside, and placed in a bottle of 95% ethanol (the same kind of bottle used for cervical Papanicolaou smears). To prevent the cells from air-drying, which might distort the nucleic parameters and impede accurate cytologic interpretation,[9,10] the radiologist must prepare the slides swiftly.

The patient undergoing FNAC may occasionally complain of discomfort, especially if she has a mass that is close to the nipple where there are more nerve endings. Nevertheless, the FNAC needle is only inside her breast for approximately 5 seconds. In fact, the entire procedure takes only 2 minutes. Virtually every patient accepts this minimal discomfort as a worthwhile tradeoff for the extra knowledge gained.

Ductography

Ductography (galactography or contrast-assisted mammography) consists of injecting an opaque contrast medium into the lactiferous ducts of the breast and then x-raying these structures.[11] This outlining of the ductal system helps determine the site, degree, and characteristics of the conditions producing a spontaneous discharge from the nipple.[12]

Indications for Ductography

A spontaneous unilateral discharge of any color or a unilateral expressed bloody discharge are indications for ductography.

Mammary secretions differ in color and consistency: they may be green or milky, sticky-purulent, or clear; they may be serous (yellow, orange, or straw-colored), serosanguinous (pink), sanguinous (bloody), or watery. Although a bloody discharge is often related to carcinoma, other processes can cause this color discharge. Carcinoma can also cause discharges of other colors.

Ductographically detected but mammographically invisible cancers account for one out of every 25 nonpalpable malignancies. If a patient has no other clinical signs of cancer, her prognosis is the same as that of any other patient with a mammographically discovered nonpalpable cancer. While ductography may not be absolutely necessary for the patient with a palpable or radiographically detected abnormality and a spontaneous unilateral discharge, nonetheless a ductogram may reveal that the breast is harboring additional foci of mammographically and clinically occult cancers. This information is particularly important because many patients now elect to have wedge resection and radiation therapy. For conservative treatment to be successful, all the perceptible tumor must be removed.

Ductography Procedure

Before performing ductography, slides of the discharge are obtained and sent for cytologic examination. However, if the secretion is sparse it should not be used up on cytology, because the fluid is the marker that identifies the correct duct to be cannulated. There are times, however, when the duct cannot be cannulated and a cancer cannot be seen on the ductogram. In these instances, cytology may be the only recourse for detecting an occult cancer. Despite cytology's relatively low yield, it saves lives and is cost-effective.

If the patient gives a history of a spontaneous discharge but no spontaneous discharge is visible during her clinic visit, she is instructed to return for a ductogram on the same day that her discharge recurs. Inasmuch as every nipple has six or seven ductal openings,[13] the telltale discharge is needed, as noted, to target the correct duct for cannulation. If the patient does have a discharge, but the opening is too small to be cannulated, she is asked to come back for a second try.

The technologist may perform the ductogram; however, the radiologist should always be available whenever a patient has a ductogram. He or she may wish to perform the procedure if the technologist has difficulty cannulating the duct.

To prepare for ductography, express a small quantity of fluid from the nipple by circumferentially stroking the breast in radial fashion from its outer perimeter toward the nipple, covering all quadrants like the spokes of a wheel. Make slides of the nipple discharge, fix them immediately in alcohol, and send them for cytologic interpretation. By expressing another tiny drop of fluid (the smaller the better), identify the correct ductal orifice to cannulate. The catheter is then introduced. Prescription-ground loupes or a small magnifying glass clipped to the edge of the eyeglasses plus a special light that illuminates the nipple enhance the ability to perceive the ductal openings.

A Ranfac or Jabczenski catheter is used. The Ranfac*30-gauge end-port, disposable, sialographic straight catheter is used if a longer catheter is necessary. This is attached to its own 27-cm (12-inch) tubing with a Luer lock hub. If the longer catheter is not required, the slightly shorter Jabczenski Ductogram† cannula is used, which is attached to its own 15-cm tubing. Each has its advantages. Because the distal 5 mm of the Jabczenski cannula is bent at a right angle it is easier to obtain leverage while introducing the catheter. However, because the Ranfac cannula can drop further into the duct, the ejection pressure through the tip of the catheter is less likely to expel it. Although several other ductographic catheters, as well as complete ductographic kits, are available commercially, their gauges are all larger, making them more difficult to introduce.

The patient is supine during ductography, so that gravity will pull the heavy contrast material down into the duct. As the catheter passes beyond the sphincter, it suddenly drops 5–10 mm into the duct's lactiferous sinus. If the resistance does not decrease suddenly in this way, the catheter probably has not passed beyond the sphincter. Not until the catheter enters the lactiferous sinus will the contrast material flow retrogradely.

When the catheter has passed the sphincter, inject full-strength contrast material until the patient feels discomfort or pressure, or until 1.5 ml has been infused, whichever comes first. The flow is slow because the material is viscous and must pass through the catheter's small 30-gauge end-port. If fluid begins to come back through the ductal orifice around the catheter, continue injecting the contrast material until the fluid is clear. When finished, tape the catheter to the nipple (so that more contrast material can be in-

jected in the event that the duct fills incompletely), tape the syringe to the patient's chest, and begin the ductogram. Because the ductal sphincter contracts around the catheter, the contrast material usually remains in the duct, but if the fluid pours out of nipple, have the patient gently compress the tip of the nipple until the films have been obtained.

First, obtain a craniocaudad mammogram with mild compression. If the duct has filled incompletely, have the patient lie down and introduce more contrast material. Not until a check film shows that the duct is well visualized on a craniocaudad projection should a lateral view be obtained. If there is extensive ductal branching, obtaining angled views may permit the overlapped ducts to be separated. If no lesion is visible on the grid views, magnification is performed.

After the ductogram, place a paper towel or nursing pad that has been dampened with water over the nipple. Cover the wet dressing with plastic wrap to protect the patient's clothing. This temporary wet dressing helps drain and dilute the salty hypertonic contrast material from the ducts. Because the high-salt content of the contrast material may irritate the duct and the nipple, the dressing is important. Instruct the patient to maintain the wet dressing for as long as 36 hours. When only a small quantity of contrast material is left in the duct, the patient usually needs the wet dressing for only 12 hours.

Preoperative Localization of a Nonpalpable Lesion

With the advent of mammography, preoperative localization of nonpalpable lesions became a necessity. Today, virtually every surgeon recognizes the need for the help provided by preoperative localization under mammographic guidance. In addition to directing the surgeon to the area requiring biopsy, localization helps the surgeon excise a smaller specimen. If the patient does not need a mastectomy, she will achieve better cosmesis if her lesion has been localized preoperatively.

Localization assists the pathologist as well. Not only does x-ray of the biopsy specimen verify that the lesion has been removed, but it also can localize the suspected lesion within the specimen. The pathologist

*Ranfac Corporation, P.O. Box 635, Avon, MA 02322.
†Cook Group, P.O. Box 489, Bloomington, IN 47402.

does not have to search through quantities of extra breast tissue to find it.

Patient Preparation

When a lesion is retrospectively nonpalpable, it is localized under mammographic direction. Before the patient comes to the office for her localization, she is asked to wear a dark blue skirt or slacks (in case the methylene blue dye leaks) and a large blouse that buttons in the front. It is also explained to her that after the procedure she will not be wearing a bra.

A surgeon may prescribe premedication with instructions to take it on the morning of surgery—which also means the morning of localization. Because active participation is needed in the procedure, the patient is asked to avoid any premedication. When the patient sets up her appointment for the localization, it is the radiologist's responsibility to caution her not to take any premedication until after her localization is completed.[14,15]

Equipment and Technique

With the greater need for preoperative localization, many localizing needle-wire sets have come on the market. Some popular types are the Homer, Frank, Kopans, Hawkins, Urrutia, and Sadowsky needles, which all have their partisans.[17–22]

A stiff trocar is more helpful than a wire; the surgeon has no trouble finding its interior tip. If the surgeon moves the outer tip back and forth, he or she can feel the inner tip of the wire seesawing back and forth and can locate the lesion. This way, the surgeon can make an incision close to the inner tip, and can avoid cutting where the trocar enters the skin and following it all the way down, a clumsier approach that leaves a larger scar.

When directed inward toward the patient's body, wires and trocars can migrate into the pectoral muscle. When the muscle contracts, its pumping motion can draw wires and trocars through the muscle toward the thorax or pericardial sac. For this reason, the trocar is always placed *parallel* to the pectoral muscle, so that it cannot enter the muscle.

To localize a lesion preoperatively, a narrow (9-cm wide) compression plate is used. The narrow plate compresses the site for localization better than a standard device that compresses the entire breast. The pa-

tient finds the small compression device less uncomfortable and less intimidating. Also, because a small device achieves greater compression of the abnormal area, the characteristics of the abnormality are more visible.

Some compression devices are designed with only a single large opening to be placed over the area requiring localization. These devices work poorly because the pressure forces breast tissue through the aperture. Not only does the protruding tissue make it radiographically difficult to see the lesion, but also the needle must pass through more tissue to reach the lesion. The narrow compression plate is perforated with multiple holes large enough to admit the hub of a needle passing through to localize the nonpalpable lesion, but small enough to prevent the tissue from bulging through the apertures.

The angle of compression depends on the site of the lesion. *The breast should always be compressed in the position in which the lesion is closest to the compression device.* If the lesion is in the upper half of the breast, begin localizing from the craniocaudad position, with the needle directed from cephalad to caudad. If the lesion is in the inferior half of the breast, begin localizing with lateral compression. If the lesion is in the lower inner quadrant, start with mediolateral compression and needle direction; if it is in the lower outer quadrant, use lateromedial compression and needle direction. By adjusting the angle of compression, the needle will travel the shortest distance from the skin to the lesion.

Standard Localization Procedure

With the patient seated at the x-ray unit, compression is applied to the breast in the position in which the lesion is closest to the compression device, a small lead marker is place over the compression device at the approximate site of the lesion. When the scout film has been developed, calculate the tumor's location by counting the number of holes between the lead marker and the aperture through which the localizing needle is inserted. Next, wipe the skin covering the lesion with an alcohol sponge, make a small (1-mm) incision in the skin with a scalpel tip, introduce the needle through the skin, and aim the needle toward the lesion. Keep the needle parallel to the collimator light, so that it is parallel to the x-ray beam. The needle should be passed beyond the lesion. This is particularly important because the needle may retract slightly after the compression plate is lifted.

With the needle in position, a check film is taken. Because the patient must sit with her breast compressed during the entire 3-minute wait for the film to be processed, only enough compression should be applied to visualize the lesion, so that she will not be so uncomfortable. Inasmuch as the compression is less, always use a grid for localization.

If the lesion is within 3 cm of the needle, the compression device is lifted up and away from the breast while making sure that the hub of the needle does not catch on the edge of the compression device. If not properly positioned, recalculate and reposition the needle. The breast is then compressed at right angles to the original film and another film is taken with moderate compression. (The patient must sit with her breast compressed until the first and second films are reviewed.) After the extent that the needle has passed beyond the lesion is determined the needle is withdrawn by that exact span, while keeping the breast compressed, until the needle is level with the lesion. To prove that the needle is in the correct position at the level of the lesion, immediately x-ray that area.

Rarely, the first two films may reveal that patient motion or other factors have resulted in positioning the needle incorrectly. If these two films show that the needle is not in the right spot, withdraw it, repeat the procedure, and obtain two more films. During all of this, an assistant, *who never leaves the patient unattended,* continues to explain what is being done and why, continues to allay the patient's fears (which do arise even though the procedure has been discussed with her before beginning), and tries to answer all her questions.

Still keeping the breast compressed, 1 ml of 1% methylene blue in a sterile solution is injected through the needle. The dye serves as a marker for locating the lesion in the event that the needle or the trocar subsequently slips out of the breast. Before injecting the dye, 1 ml of air is added and the syringe is shaken. On follow-up films, the air identifies the dye's position. First making sure that the patient is not allergic to xylocaine, 1 ml of xylocaine solution is injected to anesthetize the area until the patient undergoes her biopsy.

Once these injections have been administered, the wire trocar is set in place through the needle. The needle is then removed, leaving only the wire protruding from the skin. The wire should not be bent or taped to the skin until the patient assumes the position in which the wire *least* protrudes from the breast. If the wire is shortened and bent with the patient in the position in which the wire *most* protrudes, the bent edge could catch on the skin and yank the inner tip away from the lesion as the patient moves.

Copies (or originals) of the films are given to the patient so that she can carry them with her to the operating room. A written description of the location of the trocar and a small drawing of the breast that marks the site of the trocar and the lesion must accompany these films. A note informs the surgeon that dye has been injected for tracking purposes, in the event that the trocar is accidentally dislodged.

The technologist helps the patient dress carefully so that she does not jar the wire. She is instructed not to move her arm suddenly on the side of the localized breast.

Alternative Localization Procedures

Although some Swedish, German, and American mammographers use complex stereotactic computerized systems for localization, asserting that the stereotactic technique is more accurate, efficient, and expedient, it may be more cumbersome and time-consuming, yet no more specific, than the present method. In a comparison study, Evans and Cade reported that "standard localizing technique may be as accurate as the stereotactic technique."[23]

When a lesion is visible on only one of the two standard views, it can still be localized. Two x-ray views are obtained with the C-arm angled in both directions as far as possible from the standard view in which the lesion was originally detected, but in which the lesion is still perceptible. These two angles are often only 20–30° from each other. After obtaining the two furthest views in which the lesion can be seen, it is localized in the following fashion.

Compressing the breast in the position where the lesion is closest to the skin, the needle is introduced, a check film is taken, and the compression plate lifted up and away from the needle. Thus far, the procedure is identical to the routine localization. At this point, however, instead of obtaining a right-angle film the breast is compressed in one of the other angles in which the lesion is identifiable. Because this angle is less than 90°, the wire is not parallel to the surface of the compression device. When compression begins, the edge of the compression device is adjacent to the site at which the needle enters the skin. As compression increases the needle becomes more parallel to the surface of the compression device, so that the distance that the needle has traveled beyond the lesion can be determined. Localizing a lesion this way is possible only with a narrow compression device.

The remainder of the procedure is almost the same as the standard needle localization, with one salient exception: the final check films are again performed at the two original angled views in which the needle had been introduced and its original position checked.

Special Patient Considerations

Because each step of the localization procedure is explained, the patient understands what is happening to her and is willing to cooperate. Although a vasovagal reaction is always a possibility, compassionate technologists and assistants can do much to prevent it, while they keep a weather eye out for any untoward effects. To avoid a vasovagal reaction, Kopans recommended not letting the patient see the needle.[18] If a patient feels faint, she lies and rests until she feels better. Once she feels well enough to go on, the procedure is continued. Postponing a localization only postpones the biopsy and guarantees more sleepless nights for the patient until the next appointment arrives.

If a woman does not speak English or is deaf, the use of an interpreter or a signer for the hearing impaired is recommended so that she will understand what is happening to her.

Ultrasound or Palpation Localization

Whenever possible, localizing a lesion under sonographic guidance or by clinically palpating it is preferable to localizing it mammographically. This is quicker and is easier for the patient to tolerate the discomfort. If the lesion can be localized by palpating it, localize it in the usual way with the localizing needle, the dye, xylocaine, and the wire, with one exception to the procedure: x-ray films at each step are not necessary; only the needle's final position is verified mammographically. The surgeon often can pal-

pate such a lesion but may still prefer to localize it, because he or she is uncertain whether the lesion will be palpable through surgical gloves.

Occasionally, a lesion is clinically ill-defined, yet ultrasound reveals a definite area of attenuation. In such instances, the needle, the dye, and the xylocaine are placed in the lesion under sonographic guidance and then right-angled mammograms are taken to confirm the final position of the wire.

Localizing a lesion clinically or under sonographic guidance works particularly well with lesions in the lower half of a large breast, because mammographic guidance is more awkward and unwieldy with these lesions.

Specimen Radiography

After biopsy, the specimen should be radiographed. To x-ray the specimen, use 1.5–2× magnification, coned down to the specimen's size. Greater magnification actually blurs the lesion's outline, unless the focal spot size *measures* less than 0.15 mm (15 microns). The specimen is compressed to prevent the appearance of a "pseudomass" caused by heaped-up tissue.

Once visualized, a needle is passed through the lesion and a check film is taken to make sure that it is passing through the abnormal area. Then a thread attached to the needle is pulled through the lesion. The specimen is returned to the pathologist with the thread running through the abnormality. The lesion is circled on the x-rays, and they are sent to the pathologist with the specimen and a note describing the abnormal area.

When the specimen is x-rayed in a hospital, a small unit such as the Faxitron, which has a soft x-ray beam and is specifically designed for the pathology department, works well for specimen radiography. If the Faxitron or a reasonable facsimile is not available, a member of the hospital's radiology department can x-ray the specimen. In any event, a radiologist should oversee the specimen x-ray procedure. The radiologist should have the diagnostic mammograms in hand to compare them with the specimen radiographs. The radiologist should show the x-rays to the pathologist and make sure the pathologist knows what to look for.

References

1. Maturo VG, Zusmer NR, Gilson AJ, et al: Ultrasonic appearance of mammary carcinoma with a dedicated whole-breast scanner. *Radiology* 1982;142:713–718.

2. Logan WW: The radiologist's increasing role in breast cancer diagnosis, in Margulis AR, Gooding CA (eds): *Diagnostic Radiology*. San Francisco, University of California Printing Department, 1982, pp 471–476.

3. Logan WW: Performing the examination: Screen-film mammography, in Bassett LW, Gold RH (eds): *Mammography, Thermography, Ultrasound in Breast Cancer Detection*. New York, Grune & Stratton, 1982, pp 61–72.

4. Logan WW: Ultrasonography: Its role in the diagnosis of breast carcinoma, in Margulis AR, Gooding CS (eds): *Diagnostic Radiology*. San Francisco, University of California Printing Department, 1982, pp 457–463.

5. Logan WW: The technique of screen-film mammography, in Margulis AR, Gooding CA (eds): *Diagnostic Radiology*. San Francisco, University of California Printing Department, 1982, pp 441–455.

6. Sickles EA, Filly RA, Callen PW: Breast cancer detection with sonography and mammography: Comparison using state-of-the-art equipment. *Am J Roentgenol* 1983;140:843–845.

7. Sickles EA, Filly RA, Callen PW: Breast ultrasonography, in Feig SA, McLelland R (eds): *Breast Carcinoma, Current Diagnosis and Treatment*. New York, Masson, 1983, p 191.

8. Kopans DB: 'Early' breast cancer detection using techniques other than mammography. *Am J Roentgenol* 1984;143:465–468.

9. Layfield LJ, Glasgow BJ, Cramer H: Fine-needle aspiration in the management of breast masses. *Pathol Annu* 1989;24(2):23–62.

10. Schulte E, Wittekind C: The influence of the wet-fixed Papanicolaou and the air-dried Giemsa techniques on nuclear parameters in breast cancer cytology: A cytomorphometric study. *Diagn Cytopathol* 1987;3(3):256–261.

11. Gregl A: *Color Atlas of Galactography*. Stuttgart, F.K. Schattauer Verlag, 1980.

12. Reid AW, McKellar NJ, Sutherland GR: Breast ductography—its role in the diagnosis of breast disease. *Scottish Med J* 1989;34:497–499.

13. Kopans DB, Swann CA, White G, et al: Asymmetric breast tissue. *Radiology* 1989;171:639–643.

14. Homer MJ, Pile-Spellman ER: Needle localization of nonpalpable breast lesions: The importance of communication. *Appl Radiol* 1987;Nov:88–98.

15. Homer MJ: Breast imaging: Pitfalls, controversies, and some practical thoughts. *Radiol Clin North Am* 1985;23:466–467.

16. Horns JW, Arndt RD: Percutaneous spot localization of nonpalpable breast lesions. *AJR* 1976;127:253–256.

17. Kopans DB, Deluca S: A modified needle-hookwire technique to simplify preoperative localization of occult breast lesions. *Radiology* 1980;134:781.

18. Frank HA, Hall FM, Steel ML: Preoperative localization of nonpalpable breast lesions demonstrated by mammography. *N Engl J Med* 1976;295:259–260.

19. Homer MJ: Nonpalpable breast lesion localization using a curved-end retractable wire. *Radiology* 1985;157:259–260.

20. Hawkins IF Jr, Weaver DL, Jafri S: Wide range of applications of a new 22-gauge needle which permits placement of larger catheters or needles (including spring barb needle for breast lesion localization). Presented to the American Roentgen Ray Society, Las Vegas, April 22, 1980.

21. Urrutia EJ, Hawkins MC, Steinbach BG, et al: Retractable-barb needle for breast lesion localization: Use in 60 cases. *Radiology* 1988;169:845–847.

22. Hirsch JI, Banks WL Jr, Sullivan JS, Horsley JS III: Effect of methylene blue on estrogen-receptor activity. *Radiology* 1989;171:105–107.

23. Evans WP, Cade SH: Needle localization and fine-needle aspirations biopsy of nonpalpable breast lesions with use of standard stereotactic equipment. *Radiology* 1989;173:53–56.

Index

Numbers followed by an f indicate a figure; t following a page number indicates tabular material.

ISBN 0-397-51096-9